Sleep Related Breathing Disorders

Sleep Related Breathing Disorders

Editors

Vivek Nangia MD FCCP DLSHTM
MSc Infectious Diseases, Diploma Interventional Bronchoscopy,
Fellowship Pediatric Pulmonology, Fellowship Sleep Medicine
Director and Head
Fortis Lung Center
Fortis Flt Lt Rajan Dhall Hospital
New Delhi, India

Shivani Swami MD FSM FCCP
Consultant
Fortis Lung Center
Fortis Flt Lt Rajan Dhall Hospital
New Delhi, India

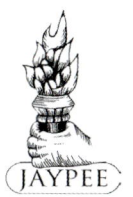

JAYPEE *The Health Sciences Publisher*

New Delhi | London | Philadelphia | Panama

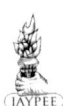
Jaypee Brothers Medical Publishers (P) Ltd

Headquarters
Jaypee Brothers Medical Publishers (P) Ltd
4838/24, Ansari Road, Daryaganj
New Delhi 110 002, India
Phone: +91-11-43574357
Fax: +91-11-43574314
Email: jaypee@jaypeebrothers.com

Overseas Offices

J.P. Medical Ltd
83 Victoria Street, London
SW1H 0HW (UK)
Phone: +44 20 3170 8910
Fax: +44 (0)20 3008 6180
Email: info@jpmedpub.com

Jaypee-Highlights Medical Publishers Inc
City of Knowledge, Bld. 237, Clayton
Panama City, Panama
Phone: +1 507-301-0496
Fax: +1 507-301-0499
Email: cservice@jphmedical.com

Jaypee Medical Inc
The Bourse
111 South Independence Mall East
Suite 835, Philadelphia, PA 19106, USA
Phone: +1 267-519-9789
Email: jpmed.us@gmail.com

Jaypee Brothers Medical Publishers (P) Ltd
17/1-B Babar Road, Block-B, Shaymali
Mohammadpur, Dhaka-1207
Bangladesh
Mobile: +08801912003485
Email: jaypeedhaka@gmail.com

Jaypee Brothers Medical Publishers (P) Ltd
Bhotahity, Kathmandu, Nepal
Phone: +977-9741283608
Email: kathmandu@jaypeebrothers.com

Website: www.jaypeebrothers.com
Website: www.jaypeedigital.com

© 2015, Jaypee Brothers Medical Publishers

The views and opinions expressed in this book are solely those of the original contributor(s)/author(s) and do not necessarily represent those of editor(s) of the book.

All rights reserved. No part of this publication may be reproduced, stored or transmitted in any form or by any means, electronic, mechanical, photocopying, recording or otherwise, without the prior permission in writing of the publishers.

All brand names and product names used in this book are trade names, service marks, trademarks or registered trademarks of their respective owners. The publisher is not associated with any product or vendor mentioned in this book.

Medical knowledge and practice change constantly. This book is designed to provide accurate, authoritative information about the subject matter in question. However, readers are advised to check the most current information available on procedures included and check information from the manufacturer of each product to be administered, to verify the recommended dose, formula, method and duration of administration, adverse effects and contraindications. It is the responsibility of the practitioner to take all appropriate safety precautions. Neither the publisher nor the author(s)/editor(s) assume any liability for any injury and/or damage to persons or property arising from or related to use of material in this book.

This book is sold on the understanding that the publisher is not engaged in providing professional medical services. If such advice or services are required, the services of a competent medical professional should be sought.

Every effort has been made where necessary to contact holders of copyright to obtain permission to reproduce copyright material. If any have been inadvertently overlooked, the publisher will be pleased to make the necessary arrangements at the first opportunity.

Inquiries for bulk sales may be solicited at: jaypee@jaypeebrothers.com

Sleep Related Breathing Disorders

First Edition: **2015**

ISBN: 978-93-5152-420-5

Printed at : Samrat Offset Pvt. Ltd.

Dedication

We would like to dedicate this book to
all the students

Contents

Contributors   ix
Preface   xiii
Acknowledgements   xv, xvii

CHAPTER 1   Normal Human Sleep   1
Vikram Sarbhai, Naveen P Shah, Poulomi Chatterjee

CHAPTER 2   Anatomy and Physiology of Obstructive Sleep
Apnea Airways   10
Ashwini Malhotra, Vivek Nangia

CHAPTER 3   Clinical Approach to Patient with
Sleep Related Breathing Disorders   22
Manoj K Goel

CHAPTER 4   Diagnostic Approach to Sleep Disordered Breathing   30
Nagarajan Ramakrishnan, Anup Bansal

CHAPTER 5   Snoring and Upper Airways Resistance Syndrome   39
Raja Dhar, Debdeep Sen

CHAPTER 6   Obstructive Sleep Apnea   46
Vivek Nangia, Shivani Swami

CHAPTER 7   Central Sleep Apnea   56
Manas K Sen

CHAPTER 8   Obesity Hypoventilation Syndrome and
Complex Sleep Apnea   67
Vivek Nangia, Shivani Swami

CHAPTER 9   Cardiac Effects of Sleep Related Breathing Disorders   79
Manish Bansal, Kapil D Mohindra

CHAPTER 10   Systemic Effects of Sleep Related Breathing
Disorders: Noncardiac   98
Gopi C Khilnani, Neetu Jain

CHAPTER 11   Positive Airway Pressure Treatment in
Obstructive Sleep Apnea   116
Vijay K Chennamchetty, Maramreddy Aparna, Praveen SV

CHAPTER 12   Pharmacotherapy   130
Shivani Swami, Vivek Nangia

CHAPTER 13 Surgical Management of Obstructive Sleep Apnea　　140
Rajeev Kumar, Alok Thakar

CHAPTER 14 Dental Sleep Medicine: An Overview　　151
Anmol S Kalha, Jayan Balakrishnan

CHAPTER 15 Obstructive Sleep Apnea in Children　　169
Praveen Khilnani, Neha Sood

CHAPTER 16 Perioperative Management of Sleep Related Breathing Disorders　　182
Roop Kaw, Vivek Nangia

Index　　*191*

Contributors

EDITORS

Vivek Nangia MD FCCP DLSHTM
MSc Infectious Diseases, Diploma Interventional Bronchoscopy,
Fellowship Pediatric Pulmonology, Fellowship Sleep Medicine
Director and Head
Fortis Lung Center
Fortis Flt Lt Rajan Dhall Hospital
New Delhi, India

Shivani Swami MD FSM FCCP
Consultant
Fortis Lung Cancer
Fortis Flt Lt Rajan Dhall Hospital
New Delhi, India

CONTRIBUTING AUTHORS

Maramreddy Aparna MD
Registrar
Department of Internal Medicine
Citizens Hospital
Hyderabad, Telangana, India

Jayan Balakrishnan MDS
Consultant
Army Dental Centre (Research and Referral)
New Delhi, India

Anup Bansal MD IDCCM IDSM
Advanced Trainee
Intensive Care Medicine Department
Westmead Hospital
Sydney, New South Wales, Australia

Manish Bansal MD DNB FASE FISCU
Senior Consultant
Department of Cardiology
Medanta - The Medicity
Gurgaon, Haryana, India

Poulomi Chatterjee MD DNB FISDA
Attending Consultant
Department of Respiratory and Sleep Medicine
Medanta - The Medcity
Gurgaon, Haryana, India

Vijay K Chennamchetty MD IDCC FSM
Interventional Pulmonologist and Sleep Disorder Specialist
Department of Pulmonary Critical Care and Sleep Sciences
Citizens Hospital
Hyderabad, Telangana, India

Raja Dhar MD MRCP CCT FCCP
Consultant Pulmonologist and Intensivist
Jadavpur University
Kolkata, West Bengal, India

Manoj K Goel MD FCCP DIP FISM FCCM
Director and Head
Department of Pulmonology
Critical Care and Sleep Medicine
Delhi Heart and Lung Institute
New Delhi, India

Neetu Jain DNB FCCP
Senior Research Associate
All India Institute of Medical Sciences
New Delhi, India

Anmol S Kalha BSc MDS Cert Lingual Orthodontics (Germany)
Director, Senior Professor
I.T.S. Dental College
Hospital and Research Center
Noida, Uttar Pradesh, India
Senior Consultant, Dental Advisor
Max Healthcare, New Delhi, India

Roop Kaw MD
Associate Professor
Departments of Hospital Medicine and Outcomes Research (Anesthesiology Institute)
Cleveland Clinic Lerner College of Medicine
Cleveland, Ohio, USA

Gopi C Khilnani MD FCCP FICCM FICP FNCCP MNAMS
Professor
Department of Pulmonary Medicine and Sleep Disorders
All India Institute of Medical Sciences
New Delhi, India

Praveen Khilnani MD Fellowship in Pediatric Critical Care
Director and Senior Consultant, Pediatric Intensivist, and Pulmonologist
BLK Superspeciality Hospital
New Delhi, India

Rajeev Kumar MS DNB MNAMS
Assistant Professor
Department of Otorhinolaryngology and Head–Neck Surgery
All India Institute of Medical Sciences
New Delhi, India

Ashwini Malhotra MBBS DNB DTCD IDCCM FICM
Consultant Pulmonology/Critical/Sleep Medicine
Bansal Hospital
Bhopal, Madhya Pradesh, India

Kapil D Mohindra PGDCC Advanced Fellowship in Non Invasive Cardiology
Associate Consultant
Department of Cardiology
Max Super Specialty Hospital
New Delhi, India

Nagarajan Ramakrishnan AB (Int Med) AB (Crit Care) AB (Sleep Med) MMM FACP FCCP FCCM FICCM FISDA
Senior Consultant, Critical Care and Sleep Medicine, Apollo Hospitals
Senior Consultant and Director, Nithra Institute of Sleep Sciences
Chennai, Tamil Nadu, India

Vikram Sarbhai MD FNCCP FCCP FISDA
Senior Consultant
Department of Respiratory and Sleep Medicine
Medanta - The Medcity
Gurgaon, Haryana, India

Debdeep Sen European Diploma in Advance Lung Function Diploma in Clinical Research
Senior Respiratory Technician
Fortis Hospitals
Kolkata, West Bengal, India

Manas K Sen MD DTCD FCCP
Consultant and Associate Professor
Department of Pulmonary, Critical Care, and Sleep Medicine
VM Medical College and Safdarjung Hospital
New Delhi, India

Naveen P Shah MD
Fellow
Department of Respiratory and Sleep Medicine
Medanta - The Medcity
Gurgaon, Haryana, India

Neha Sood MBBS DNB MNAMS
Consultant, ENT Surgeon, Department of ENT
BLK Superspeciality Hospital
New Delhi, India

Praveen SV MD MRCP
Head, Department of Internal Medicine
Citizens Hospital
Hyderabad, Telangana, India

Alok Thakar MS FRCSed
Professor of Otorhinolaryngology and Head-Neck Surgery
All India Institute of Medical Sciences
New Delhi, India

Preface

Although we spend nearly one-third of our lifetime (i.e., almost 8 out of 24 hours daily) in sleeping, yet there is so little we know about our sleep. As clinicians, we ask our patients about their present, past, personal, and family history but never do we, as a routine, ask about their sleep history.

The earliest mention about sleep also having stages, can be found in the *Panchratra Agamas*, in the Hindu mythology, which were composed sometime between 3000 BC and 800 AD. They describe two stages of sleep: *Sushupti*, the stage of deep sleep in which the individual is self-oblivion, unaware as the mind is also at rest along with the five senses and *Swapna*, the dreaming stage in which the individual enjoys the five objects of senses while all the five sense organs are at rest and only the mind is working. Insomnia and poppy seeds (opium) as its treatment, finds mention in the ancient Egyptian texts. Hippocrates has made a reference to disordered sleep and dreams. However, sleep was considered a passive process and wakefulness an active state until the scientific discoveries of early 20th century. The development of electroencephalography in 1930s enabled scientists to study the characteristic high amplitude slow waves during sleep and led them to question the basic view that sleep is a passive process.

The modern day knowledge of sleep has evolved, largely, over the last 3–4 decades. Sleep disorders can be classified into: insomnia, parasomnia, hypersomnia, and circadian rhythm disorders. While insomnia refers to lack of sleep, parasomnia refers to abnormal movements, behaviors, emotions, perceptions, and dreams that occur while falling asleep, sleeping, between sleep stages, or during arousal from sleep. Sleep walking (somnambulism), sleep terror (night terror), sleep sex (sexsomnia), bruxism, sleep related eating disorder, restless leg syndrome, and periodic limb movement, and REM sleep behavior disorder are the common examples of parasomnias. Hypersomnia, as the name suggests, refers to excessive sleepiness and is most commonly caused by fragmented sleep while insufficient sleep and excessive sleep drive are the other causes. Fragmented sleep often results from an abnormal respiratory pattern and this group of disorders is collectively referred to as the *sleep related breathing disorders* or *sleep disordered breathing* (SDB).

The current manuscript focuses on this group of disorders as they are now known to be widely prevalent in the general population and have been identified to have far reaching adverse consequences on the cardiovascular and metabolic systems and the neurocognitive and renal functions of the individual. Sleep disordered breathing also has major socioeconomic consequences for the individual as well as for the society at large. The main objective is to provide a detailed description of the various aspects of SDB in a simple and comprehensible format which can be easily mastered by a novice and an expert, alike.

Time has come when sleep medicine should be included in the undergraduate medical curriculum and sleep history be included in every patient record.

Vivek Nangia
Shivani Swami

Acknowledgements

I am indebted to many people who have contributed directly or indirectly to this book but would like to acknowledge a few individuals.

At the outset, I would like to express my sincere gratitude towards Jaypee Brothers Medical Publishers (P) Ltd. for providing me this unique opportunity of compiling this book. Many thanks to my co-editor, Dr Shivani Swami, for working tirelessly on the manuscripts. I am grateful to all the contributors for having taken out time from their busy schedules to pen down their respective chapters. I owe it to my family and friends, who stood by me throughout the long drawn period of compiling this book.

My main inspiration for dissemination of knowledge comes from my deceased mother, Kusum Nangia and my guide and guru, Professor Premendra Bahadur.

Vivek Nangia

Acknowledgements

There are few well deserved acknowledgments I would like to extend. Firstly, I would sincerely thank Dr Vivek Nangia, for giving me the opportunity to assist him in compiling this book. I would like to thank the publishers, Jaypee Brothers Medical Publishers (P) Ltd., for the conceptualization of the book. A special thanks to my family, specially my parents, for extending unconditional support in all my endeavors. I would also like to thank my teacher, Dr Girija Nair, who laid the foundation stone of my journey in pulmonology. Last but not the least, I would like to thank all my teachers, colleagues, and patients who have taught me at every step.

Shivani Swami

CHAPTER 1

Normal Human Sleep

Vikram Sarbhai, Naveen P Shah, Poulomi Chatterjee

NORMAL HUMAN SLEEP

Normal human sleep can probably be described as "a reversible behavioral state of perceptual disengagement and unresponsiveness to the environment". It is also true that sleep is a complex amalgam of physiologic and behavioral processes. Typically, sleep is usually accompanied by postural recumbence, involuntary behavioral quiescence usually get closed eyes, along with physiological alterations one commonly associates with sleeping.

It is certain that sleep is essential, not only for humans but for almost all animals. Physiologically, sleep is a complex neural process that is essential for the restoration and renewal of body functions, which seems to be necessary for life. Scientists still do not have a definitive explanation for why there seems to be an essentiality of the phenomenon of sleep in almost all living forms besides humans as well. We do know that sleep is not a passive process or "switching off" of body functions. In fact, sleep is believed to be important for many physiologic functions including the processing of experiences and the consolidation of diverse neural processes and its manifestations.

Important things to know about normal human sleep:
- Sleep duration and characteristics decrease with age—sleep characteristics stabilizes until around 20 years of age
- Sleep differentiation is highly individualized
- It is normal for children to have daytime naps until 3–5 years old
- If a child takes naps often past this age, he or she might not be sleeping enough at night
- Teenagers will tend to go to bed later
- Older people spend more time in bed, but their sleep requirement is normally similar to that of early adult life.

Age Related Sleep Alterations

It is well known that, as children get older their sleep duration is reduced. Different people have different sleep duration requirements. The average sleep durations in different age groups according to Sleep Health Foundation (2011) is described in table 1. Daytime functioning and actions of people can be an indicator to assume their adequacy of sleep at night.

Table 1: Average sleep requirement (Sleep Health Foundation, 2011)			
Age group	Total sleep (hours/day)	Sleep at night (hours)	Sleep during day (hours)
Newborns (0–2 months)	12–18	6–9	6–9
Infants (2–12 months)	14–15	9–12	2.5–5
Toddlers (1–3 years)	12–15	9.5–11.5	1.5–3.5
Preschool (3–5 years)	11–13	Most sleep is at night	Daytime naps become rarer. A child tends to stop napping at this age
School-age (5–12 years)	9–11	All sleep should be at night	Naps at this age tend to be from not getting enough sleep at night
Teenagers (12–18 years)	8.5–9.5	All sleep should be at night	Naps at this age tend to be from not getting enough sleep at night
Adults	7–9	All sleep should be at night	Naps at this age tend to be from not getting enough sleep at night

Note that these are average sleep requirements: some people require more and others less.

Age Related Sleep Changes

From birth to two months of age, one period of sleep can vary from 30 minutes to 3–4 hours both during day as well as night. Bottle-fed babies tend to sleep longer than breast-fed babies (3–4 hours vs. 2–3 hours). Two months onwards babies start to sleep longer at a time. This is especially so at night between 12 midnight and 5 AM. This is possibly because babies start to develop their internal circadian (day-night) rhythm around this time. This circadian rhythm favors sleep at night and being more awake during the day. *By 6 months*, babies can get 5–8 hours of sleep at night. However, in around 25–50% cases, 6 month old children still wake up at night. There are behavioral strategies that can be done to improve and increase night-time sleep, including training babies learn to go to sleep in their cot by themselves. With these measures, they are able to self-soothe themselves back to sleep after waking up during the night. From 2 months to 12 months, the number of daytime naps gets reduced from 3–4 naps to 2 naps. Usually by 12–18 months of age, morning naps stop. It is preferred to allow an afternoon nap after lunch and before 4 pm. Daytime naps become less common from about 2 or 3 years onwards. Persistent daytime naps beyond 5 years of age are not considered normal. It usually means, the child might not be getting enough sleep at night and is suffering from sleep deprivation, quantitative or qualitative. This may be due to poor sleep routines, sleep problems, or sleep disorders.

Adult Sleep

Sleep requirements tends to stabilize by 20 years of age. Most adults require between 7 hours and 9 hours a night to feel properly refreshed and function optimally the next day, however, individuals may vary in their sleep needs.

Some people are genuine short sleepers while others may require considerably more than the average sleep time. Several people try to get away with less sleep.

The reasons for this individual variability in sleep requirement are not well understood. Sleep requirements get reduced with age and older adults spend more time in bed but tend to sleep less. There is a constant reduction in share of rapid eye movement (REM) sleep as compared to non-rapid eye movement (NREM) sleep with age.

STAGES OF SLEEP

Sleep time is classified into stages (Figure 1). For scientific applications, sleep is typically scored in recording of 30 seconds (termed as Epoch) with stages of sleep defined by the visual scoring of three parameters: (i) electroencephalogram (EEG); (ii) electrooculogram (EOG); and (iii) electromyogram (EMG) recorded beneath the chin. Sleep can be classified as NREM sleep and REM sleep. During wakefulness, the EEG shows a low voltage fast activity or activated pattern. Voluntary eye movements and eye blinks are obvious. The EMG has a high tonic activity with additional phasic activity sleep related to voluntary movements. As the eyes are closed in sleep preparation, alpha waves [8–13 cycles per second (cps)] become prominent, particularly in occipital regions. NREM sleep, which usually precedes REM sleep, is divided into three stages [namely stage 1, 2, and slow wave sleep (SWS)]. Sleep is usually entered through a transitional state, stage 1 sleep. Stage 1 sleep is characterized by loss of alpha activity and the appearance of a low voltage mixed frequency EEG pattern with prominent theta activity (3–7 cps) and occasional vertex sharp waves. Eye movements become slow and rolling, and skeletal muscle tone relaxes. Subjectively, stage 1 may not be perceived as sleep, however, there is a reduced sensory stimuli, especially visual and mental activity is more dream-like. There may be persistence of

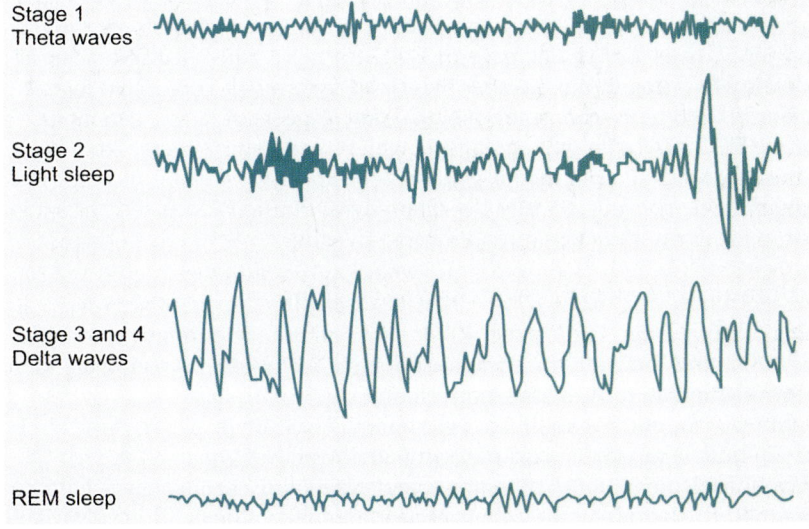

REM, rapid eye movement

Figure 1: Various stages of sleep.

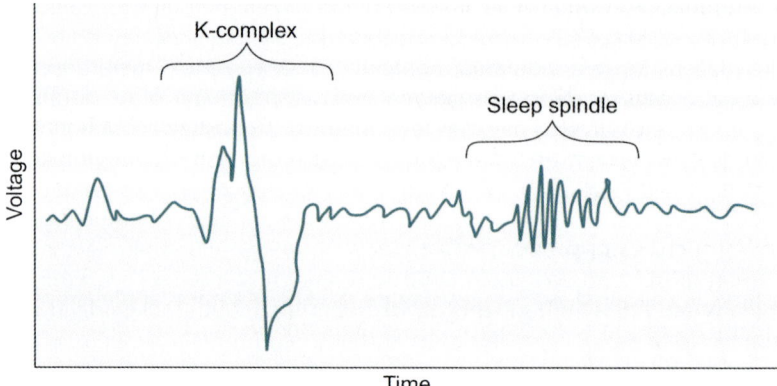

Figure 2: Sleep spindle (12-14 cps) and K-complex (high amplitude negative sharp wave followed by positive slow waves).

motor activity for a number of seconds during stage 1 NREM sleep. Sometimes, individuals may experience sleep jerks, which are sudden muscle contractions, accompanied by a sense of falling and/or dream-like imagery. Such hypnic (hypnosis = mental state like sleep) jerks are generally benign and may be exaggerated by sleep deprivation. After a few minutes of stage 1 NREM, sleep usually progresses to stage 2 NREM, which is characterized by the appearance of sleep spindles (12–14 cps) and K-complexes (high amplitude negative sharp waves followed by positive slow waves) in the EEG (Figure 2). NREM sleep stages 2, SWS, and REM sleep are all subjectively perceived as sleep. Generally, stage 2 NREM is followed by SWS, predominantly more in the first one-third of the night. Delta waves (<2 cps in humans) are characteristic of SWS. In the earlier classification, SWS was subdivided into NREM stage 3 and 4. SWS is also known as deep sleep. The threshold (i.e., sleep intensifies) of arousals increases incrementally from stage 1 through SWS. Eye movements cease during stages 2 and SWS, with further decrease in EMG (muscle) activity. REM sleep is not subdivided into stages, but is rather described in terms of Tonic REM (persistent) and Phasic REM (episodic) components. Tonic aspects of REM sleep include the activated EEG similar to that of stage 1, which may exhibit increased activity in the theta band (3–7 cps), and a generalized atonia of skeletal muscles except for the extra-ocular muscles and the diaphragm. Phasic REM is seen as irregular bursts of rapid eye movements and muscle twitches.

Physiological Changes Associated with Sleep

During NREM sleep and tonic REM sleep, there is a relative increase in parasympathetic activity. In comparison to wakefulness, autonomic nervous system reaches its most stable state during SWS. The autonomic system gets unstable (autonomic instability) during phasic REM sleep, where there are brief surges in both sympathetic and parasympathetic activity.

Physiologically, blood pressure, heart rate, and cardiac output decrease during NREM sleep, reaching their lowest average values and least variability in SWS. Although these parameters remain reduced on average, during REM sleep in comparison to waking, they attain their peak values during

REM. Irregularity in heart rhythm and arrhythmias are more prevalent in REM sleep.

Physiologically, onset of sleep may show temporary breathing instability and/or periodic breathing. The respiratory rate and minute ventilation also decrease during sleep. Muscle relaxation during sleep results in increase in upper airway resistance, most significantly during REM sleep.

These changes contribute to exacerbation of underlying pulmonary disease as well as sleep related breathing disorders due to sleep related upper airway instability such as obstructive sleep apnea.

During NREM sleep, brain and body temperature are downregulated, particularly in NREM SWS, as a result of a decreased hypothalamic temperature set point. There is additional active heat loss through perspiration because of increased cutaneous blood flow (vasodilation). It is usual to experience this phenomenon when people go to sleep feeling somewhat cold and later wish to remove their extra covers as they feel too warm on waking up several hours later. During REM sleep, there is a decreased ability to regulate body temperature through sweating and shivering.

Sleep Influence on Endocrine System

Most hormones also show significant interactions with sleep-wakefulness patterns.

Growth hormone (GH) is released during the early part of the sleep and its secretion gets enhanced by NREM SWS. Sleep also stimulates *prolactin* secretion. Prolactin usually peaks after GH, usually during the middle portion of the sleep cycle. Pulses of GH and prolactin releases can occur after the onset of sleep, regardless of its timing. Both GH and prolactin may have feedback effects on sleep as well; GH seems to enhance SWS, whereas prolactin may increase REM sleep. Contrastingly, thyroid stimulating hormone (TSH) reaches its peak level in the evening just prior to sleep onset; its secretion is inhibited by sleep and gets stimulated by sleep deprivation. On sleep onset, the hypothalamic-pituitary-adrenal axis (HPA axis) is usually at its most inactive state. Sleep onset inhibits cortisol release, however, adrenocorticotrophic hormone (ACTH) and cortisol levels rise at the end of the sleep period, just before awakening and are presumed to contribute to morning awakening. Severe sleep fragmentation or sleep deprivation may have significant clinical consequences on the endocrine system. GH and prolactin levels are decreased in patients with obstructive sleep apnea. Sleep deprivation produces evidence of HPA axis activation in the evening of the day following deprivation. Phenomenon of penile reactions, right from infancy till old age, is one of the characteristics of REM sleep in men. Nocturnal penile tumescence studies are, therefore, helpful in determining whether cases of impotence are related to organic or psychogenic reasons. Similarly, in women, REM sleep produces increased vaginal blood flow and clitoral erection. These changes are not necessarily linked to sexual content in associated dreams.

How Sleep Problems are Diagnosed?

Several different medical tests are there to evaluate sleep and assess whether a sleep disorder is present. Most important is a carefully obtained medical history and physical examination to identify a medical conditions that may be interfering with the person's sleep. History of use of prescription and non-prescription medications as well as alcohol, tobacco, and caffeine use is important. Laboratory tests may also be used to help diagnose any medical conditions that may cause sleep problems.

Specialized testing of sleep is termed as sleep study, which are performed to identify a sleep disorder. A sleep study is called polysomnography (PSG). The most common sleep tests include the following:

- Polysomnography: In this test/study, electrodes are attached to the face, eyes, and scalp to measure brain waves such as EEG, EOG, and muscle tone (EMG) during a night's sleep. Other body functions parameters such as airflow, breathing effort, blood oxygen levels, leg movements, electrocardiogram (ECG), and body position are also be measured. Sleep studies are most commonly conducted in specially designed labs in hospitals or sleep clinics
- The multiple sleep latency test (MSLT) are a series of sleep studies (PSG) designed to measure daytime sleepiness. The test is based upon the fact that the sleepier an individual is, the faster he or she will fall asleep. During this test, the patient is given 4–5 opportunities to nap in a quiet, dark room, usually at 2 hour intervals during the daytime. Body functions such as EEG, EOG, and muscle tone are studied as in PSG. The time period of sleep onset from wakefulness is measured to determine the "sleep latency". Similar PSG are repeated during each of the 4–5 naps, and an average time for sleep latency across all the naps is calculated. Usually, sleep latency of 5 minutes or less is marked as significant to suggest severe daytime sleepiness
- Maintenance of wakefulness test (MWT) is similar to the MSLT and is conducted to assess the individual's ability to stay awake when reclining in a quiet, darkened room
- The Epworth sleepiness scale is the most popular questionnaire that is given to patients, as part of clinic visit by the patient. The test comprises of several questions to rate how likely they would be to fall asleep in a number of diverse situations (such as travel in a car, sitting quietly after lunch, etc.).

SLEEP HYGIENE

Nonmedical lifestyle behavioral practices that are believed to help in sleep are referred to as sleep hygiene. These lifestyle adjustments offer the maximum potential for restorative and sound sleep. Good sleep hygiene practices include:

- Avoid caffeine, nicotine, and alcohol before bedtime. Caffeine consumed early in the day can also have an effect on the ability to fall asleep at night
- Adhere to a regular bedtime and waking schedule
- Maintain a comfortable sleep environment, including a comfortable temperature of the room
- Do not lie in bed awake or worry about not sleeping (or anything else negative) while in bed. This produces anxiety and can make the problem of sleeplessness worse
- Get regular daily exercise in the morning, however, avoid exercise 2 hours prior to bedtime.

SLEEP MYTHS

Myth 1: *Sleep is a time when our body and brain stops working for rest and relaxation.* Evidence, in fact, shows some physiological processes actually become more active while one sleeps proving the belief of organ shut down wrong. For example, secretion of certain hormones is boosted, the pathways in the brain linked to learning and memory shows an increased activity.

Myth 2: *Sleeping one hour less won't affect your normal daytime functioning.* One hour of less sleep may not make one sleepy, but one's ability to think and decide quickly may be affected, if lack of sleep continues, cardiovascular health and energy balance as well as one's ability to fight infections declines. If one consistently does not get enough sleep, a sleep debt builds up that one can never repay. This sleep debt affects one's health and quality of life and makes one feel tired during the day.

Myth 3: *One's body adjusts quickly to different sleep schedules.* Normally, one's biological clock makes one most alert during the daytime and least alert at night. Thus, even if one works in night shift he will feel sleepy during night. Most people can reset their biological clock, but by 1–2 hours per day at maximum. Thus, at least more than a week time is required for one to adjust to a substantial change in ones sleep–wake cycle—for example, when traveling across several time zones or switching from working the day shift to the night shift.

Myth 4: *People need less sleep as they get older.* Physiologically, as people age, the quality of their sleep changes. They find their sleep less refreshing and insomnia or medical conditions disrupting their sleep which is quite common, but they don't need less sleep.

Myth 5: *Extra sleep for one night can cure one with excessive daytime tiredness.* The quality of sleep is as important as the quantity of sleep. This explains why some people may sleep 8 or 9 hours a night but don't feel well rested as their quality of sleep is poor. The quality of sleep is affected by a number of sleep disorders and some medical conditions, unless these conditions are corrected, excessive daytime fatigue won't be lessened. Adequate behavioral changes or medical therapy can treat most of these conditions.

Myth 6: *By sleeping more on the weekends one can make up for lost sleep during the week.* Inadequate sleep of many days can't be met by sleeping more on weekends even though one may feel more rested. On the other hand it further complicates ones biological clock and it is much harder to go to sleep at the right time on Sunday nights and get up early on Monday mornings.

Myth 7: *Naps wastes ones time.* Although naps can never substitute a good night's sleep, but can be refreshing and can be restorative. But one should avoid taking naps later than 3 PM, especially if one has difficulty falling asleep at night, as late naps can make it harder for you to fall asleep when you go to bed. Naps longer than 20 minutes should be avoided as it is more difficult to get into the swing of things after a long nap. A hidden sleep disorder should be suspected if one takes too many naps during the day.

Myth 8: *Snoring implies sound sleep.* As one gets older snoring during sleep is common. It is established that snoring on a regular basis can increase the risk for diabetes and heart disease and make one tired during the day. Child snorers have been established as poor achievers in school in studies. In fact loud snoring may signify obstructive sleep apnea which is a serious sleep disorders and warrants treatment.

Myth 9: *Children who don't sleep enough at night are sleepy during the day.* In contrast to adults, children not getting enough sleep at night are not sleepy but become hyperactive, irritable, and inattentive during the day. They also have increased risk of behavioral problems, are prone to injuries, and may have impaired growth rate. Sleep debt appears to be quite common during young age and at times misdiagnosed as attention-deficit hyperactivity disorder.

Myth 10: *Insomnia is most commonly caused by worry.* True, stress and worry may be a cause for temporary insomnia, but a persistent insomnia should be prodded more deeply. Certain medications and sleep disorders are known to cause insomnia. Depression, anxiety disorders and asthma, arthritis, or other medical conditions are known to cause insomnia.

REFERENCES

1. National Transportation Safety Board. Grounding of the U.S. Tankship EXXON VALDEZ on Bligh Reef, Prince William Sound near Valdez, AK March 24, 1989. Washington, DC. National Transportation Safety Board; 1990. NTIS Report Number PB90-916405.
2. Report of the Presidential Commission on the Space Shuttle Challenger Accident. Vol. 2. Appendix G. Human Factors Analysis. Washington, DC. U.S. Government Printing Office; 1986.
3. Knipling R, Wang J. Revised estimates of the U.S. Drowsy driver crash problem size based on general estimates system case reviews. Thirty-Ninth Annual Proceedings of the Association for the Advancement of Automotive Medicine. Des Plaines, IL: Association for the Advancement of Automotive Medicine; 1995:415-66.
4. Stoller MK. Economic effects of insomnia. *Clin Ther*. 1994;16:873-97.
5. National Sleep Foundation. Survey: Sleep in America. Washington, DC. National Sleep Foundation; 2000.
6. Scammell TE. The Regulation of Sleep and Circadian Rhythms. *Sleep Medicine Alert*. (National Sleep Foundation). 2004;8:1-6.
7. Iber C, Ancoli-Israel S, Chesson AL, et al. The AASM Manual for the Scoring of Sleep and Associated Events: Rules, Terminology and Technical Specifications. Westchester, IL: American Academy of Sleep Medicine; 2007.
8. Kryger MH, Roth T, Dement WC, editors. Principals and Practice of Sleep Medicine. Philadelphia, Pa: Saunders; 2005.
9. Siegel JM. Clues to the functions of mammalian sleep. *Nature*. 2005;437(7063):1264-71.
10. Siegal JM, Moore R, Thannickal T, et al. A Brief History of Hypocretin/Orexin and Narcolepsy. *Neuropsychopharmacology*. 2001;25:S14-20.
11. España RA, Scammell TE. Sleep neurobiology for the clinician. *Sleep*. 2004;27:811-20.
12. Chokroverty S. Physiologic changes in sleep. In: Sleep Disorders Medicine. Boston: Butterworth-Heinemann; 1999. pp. 95-126.
13. Saper CB, Scammell TE, Lu J. Hypothalamic regulation of sleep and circadian rhythms. *Nature*. 2005;437(7063):1257-63.
14. Morrison AR. Coming to grips with a "new" state of consciousness: the study of rapid-eye-movement sleep in the 1960s. *J Hist Neurosci*. 2013;22(4):392-407.
15. Tobaldini E, Nobili L, Strada S, et al. Heart rate variability in normal and pathological sleep. *Front Physiol*. 2013;4:294.
16. Braun AR, Balkin TJ, Wesensten NJ, et al. Regional cerebral blood flow throughout the sleep-wake cycle. An H2(15)O PET study. *Brain*. 1997;120(Pt 7):1173-97.
17. Desseilles M, Dang-Vu T, Schabus M, et al. Neuroimaging insights into the pathophysiology of sleep disorders. *Sleep*. 2008;31(6):777-94.
18. Anderson KN, Catt M, Collerton J, et al. Assessment of sleep and circadian rhythm disorders in the very old: the Newcastle 85+ Cohort Study. *Age Ageing*. 2014;43:57-63.
19. Czeisler CA, Duffy JF, Shanahan TL, et al. Stability, precision, and near-24-hour period of the human circadian pacemaker. *Science*. 1999;284(5423):2177-81.

20. Tosini G, Pozdeyev N, Sakamoto K, et al. The circadian clock system in the mammalian retina. *Bioessays.* 2008;30(7):624-33.
21. Sack RL, Auckley D, Auger R, et al. Circadian rhythm disorders: Part 1, Basic Principles, Shift Work and Jet Lab Disorders. *Sleep.* 2007;30(11):1460-83.
22. Sack RL, Auckley D, Auger RR, et al. Circadian rhythm sleep disorders: Part II, advanced sleep phase disorder, delayed sleep phase disorder, free-running disorder and irregular sleep-wake rhythtm. *Sleep.* 2007;30(11):1484-501.
23. Banks S, Dinger DF. Behavioral and physiological consequences of sleep restriction. *J Clin Sleep Med.* 2007;3(5):519-28.
24. Bonnet MH, Arand DL. We are chronically sleep deprived. *Sleep.* 1995;18(10):908-11.
25. Moldofsky H. Sleep and the immune system. *Int J Immunopharmacol.* 1995;17(8):649-54.
26. Gomes AA, Tavares J, de Azevedo MH. Sleep and academic performance in undergraduates: a multi-measure, multi-predictor approach. *Chronobiol Int.* 2011;28(9):786-801.
27. Thorne D, Thomas M, Russo M, et al. Performance on a driving-simulator divided attention task during one week of restricted nightly sleep. *Sleep.* 1999;22(Suppl 1):301.
28. Boto LR, Crispim JN, de Melo IS, et al. Sleep deprivation and accidental fall risk in children. *Sleep Med.* 2011;13:88-95.
29. Howard ME, Jackson ML, Berlowitz D, et al. Specific sleepiness symptoms are indicators of performance impairment during sleep deprivation. *Accid Anal Prev.* 2013;62C:1-8.
30. Veauthier C. Younger age, female sex, and high number of awakenings and arousals predict fatigue in patients with sleep disorders: a retrospective polysomnographic observational study. *Neuropsychiatr Dis Treat.* 2013;9:1483-94.
31. Baird AL, Coogan AN, Siddiqui A, et al. Adult attention-deficit hyperactivity disorder is associated with alterations in circadian rhythms at the behavioural, endocrine and molecular levels. *Mol Psychiatry.* 2011;
32. Thorne D, Thomas M, Sing H, et al. Driving-simulator accident rates before, during, and after one week of restricted night sleep. *Sleep.* 1998;21(Suppl 3):235.
33. Knutson KL, Ryden AM, Mander BA, et al. Role of sleep duration and quality in tihe risk and severity of type 2 diabetes mellitus. *Arch Inter Med.* 2006;166(16):1768-74.

CHAPTER 2

Anatomy and Physiology of Obstructive Sleep Apnea Airways

Ashwini Malhotra, Vivek Nangia

INTRODUCTION

The airways form the connection between the outside world and the terminal respiratory units. They are of central importance to our understanding of lung function in health and disease (Figure 1). Intrapulmonary airways are divided into three major groups: bronchi, membranous bronchioles, and respiratory bronchioles/gas exchange ducts.

Bronchi, by definition, have cartilage in their wall. Respiratory bronchioles serve a dual function as airways and as part of the alveolar volume (gas exchange). The membranous bronchioles (non-cartilaginous airways of approximately 1 mm diameter or less), although exceedingly numerous, are short in length. They consist of about five branching generations and end at the terminal bronchioles. In contrast to the bronchi, the membranous bronchioles are tightly embedded in the connective tissue framework of the lung and, therefore, enlarge passively as lung volume increases

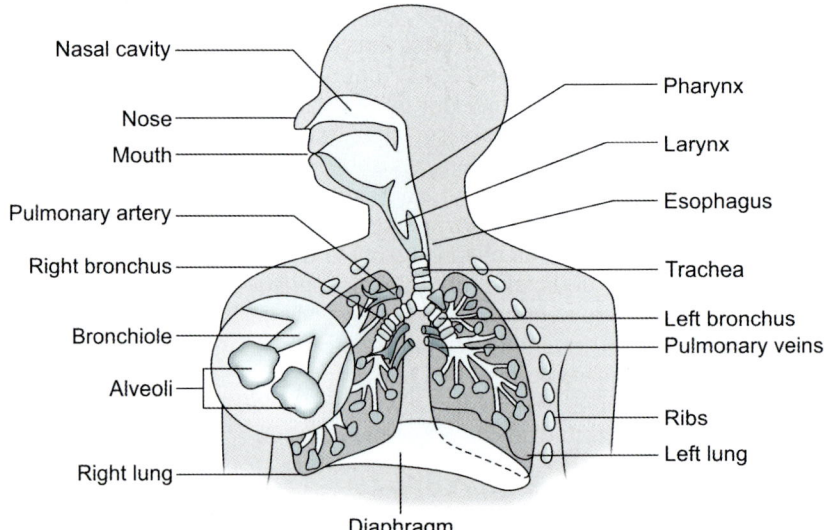

Figure 1: Respiratory system.

Most airway resistance resides in the upper airways and bronchi. Normally, the large airways maintain partial constriction due to bronchomotor tone. Minimal airway diameter in the human lung, about 0.5 mm, is reached at the level of the terminal bronchioles; succeeding generations of exchange ducts (respiratory bronchioles and alveolar ducts) are of constant diameter.

ANATOMY OF UPPER AIRWAY OBSTRUCTION

Obstructive sleep apnea (OSA) is known to be associated with alterations in upper airway anatomy. With a change in state comes a change in upper airway collapsibility.

Patency of pharyngeal airway is maintained by opposing forces: the activity of upper airway muscles, which dilates and stiffens the airways and negative intraluminal pressure, which tends to collapse them. This balance can be disturbed by abnormalities involving neural control and/or upper airway anatomy. Patients with OSA have been shown to have a narrowed, more collapsible pharyngeal airway. Sleep related decrease in upper airway dilating muscle activity can lead to greater negative intraluminal pharyngeal pressure, which leads in turn to further narrowing and complete closure of the airway.

Possible Sites of Upper Airway Obstruction

- Nose
  - Blocked nose due to choanal atresia/foreign body/polyps/allergy
- Oropharynx
  - Adenoidal hypertrophy, micrognathia, craniofacial abnormalities, large tongue
- Supraglottis
  - Epiglottitis: *H. influenzae* type B
- Larynx
  - Laryngomalacia due to obstruction, laryngeal papillomata
- Subglottis
  - Laryngotracheobronchitis (Croup).

The upper airway is a common passage for digestive, respiratory, and phonatory systems. Traditionally, it is divided to three sections: (1) the nasopharynx; (2) oropharynx; and (3) hypopharynx (Figure 2).

Nasopharynx

Nasopharynx extends from the posterior margin of the nasal turbinates; it lies above the soft palate and continues inferiorly with the oropharynx. Adenoids occupy the posterior wall, which when inflamed can partially obstruct the upper airway.

Soft palate is nearly a vertical flap which extends from the posterior edge of hard palate and terminates in the uvula. All the muscles of the soft palate are innervated by the pharyngeal branch of vagus nerve except the tensor veli palatini, which is innervated by the medial pterygoid nerve. A posterior elevation of the soft palate toward the posterior pharyngeal wall can cause enlargement of the oral cavity during swallowing and produce narrowing of the nasopharynx. Adenotonsillar disease can lead to sleep-disordered breathing. Polysomnography

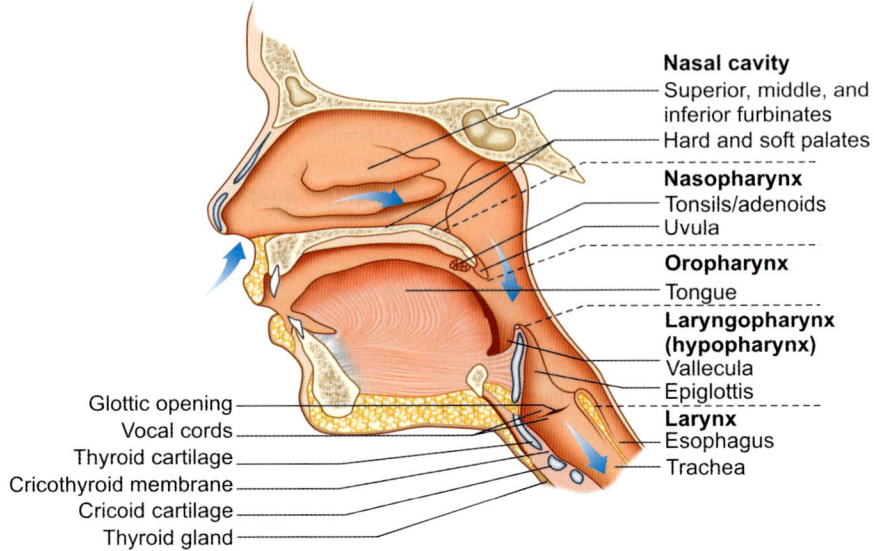

Figure 2: Nasal cavity.

in children with allergic rhinitis and adenoidal hypertrophy found that 2/3rd of such have mild apnea during sleep.[1] Amongst children, tonsillectomy and/or adenoidectomy is the first therapeutic modality to be considered for the treatment of OSA.[2]

Natural breathing in humans is through nose, particularly during sleep, when the daily oral fraction of breathing, estimated at 7%, drops to 4% during sleep.[3] Nasal and oral resistances are equal during wakefulness, but nasal resistance is lower than the oral at night[4] but increases in the supine position.[5]

Connection between the nose and breathing in sleep was first mentioned by Hippocrates[6] when he described a role of nasal polyps in restless sleep. Nasal obstruction can occur secondary to deviated nasal septum, chronic rhinosinusitis, and nasal polyps. Nasal congestion has been associated with a threefold increase in the incidence of snoring and daytime sleepiness.[7] Few earlier studies have indicated that acute nasal obstruction could increase apnea-hypopnea index, prolong rapid eye movement (REM) latency, and increase non-REM sleep.[8] However, nasal obstruction alone is not thought to cause any moderate or severe OSA.[6,9]

Oropharynx

The roof of the oral cavity is formed by *hard and soft palate* (Figure 3) and the lingual mucosa covers the floor. Buccal mucosa and anterior pillars of palatine tonsils covers the lateral part of the oral cavity, which define the junction with oropharynx. The oropharynx extends from the soft palate to the epiglottis (Figure 4). The anterior part of oropharynx is formed by the posterior part of the tongue and the soft palate, whereas the posterior part is formed by the pharyngeal constrictor muscles. The lateral pharyngeal walls are formed by the pharyngeal constrictors, muscles of the extrinsic muscles of the soft palate, and the larynx.

Anatomy and Physiology of Obstructive Sleep Apnea Airways

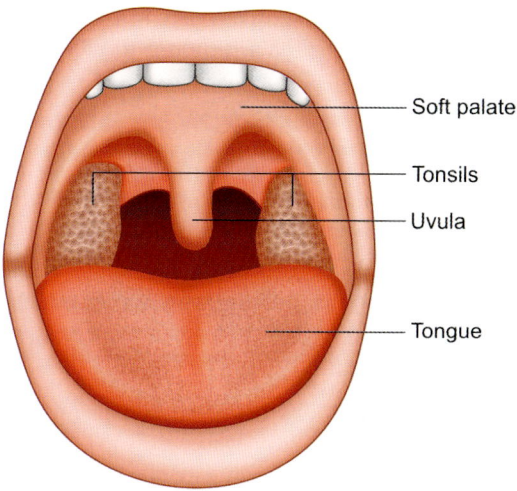

Figure 3: Tonsils.

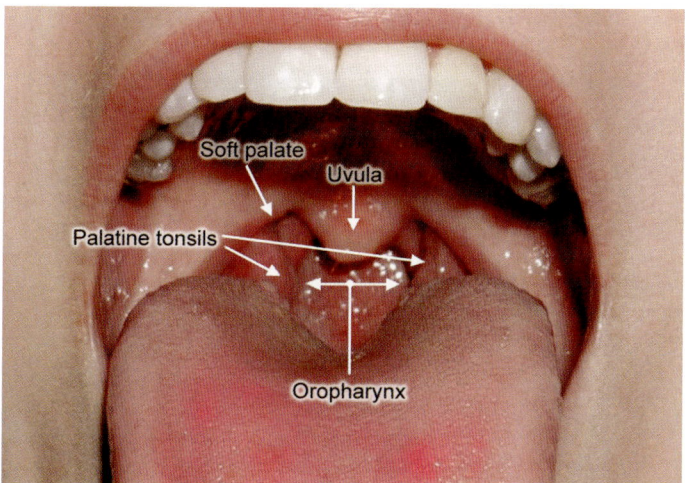

Figure 4: Oropharynx.

Other structures that contribute to upper airway lume, located in the retropalatal area, are the palatine tonsils and parapharyngeal fat pads.

The *tongue* occupies the major part of the oral cavity and has both extrinsic and intrinsic muscle groups. The four extrinsic tongue muscles are (1) genioglossus; (2) hyoglossus; (3) palatoglossus; and (4) styloglossus. The genioglossus is the largest and most-studied pharyngeal dilator muscle. All of these muscles are innervated by the hypoglossal nerve except the palatoglossus, which is innervated by the vagus nerve. The intrinsic muscles of the tongue (superior and inferior longitudinal, transverse, and vertical muscles) are confined to the tongue. The anterior two-thirds of the tongue is innervated by the facial nerve, whereas the posterior one-third is innervated by cranial nerve IX. The size of the tongue is an important risk factor for OSA.[10]

An increase in the size of type II muscle fibers is seen in OSA compared with normal subjects, which could represent a response to vibratory strain or perhaps neuronal activity.[11,12] The hypoglossal nerve is a critical component in the motor control of upper airway dilatation. The muscle fibers in the posterior part of the tongue are fatigue-resistant, thereby sustaining the forward tongue position and preventing its collapse into the retroglossal area. Using this mechanism, the therapeutic effect of proximal hypoglossal nerve stimulation can be used to treat OSA.[13]

It was found that there is a smaller minimum airway area in patients with OSA in the retropalatal region, and particularly in the lateral dimension, compared with individuals with normal breathing.[14] Independent risk factors of OSA are the volume of the tongue and lateral walls.[15]

Most common site of airway collapse in patients with OSA is oropharynx,[16] which is more likely to occur during REM sleep.[17] The role of parapharyngeal fat in the predisposition to OSA has been studied using magnetic resonance imaging (MRI).

Those patients with retropalatal airway closure had a more parapharyngeal and soft palate fat, whereas patients with retroglossal airway closure had more of the tongue and parapharyngeal fat pad.[18]

Hypopharynx

Hypopharynx is the caudal portion of upper airways, which extends from the superior border of the epiglottis to the inferior border of the cricoid cartilage.

Obstruction at the level of the hypopharynxis is less common than at the oropharynx. The structures in the hypopharynx, such as the lingual tonsils, can have a potential role in OSA.[19] In children with tonsillar hypertrophy, tonsillectomy is an effective treatment for snoring and OSA.[20]

Epiglottic prolapse (Figure 5) during inspiration has been described as a cause of OSA, with a partial laser epiglottidectomy reported as a cure.[21,22]

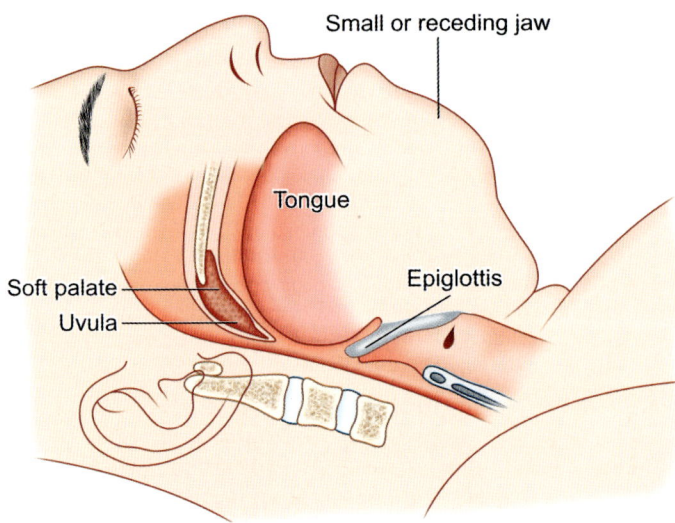

Figure 5: Epiglottic prolapse.

PHYSIOLOGY

The goals of respiration are to provide oxygen to the tissues and to remove carbon dioxide. To achieve these goals, respiration can be divided into four major functions: (1) pulmonary ventilation, which means the inflow and outflow of air between the atmosphere and the lung alveoli; (2) diffusion of oxygen and carbon dioxide between the alveoli and the blood; (3) transport of oxygen and carbon dioxide in the blood and body fluids to and from the body's tissue cells; and (4) regulation of ventilation and other facets of respiration.

The lungs can be expanded and contracted in two ways: (1) by downward and upward movement of the diaphragm to lengthen or shorten the chest cavity and (2) by elevation and depression of the ribs to increase and decrease the anteroposterior diameter of the chest cavity.

The lung is an elastic structure that collapses like a balloon and expels all its air through the trachea whenever there is no force to keep it inflated. Also, there are no attachments between the lung and the walls of the chest cage, except where it is suspended at its hilum from the mediastinum. Instead, the lung "floats" in the thoracic cavity, surrounded by a thin layer of pleural fluid that lubricates movement of the lungs within the cavity.

PATHOPHYSIOLOGY

Obstructive sleep apnea is characterized by recurrent collapse of the pharyngeal airway during sleep, resulting in substantially reduced (hypopnea) or complete cessation (apnea) of airflow despite ongoing breathing efforts. These disruptions to breathing lead to intermittent blood gas disturbances (hypercapnia and hypoxemia) and surges of sympathetic activation. Loud snoring is a typical feature of OSA and in most cases the culmination of a respiratory event is associated with a brief awakening from sleep (arousal). These events result in a cyclical breathing pattern and fragmented sleep as the patient oscillates between wakefulness and sleep. In severe cases, respiratory events can occur more than 100 times per hour and typically each event lasts 20–40 seconds.

The multifactorial pathophysiology of OSA comes with individual variability. The complex interaction among pharyngeal dilator tone, arousal threshold, respiratory control instability, and changes in lung volume during sleep plays an important role in OSA.

Collapsibility of Upper Airways

Although the ability of the upper airway to change shape and momentarily close is essential for speech and swallowing during wakefulness, this feature also provides the opportunity for collapse at inopportune times such as during sleep.

From a purely anatomic perspective, a narrow upper airway is generally more prone to collapse than a larger one.

Due to changes in transmural pressure, the vulnerable airway which is from the hard palate to the larynx, can collapse while sleeping.

Apneic airway has thicker lateral pharyngeal walls with an anteroposterior elliptical configuration, in contrast to the horizontal configuration of normal airways. This fact of thickened airways is more important than the enlargement of parapharyngeal fat pads for causing airway narrowing in apneic patients.[14]

The minimal airway area is also smaller in apneic patients, contributing to the airway collapse. Threshold pressure required to maintain patency of the upper airways is called pharyngeal critical closing pressure (Pcrit). Pcrit has been shown to correlate with OSA severity.[23]

Pharyngeal airway is a collapsible tube surrounded by tissue within a bony box.[24] The luminal size is determined by the properties of the tube and the transmural pressure. Increase in the pressure outside the tube will promote luminal narrowing.

Pharyngeal closing pressure increases as the tissue pressure increases, which can happen in following conditions—a high-arched palate, midface hypoplasia, reduction in size of the bony box from micrognathia or from soft tissue crowding caused by macroglossia, adenotonsillar hypertrophy, and central adiposity.[25] Obesity acts synergistically with narrowing of the bony box. The receded mandibles in apneic patients contribute to increased tissue pressure[26] and, consequently, pharyngeal collapse. Conversely, weight loss has been shown to reduce Pcrit[27] and the resolution of sleep disordered breathing depends on the degree of Pcrit reduction. Similarly, a stepwise advancement of the mandible in apneic patients leads to dose dependent reductions in Pcrit.[28]

Effects of Lung Volumes

The interaction between pharyngeal patency and lung volume is believed to be an important contributor to OSA pathogenesis.

Caudal traction and elongation of the airway reduces Pcrit through stiffening the airway and mitigating the surrounding tissue pressures.[29,30]

Lung volumes are reduced in supine position in apneic patients, which decreases caudal traction on the airway. By increasing end-expiratory lung volume using continuous positive airway pressure (CPAP) apnea severity is reduced and sleep architecture is improved.[31] While sleeping in the semi-recumbent position also reduces apnea severity.[32]

Upper Airway Dilator Muscle Activity and Reflex Responsiveness

Pharyngeal dilator muscle activity is offset by collapsing forces related to tissue pressure and intraluminal negative pressure. Genioglossus, the largest and most extensively studied upper airway dilator muscle in humans, has higher activity in patients with OSA compared with control subjects.[33] During wakefulness, upper airway dilator tone is high, and this maintains an open airway. With sleep onset, a decrease in the tone of the genioglossus muscle occurs. Airway instability occurs in apneic patients who rely on heightened genioglossus tone to support the airway.[34] The degree to which this occurs also depends on the sleep stage. Heightened genioglossus tone is present in slow wave sleep, which might be protective against OSA.[35] During REM sleep, a reduction in tonic genioglossus activity occurs, which potentiates further apneas.[36] Genioglossus and tensor palatine tone increases with local reflexes generated by negative pharyngeal pressure during sleep, especially in the supine position.[37,38] Genioglossus activity increases during inspiration but decreases during expiration.[33] The genioglossus has both excitatory and inhibitory responses to airway collapse, but the response is variable.[39]

AROUSAL RESPONSE IN OBSTRUCTIVE SLEEP APNEA

Arousal from sleep at the cessation of a hypopnea or an apnea has long been believed to be an important protective mechanism for airway re-opening. Most apneic episodes are followed by arousals, which are thought to be mediated via negative intrathoracic pressure generation.[40] With the accumulation of stimuli, such as chemical drive and negative intrapharyngeal pressures, apnea termination can occur without arousals.[41-43] OSA impairs the arousal threshold, and therefore apneic patients need greater inspiratory efforts to trigger an arousal.[44]

Heightened arousal threshold in apneic patients is reduced with the treatment using CPAP.[45] Slow-wave sleep may stabilize the breathing in apneic patients via the arousal threshold. Ratnavadivel and colleagues[46] showed that the arousal threshold is further increased in slow-wave sleep compared with N2 sleep, but they did not find evidence supporting increased ventilatory drive or increased upper airway responses during slow-wave sleep compared with N2 sleep.

Ventilatory Control Stability and Pharyngeal Neuropathy

Typical feature of OSA is the cyclical breathing pattern that develops whereby the patient oscillates between obstructive breathing events (sleep) and arousal (wakefulness).

Ventilatory control stability contributes to OSA pathogenesis but is incompletely understood.[22] Loop gain is the feedback loop that controls the respiratory response to airway collapsibility and arousal, and which refers to the magnitude of the response relative to the intensity of the input.[47] Elevated loop gain is found in apneic patients, particularly those with severe OSA,[48,49] which leads to excessive increase of ventilatory response to apneas and arousal, leading to disproportionately lowered carbon dioxide (CO_2).

In a recent study, Yuan and colleagues[50] found that obese adolescents with OSA had a higher CO_2 sensitivity during wakefulness compared with the lean control group. In few studies, the ventilatory response during wakefulness in OSA has been inconsistent.[51] Importantly, the sensitivity decreased during sleep in the apneic adolescents. This blunting would lead to prolonged obstructive events. However, the magnitude of the ventilatory response to spontaneous arousal may promote driving the CO_2 below the apneic threshold, leading to further sleep-disordered breathing.[50] In a study by Edwards and colleagues,[52] acetazolamide reduced the ventilator response to spontaneous arousal in patients with OSA treated with CPAP, and improved this ventilatory instability.

Pharyngeal neuropathy is well described in OSA patients.[53-55] Two-point discrimination and vibratory tests are used to show the selective impairment of the ability to detect mechanical stimuli in the upper airway of patients with OSA and snorers.[53] Air pressure pulses during endoscopy is used to show the abnormal laryngeal sensation in patients with OSA.[54] Inflammation and denervation affect the oral mucosa and upper airway muscles in patients with OSA.[55] Whether it is the vibratory strain[56] or intermittent hypoxia[57] that plays a major role in promoting the pharyngeal neuropathy is still not clear. A recent study found neurogenic changes in the genioglossus[58] using measurements of motor unit potentials.

Saboisky and colleagues[58] reported evidence of collateral sprouting and re-innervation in the genioglossus, which correlated with lowest oxygen desaturation in patients with OSA. How this neuropathy affects upper airway function during sleep remains to be determined.

Increased fat deposits in the soft tissue surrounding the upper airway is found in obese patients, including in the soft palate.[59,60] Obesity is a major risk factor in OSA. Finding of a small increase in upper airway soft tissue volume in apneic patients compared with normal controls was confirmed in Japanese patients.[61]

Furthermore, a small decrease of 17 cm^3 in upper airway volume from overall weight loss (average of 7.8 kg) led to a 31% decrease in the AHI.[62] A reduction in functional residual capacity (FRC) is seen in obese individuals[63] and decreased upper airway patency from low FRC is an additional mechanism contributing to OSA in obese patients.[64] Consequently, weight loss and improvement in FRC would augment upper airway patency.

CONCLUSION

Understanding of the pathogenesis of OSA is evolving. Airway obstruction can occur at several sites in the upper airway, with the oropharynx being the most common. The hypoglossal nerve is a key player in upper airway dilator function. Retrognathia, adenotonsillar hypertrophy, enlarged tongue, lateral pharyngeal wall thickening, and parapharyngeal fat pads are important anatomic risk factors. The arousal response is heightened in apneic patients. Elevated loop gain leads to an overshoot of ventilator response in OSA, contributing to ventilator instability. The role of pharyngeal neuropathy in the pathophysiology of OSA is being investigated.

REFERENCES

1. Ramos RT, Da Cunha Daltro CH, et al. OSAS in children: clinical and polysomnographicrespiratory profile. *Braz J Otorhinolaryngol.* 2006;72(3):355-61.
2. Marcus CL, Brooks LJ, Ward SD, et al. Diagnosis and management of childhood obstructive sleep apnea syndrome. *Pediatrics.* 2012;130(3):714-55.
3. Fitzpatrick MF, Driver HS, Chatha N, et al. Partitioning of inhaled ventilation between the nasal and oral routes during sleep in normal subjects. *J Appl Physiol.* 2003;94(3):883-90.
4. Fitzpatrick MF, McLean H, Urton AM, et al. Effect of nasal or oral breathing route on upper airway resistance during sleep. *Eur Respir J.* 2003;22(5):827-32.
5. Duggan CJ, Watson RA, Pride NB. Postural changes in nasal and pulmonary resistance in subjects with asthma. *J Asthma.* 2004;41(7):701-7.
6. Georgalas C. The role of the nose in snoring and obstructive sleep apnoea: an update. *Eur Arch Otorhinolaryngol.* 2011;268(9):1365-73.
7. Young T, Finn L, Palta M. Chronic nasal congestion at night is a risk factor for snoring in a population based cohort study. *Arch Intern Med.* 2001;161(12):1514-9.
8. Olsen KD, Kern EB, Westbrook PR. Sleep and breathing disturbance secondary to nasal obstruction. *Otolaryngol Head Neck Surg.* 1981;89(5):804-10.
9. McNicholas WT. The nose and OSA: variable nasal obstruction may be more important in pathophysiology than fixed obstruction. *Eur Respir J.* 2008;32(1):3-8.
10. Schwab RJ, Pasirstein M, Pierson R, et al. Identification of upper airway anatomic risk factors for obstructive sleep apnea with volumetric magnetic resonance imaging. *Am J Respir Crit Care Med.* 2003;168(5):522-30.
11. Series F, Cote C, Simoneau JA, et al. Physiologic, metabolic, and muscle fiber type characteristics of musculus uvulae in sleep apnea hypopnea syndrome and in snorers. *J Clin Invest.* 1995;95:20-5.
12. Lindman R, Stal PS. Abnormal palatopharyngeal muscle morphology in sleep-disordered breathing. *J Neurol Sci.* 2002;195:11-23.

13. Zaidi FN, Meadows P, Jacobowitz O, et al. Tongue anatomy and physiology, the scientific basis for anovel targeted neuro stimulation system designed for the treatment of obstructive sleep apnea. *Neuromodulation.* 2013;16(4):376-86.
14. Schwab RJ, Gupta KB, Gefter WB, et al. Upper airway and soft tissue anatomy in normal subjects and patients with sleep-disordered breathing. Significance of the lateral pharyngeal walls. *Am J Respir Crit Care Med.* 1995;152:1673-89.
15. Katsantonis GP, Moss K, Miyazaki S, et al. Determining the site of airway collapse in obstructive sleep apnea with airway pressure monitoring. *Laryngoscope.* 1993;103(10):1126-31.
16. Schwab RJ, Gefter WB, Hoffman EA, et al. Dynamic upper airway imaging during awake respiration in normal subjects and patients with sleep disordered breathing. *Am Rev Respir Dis.* 1993;148(5):1385-400.
17. Boudewyns AN, Van de Heyning PH, DeBacker WA. Site of upper airway obstruction in obstructive apnoea and influence of sleep stage. *Eur Respir J.* 1997;10(11):2566-72.
18. Li Y, Lin N, Ye J, et al. Upper airway fat tissue distribution in subjects with obstructive sleep apnea and its effect on retropalatal mechanical loads. *Respir Care.* 2012;57(7):1098-105.
19. Suzuki K, Kawakatsu K, Hattori C, et al. Application of lingual tonsillectomy to sleep apnea syndrome involving lingual tonsils. *Acta Otolaryngol Suppl.* 2003;550:65-71.
20. Abdel-Aziz M, Ibrahim N, Ahmed A, et al. Lingual tonsils hypertrophy; a cause of obstructive sleep apnea in children after adenotonsillectomy: operative problems and management. *Int J Pediatr Otorhinolaryngol.* 2011;75(9):1127-31.
21. Catalfumo FJ, Golz A, Westerman ST, et al. The epiglottis and obstructive sleep apnoea syndrome. *J Laryngol Otol.* 1998;112(10):940-3.
22. Eckert DJ, Malhotra A. Pathophysiology of adult obstructive sleep apnea. *Proc Am Thorac Soc.* 2008;5:144-53.
23. Issa FG, Sullivan CE. Upper airway closing pressures in obstructive sleep apnea. *J Appl Physiol.* 1984;57:520-7.
24. Smith PL, Wise RA, Gold AR, et al. Upper airway pressure-flow relationships in obstructive sleep apnea. *J Appl Physiol.* 1988;64(2):789-95.
25. Schwartz AR, Smith PL, Schneider H, et al. Invited editorial on "Lung volume and upper airway collapsibility: what does it tell us about pathogenic mechanisms?" *J Appl Physiol.* 2012;113:689-90.
26. Watanabe T, Isono S, Tanaka A, et al. Contribution of body habitus and craniofacial characteristics to segmental closing pressures of the passive pharynx in patients with sleep-disordered breathing. *Am J Respir Crit Care Med.* 2002;165:260-5.
27. Schwartz AR, Gold AR, Schubert N, et al. Effect of weight loss on upper airway collapsibility in obstructive sleep apnea. *Am Rev Respir Dis.* 1991;144:494-8.
28. Kato J, Isono S, Tanaka A, et al. Dose-dependent effects of mandibular advancement on pharyngeal mechanics and nocturnal oxygenation in patients with sleep-disordered breathing. *Chest.* 2000;117:1065-72.
29. Thut DC, Schwartz AR, Roach D, et al. Tracheal and neck position influence upper airway airflow dynamics by altering airway length. *J Appl Physiol.* 1993;75:2084-90.
30. Kairaitis K, Byth K, Parikh R, et al. Tracheal traction effects on upper airway patency in rabbits: the role of tissue pressure. *Sleep.* 2007;30:179-86.
31. Heinzer RC, Stanchina ML, Malhotra A, et al. Effect of increased lung volume on sleep disordered breathing in patients with sleep apnoea. *Thorax.* 2006;61:435-9.
32. McEvoy RD, Sharp DJ, Thornton AT. The effects of posture on obstructive sleep apnea. *Am Rev Respir Dis.* 1986;133:662-6.
33. Jordan AS, White DP. Pharyngeal motor control and the pathogenesis of obstructive sleep apnea. *Respir Physiol Neurobiol.* 2008;160:1-7.
34. Mezzanotte WS, Tangel DJ, White DP. Influence of sleep onset on upper-airway muscle activity in apnea patients versus normal controls. *Am J Respir Crit Care Med.* 1996;153:1880-7.
35. Basner RC, Ringler J, Schwartzstein RM, et al. Phasic electromyographic activity of the genio-glossus increases in normals during slow-wave sleep. *Respir Physiol.* 1991;83:189-200.

36. Jordan AS, White DP, Lo YL, et al. Airway dilator muscle activity and lung volume during stable breathing in obstructive sleep apnea. *Sleep.* 2009;32(3):361-8.
37. Malhotra A, Trinder J, Fogel R, et al. Postural effects on pharyngeal protective reflex mechanisms. *Sleep.* 2004;27:1105-12.
38. Wheatley JR, Tangel DJ, Mezzanotte WS, et al. Influence of sleep on response to negative airway pressure of tensor palatini muscle and retropalatal airway. *J Appl Physiol.* 1993;75:2117-24.
39. Eckert DJ, Saboisky JP, Jordan AS, et al. A secondary reflex suppression phase is present in genioglossus but not tensor palatini in response to negative upper airway pressure. *J Appl Physiol.* 2010;108(6):1619-24.
40. Gleeson K, Zwillich CW, White DP. The influence of increasing ventilatory effort on arousal from sleep. *Am Rev Respir Dis.* 1990;142:295-300.
41. Younes M. Role of arousals in the pathogenesis of obstructive sleep apnea. *Am J Respir Crit Care Med.* 2004;169:623-33.
42. Lo YL, Jordan AS, Malhotra A, et al. Genioglossal muscle response to CO_2 stimulation during NREM sleep. *Sleep.* 2006;29:470-7.
43. Horner RL, Innes JA, Murphy K, et al. Evidence for reflex upper airway dilator muscle activation by sudden negative airway pressure in man. *J Physiol.* 1991;436:15-29.
44. Berry RB, Kouchi KG, Der DE, et al. Sleep apnea impairs the arousal response to airway occlusion. *Chest.* 1996;109:1490-6.
45. Haba-Rubio J, Sforza E, Weiss T, et al. Effect of CPAP treatment on inspiratory arousal threshold during NREM sleep in OSAS. *Sleep Breath.* 2005;9:12-9.
46. Ratnavadivel R, Stadler D, Windler S, et al. Upper airway function and arousability to ventilatory challenge in slow wave versus stage 2 sleep in obstructive sleep apnoea. *Thorax.* 2010;65:107-12.
47. Khoo MC, Kronauer RE, Strohl KP, et al. Factors inducing periodic breathing in humans: a general model. *J Appl Physiol.* 1982;53:644-59.
48. Ryan CM, Bradley TD. Pathogenesis of obstructive sleep apnea. *J Appl Physiol.* 2005;99:2440-50.
49. Younes M, Ostrowski M, Thompson W, et al. Chemical control stability in patients with obstructive sleep apnea. *Am J Respir Crit Care Med.* 2001;163:1181-90.
50. Yuan H, Pinto SJ, Huang J, et al. Ventilatory responses to hypercapnia during wakefulness and sleep in obese adolescents with and without obstructive sleep apnea syndrome. *Sleep.* 2012;35(9):1257-67.
51. Foster GE, Hanly PJ, Ostrowski M, et al. Ventilatory and cerebrovascular responses to hypercapnia inpatients with obstructive sleep apnoea: effect of CPAP therapy. *Respir Physiol Neurobiol.* 2009;165:73-81.
52. Edwards BA, Connolly JG, Campana LM, et al. Acetazolamide attenuates the ventilatory response to arousal in patients with obstructive sleep apnea. *Sleep.* 2013;36(2):281-5.
53. Kimoff RJ, Sforza E, Champagne V, et al. Upper airway sensation in snoring and obstructive sleep apnea. *Am J Respir Crit Care Med.* 2001;164:250-5.
54. Nguyen AT, Jobin V, Payne R, et al. Laryngeal and velopharyngeal sensory impairment in obstructive sleep apnea. *Sleep.* 2005;28:585-93.
55. Boyd JH, Petrof BJ, Hamid Q, et al. Upper airway muscle inflammation and denervation changes in obstructive sleep apnea. *Am J Respir Crit Care Med.* 2004;170:541-6.
56. Friberg D, Ansved T, Borg K, et al. Histological indications of a progressive snorers disease in an upper airway muscle. *Am J Respir Crit Care Med.* 1998;157:586-93.
57. Mayer P, Dematteis M, Pepin JL, et al. Peripheral neuropathy in sleep apnea: a tissue marker of the severity of nocturnal desaturation. *Am J Respir Crit Care Med.* 1999;159:213-9.
58. Saboisky JP, Stashuk DW, Hamilton-Wright A, et al. Neurogenic changes in the upper airway of patients with obstructive sleep apnea. *Am J RespirCrit Care Med.* 2012;185(3):322-9.
59. Shelton KE, Woodson H, Gay S, et al. Pharyngeal fat in obstructive sleep apnea. *Am Rev Respir Dis.* 1993;148:462-6.

60. Horner RL, Mohiaddin RH, Lowell DG, et al. Sites and sizes of fat deposits around the pharynx in obese patients with obstructive sleep apnoea and weight matched controls. *Eur Respir J*. 1989;2:613-22.
61. Saigusa H, Suzuki M, Higurashi N, et al. Three dimensional morphological analyses of positional dependence in patients with obstructive sleep apnea syndrome. *Anesthesiology*. 2009;110:885-90.
62. Sutherland K, Lee RW, Phillips CL, et al. Effect of weight loss on upper airway size and facial fat in men with obstructive sleep apnoea. *Thorax*. 2011;66:797-803.
63. Jones RL, Nzekwu MM. The effects of body mass index on lung volumes. *Chest*. 2006;130:827-33.
64. Hoffstein V, Zamel N, Phillipson EA. Lung volume dependence of pharyngeal cross-sectional area in patients with obstructive sleep apnea. *Am Rev Respir Dis*. 1984;130:175-8.

CHAPTER 3

Clinical Approach to Patient with Sleep Related Breathing Disorders

Manoj K Goel

INTRODUCTION

Sleep related breathing disorders (SRBD), formerly called as sleep disordered breathing, are characterized by an abnormality in respiratory pattern such as apneas, hypopneas, or respiratory effort related arousals during sleep. There may be an abnormal reduction in gas exchange in the form of hypoventilation during sleep. The abnormality in respiration tends to repetitively alter sleep architecture, may cause excessive daytime sleepiness (EDS), and may be associated with features of organ system dysfunction.[1,2] Obstructive sleep apnea (OSA) is the most common type of SRBD with a prevalence of 2% in women and 4% in men between 30 years and 60 years.[2]

Sleep related breathing disorders may result in significant negative outcome on the physical as well as mental well being as some of the sequelae are irreversible. Therefore, early treatment of SRBD is important to avoid the occurrence of various comorbidities. Hence, it is reasonable to make early diagnosis for OSA. This is even more important as at least 75% of adult OSA-patients are not yet diagnosed.[3]

CLASSIFICATION

According to the most recent classification[4] entitled "International Classification of Sleep Disorders: Diagnostic and Coding Manual (ICSD- 2)" published in year 2005, there are four major types of sleep related breathing disorders (Box 1).

This chapter will focus on OSA in adults, which is SRBD with the highest prevalence. However, different patterns of SRBD can be found in the same patient influencing both diagnosis and treatment.

HISTORY

It is difficult to take a history of a sleep disorder from the patient because many symptoms occur during sleep. The patient often has a little or no awareness of the problem; and it is therefore important to obtain the bed partner's view of the events during sleep and during wakefulness.

Obstructive sleep apnea is characterized by a recurrent partial or complete collapse of pharynx causing cessation or impairment of breathing such as apneas

> **Box 1: Classification of sleep related breathing disorders**
>
> **Central apnea syndromes**
> - Primary central apnea
> - Cheyne-Stokes respiration
> - Periodic respiration of high altitude
> - Central apneas without Cheyne-Stokes respiration secondary to other disorders (vascular, malignant, degenerative or traumatic disorders of the central nervous system, cardiac/renal disorders)
> - Central apneas caused by medicine or other substances
> - Primary sleep apnea of newborn
>
> **Obstructive apnea syndromes**
> - Obstructive apnea in adults
> - Obstructive apnea in children
>
> **Hypoventilation/hypoxemia syndromes associated with sleep**
> - Non-obstructive alveolar hypoventilation, idiopathic
> - Congenital central hypoventilation
> - Hypoventilation/hypoxemia secondary to other disorders: lung parenchymal, airway (e.g., COPD), or vascular (e.g., pulmonary hypertension) disorders; neuromuscular disorders; thoracic wall abnormalities; obesity.
>
> **Undefined/nonspecific sleep disorders**
> - Disorders without specific characteristics to allow their classification in any of the previous categories. Further investigation is required.
>
> *Source:* American Academy of Sleep Medicine. International classification of sleep disorders. Diagnostic and coding manual, 2nd edition. Westchester: American Academy of Sleep Medicine; 2005.

and hypopneas. Impaired breathing spells are terminated by arousals lasting a few seconds, which reopen the upper airway to normalize the ventilation. This causes loud snoring, sleep fragmentation with inadequate deep stages of sleep including the rapid eye movement (REM) sleep and recurrent oxygen desaturation in blood leading to development of other cardinal symptoms of OSA. The symptoms of obstructive sleep apnea syndrome can be divided into two groups; those occurring during sleep and those occurring during waking hours (Box 2).[5] The two most cardinal symptoms of OSA are loud snoring and excessive daytime sleepiness. These two symptoms are most useful for the screening of patients with SRBD.

Loud snoring may be accompanied by mouth breathing, unusual body positions, or visible restlessness during sleep. Respiratory pauses are sometimes witnessed by bed partners or family members. Such symptoms are most informative when present. Conversely, the absence of observed apnea and even snoring does not rule out the possibility of an obstructive SRBD.

Excessive daytime sleepiness, defined as sleepiness that interferes with daytime activities, productivity, or enjoyment, or occurs at inappropriate times is almost always abnormal, particularly if the somnolence is chronic, recurrent, or severe.

In many cases simple snoring is the only symptom for years. As other features of OSA may develop slowly, diagnosis is delayed and treatment is often initiated when cardiovascular and other comorbidities have already appeared. Therefore, it is necessary to recognize patients at high risk for screening for OSA. Likely candidates for SRBD are those who exhibit snoring and fall asleep at inappropriate

> **Box 2: Signs and symptoms in obstructive sleep apnea syndrome**
>
> **Nocturnal symptoms during sleep**
> - Loud snoring (often with a long history)
> - Choking during sleep
> - Cessation of breathing (apneas witnessed by bed partner)
> - Sitting up or fighting for breath
> - Abnormal motor activities (e.g., thrashing about in bed)
> - Severe sleep disruption
> - Gastroesophageal reflux causing heartburn
> - Nocturia and nocturnal enuresis (mostly in children)
> - Insomnia (in some patients)
> - Excessive nocturnal sweating (in some patients)
>
> **Daytime symptoms**
> - Excessive daytime somnolence
> - Forgetfulness
> - Personality changes
> - Decreased libido and impotence in men
> - Dryness of mouth on awakening
> - Morning headache (in some patients)
> - Automatic behavior with retrograde amnesia
> - Hyperactivity in children
> - Hearing impairment (in some patients)

Source: Chokroverty S. Overview of sleep & sleep disorders. *Indian J Med Res*. 2010;131:126-40.

> **Box 3: Patients at high risk for OSA who should be evaluated for OSA symptoms**
>
> - Obesity (BMI >35)
> - Congestive heart failure atrial fibrillation
> - Treatment refractory hypertension
> - Type 2 diabetes
> - Nocturnal dysrhythmias stroke
> - Pulmonary hypertension high-risk driving populations
> - Preoperative for bariatric surgery

OSA, obstructive sleep apnea; BMI, body mass index.
Source: Epstein LJ, Kristo D, Strollo PJ, et al. Clinical guideline for the evaluation, management and long-term care of obstructive sleep apnea in adults. *J Clin Sleep Med*. 2009;5:263-76.

times and places, e.g., during conversation, while at work, lecturing, and driving. People who are overweight, or those who have some physical abnormality, in the nose, throat, or other parts of the upper airway are also at high risk. The other important risk factors are habitual consumption of alcohol, drug abuse, depression, and other psychotic disorders (Box 3).[6]

A patient suspected of OSA must be evaluated for the history of snoring, witnessed apneic spells, choking episodes during sleep, disturbed fragmented or lack of refreshing sleep, nocturia, and morning headache. An evaluation of consequences of SRBD including cardiovascular comorbidities such as hypertension, cardiovascular accidents, myocardial infarction, cor pulmonale, and other secondary effects such as decreased daytime alertness, decreased concentration and memory impairment, irritability and impairment of libido and motor vehicle accidents, should also be obtained.

QUESTIONNAIRES

The sleep questionnaires are a set of questions to be self answered by the patients themselves or by their spouses. The questionnaires are used to provide a reliable, valid, and standardized measure of sleep quality. The two most commonly used questionnaires which provide an index that is easy for subjects to use and for clinicians and researchers to interpret are as follows:
- Epworth Sleepiness Score (ESS)
- Berlin Sleep Questionnaire.

Epworth Sleepiness Score

The ESS is used to objectively quantify subjective daytime sleepiness.[7] Patients are asked to score the possibility of dozing off or falling asleep in eight different situations. The scale (Box 4)[7] is used to choose the most appropriate number for each situation. Scores above 10 are indicative for hypersomnia.

Box 4: The Epworth sleepiness scale

Name:

Today's date:

Your age (years): _____ Your sex (male = M; female = F): _____

How likely are you to doze off or fall asleep in the following situations, in contrast to feeling just tired?

This refers to your usual way of life in recent times. Even if you have not done some of these things recently try to work out how they would have affected you. Use the following scale to choose the most appropriate number for each situation:

0 = would never doze
I = slight chance of dozing
2 = moderate change of dozing
3 = high chance of dozing

Situation	Chance of dozing
Sitting and reading	_____
Watching TV	_____
Sitting, inactive in a public place (e.g., a theater or a meeting)	_____
As a passenger in a car for an hour without a break	_____
Lying down to rest in the afternoon when circumstances permit	_____
Sitting and talking to someone	_____
Sitting quietly after a lunch without alcohol	_____
In a car, while stopped for a few minutes in the traffic	_____

Thank you for your cooperation

Source: Johns MW. A new method for measuring daytime sleepiness: the Epworth sleepiness scale. *Sleep.* 1991;14:540-45.

The ESS quantifies a nonspecific symptom of EDS which can be found not only in OSA but also in many other sleep disorders. Sensitivity of and specificity of an ESS with a cut-off value of 12 have been reported in only 42% and 68%, respectively, which is suggestive of its overall poor correlation with apnea/hypopnea index (AHI).[8] Therefore, ESS may not be suitable for the early diagnosis of OSA.[9] However, it is useful to assess and monitor sleepiness during the course of SRBD, e.g., before and after therapy. A combination of symptoms such as loud snoring and EDS as assessed by ESS in patients at risk can be used for the screening and early diagnosis of SRBD.

Berlin Questionnaire

Berlin questionnaire[10] includes a set of questions concerning various known risk factors and symptoms of OSA (Box 5). The Berlin questionnaire is simple and very easy for the screening of large populations. It does not require any extensive medical training to help patients to fill up as well as to analyze the questionnaire. Its sensitivity, specificity, and predictive values are sufficient for early diagnosis of OSA.[11,12]

Sharma et al.[13] validated the Berlin questionnaire in comparison to polysomnography in 320 consecutive outpatients. They also made Indian

---

Box 5: Berlin questionnaire

The questionnaire consists of three categories related to the risk of having sleep apnea. Patients can be classified into high risk or low risk based on their responses to the individual items and their overall scores in the symptom categories

Categories and scoring:

Category 1: items 1, 2, 3, 4, 5.

Item 1: if "Yes", assign 1 point

Item 2: if "c" or "d" is the response, assign 1 point

Item 3: if "a" or "b" is the response, assign 1 point

Item 4: if "a" is the response, assign 1 point

Item 5: if "a" or "b" is the response, assign 2 points

Add points

Category 1 is positive if the total score is 2 or more points

Category 2: items 6, 7, 8 (item 9 should be noted separately)

Item 6: if "a" or "b" is the response, assign 1 point

Item 7: if "a" or "b" is the response, assign 1 point

Item 8: if "a" is the response, assign 1 point

Add points

Category 2 is positive if the total score is 2 or more points

Category 3 is positive if the answer to item 10 is "Yes" OR if the BMI of the patient is greater than 30 kg/m²

(BMI must be calculated. BMI is defined as weight (kg) divided by height (m) squared, i.e., kg/m²)

High Risk: if there are two or more Categories where the score is positive

Low Risk: if there is only one or no Categories where the score is positive

Additional question: item 9 should be noted separately

Berlin Questionnaire

Height (m) _____ Weight (kg) _____ Age _____ Male/Female

Contd....

Contd....

Please choose the correct response to each question

Category 1
1. Do you snore?
   a. Yes
   b. No
   c. Don't know

If you snore:
2. Your snoring is:
   a. Slightly louder than breathing
   b. As loud as talking
   c. Louder than talking
   d. Very loud—can be heard in adjacent rooms
3. How often do you snore?
   a. Nearly every day
   b. 3–4 times a week
   c. 1–2 times a week
   d. 1–2 times a month
   e. Never or nearly never
4. Has your snoring ever bothered other people?
   a. Yes
   b. No
   c. Don't know
5. Has anyone noticed that you quit breathing during your sleep?
   a. Nearly every day
   b. 3–4 times a week
   c. 1–2 times a week
   d. 1–2 times a month
   e. Never or nearly never

Category 2
6. How often do you feel tired or fatigued after your sleep?
   a. Nearly every day
   b. 3–4 times a week
   c. 1–2 times a week
   d. 1–2 times a month
   e. Never or nearly never
7. During your waking time, do you feel tired, fatigued or not up to par?
   a. Nearly every day
   b. 3–4 times a week
   c. 1–2 times a week
   d. 1–2 times a month
   e. Never or nearly never
8. Have you ever nodded off or fallen asleep while driving a vehicle?
   a. Yes
   b. No

If yes:
9. How often does this occur?
   a. Nearly every day
   b. 3–4 times a week
   c. 1–2 times a week
   d. 1–2 times a month
   e. Never or nearly never

Category 3
10. Do you have high blood pressure?
    a. Yes
    b. No
    c. Don't know

Source: Netzer NC, Stoohs RA, Netzer CM, et al. Using the Berlin Questionnaire to identify patients at risk for the sleep apnea syndrome. *Ann Intern Med.* 1999;131:485-91.

modification in category III, which is already considered positive if the body mass index (BMI) is above 25 kg/m². In category II, the item "driving a car" is replaced by monotonous situations every Indian is acquainted with like waiting at a doctor's clinic or watching TV.

CLINICAL EXAMINATION

Evaluation and physical examination of a patient with SRBD may require multi-specialty approach. This involves necessary clinical examination not only for OSA but also for risks and consequences of the disease process. Since pharyngeal obstructions play an important role, an examination by an ENT colleague may be of particular importance apart from general findings such as BMI or neck circumference while screening for OSA. The comprehensive physical examination must also include the respiratory, cardiovascular, and neurologic systems. Physical examination may reveal obesity in approximately 70% of cases.[4]

Features that may suggest the presence of OSA include increased neck circumference (>7 inches in men, >16 inches in women), BMI more than 30 kg/m², a modified Mallampati score of 3 or more.[14] The anatomical abnormalities to be carefully looked for include retrognathia, lateral peritonsillar narrowing, macroglossia, tonsillar hypertrophy, elongated or enlarged uvula, high arched or narrow hard palate, and nasal abnormalities such as polyps, gross deviation of nasal septum, and hypertrophy of turbinates.

Clinical examination of the upper airway requires experience and training in order to come to a correct assessment. However, the statistical data in the literature at present is too limited to ascertain the importance of clinical examination for early diagnosis of OSA.[15,16] Dreher et al. did not find significant difference in the measurement findings of nose, tonsils, palate, and tongue base in 52 patients of OSA with an AHI more than 10 and 49 subjects with an AHI less than 10.[17] Even the Mallampati index did not show relevant difference between patients with or without OSA.[18] The same is true for a cut-off BMI less than 28 kg/m² which could detect an AHI less than 20/h only with a sensitivity of 39%.[19]

CONCLUSION

Various methods for diagnosis of SRBD include history, clinical examination, standardized questionnaires, and unattended and attended polysomonography. Attended polysomnography is the gold standard, which can even detect minor and very discrete forms of SRBD. However, detection of mild forms of SRBD by attended polysomnography usually does not involve major therapeutic interventions such as application of continuous positive airway pressure device and would also add to the cost tremendously. Therefore, clinical parameters such as history, physical examination, and questionnaire are very important tools for screening for moderate to severe cases of SRBD who can be subjected to full attended polysomnography in order to make the diagnosis very cost effective. General physicians should have a high index of clinical suspicion about the presence of sleep related breathing disorders, which are prevalent in the society. Timely referral on clinical suspicion to sleep specialists can help in early diagnosis and treatment of these patients.

REFERENCES

1. Iber C, Ancoli-Israel S, Chesson AL, et al. The AASM Manual for the Scoring of Sleep and Associated Events, American Academy of Sleep Medicine, West Chester, IL: 2007.
2. Young T, Palta M, Dempsey J, et al. The occurrence of sleep-disordered breathing among middle-aged adults. *N Engl J Med.* 1993;328:1230-35.
3. Young T, Evans L, Finn L, et al. Estimation of the clinically diagnosed proportion of sleep apnea syndrome in middle-aged men and women. *Sleep.* 1997;20:705-6.
4. American Academy of Sleep Medicine. International classification of sleep disorders. Diagnostic and coding manual, 2nd edition. Westchester: American Academy of Sleep Medicine; 2005.
5. Chokroverty S. Overview of sleep & sleep disorders. *Indian J Med Res.* 2010;131:126-40.
6. Epstein LJ, Kristo D, Strollo PJ, et al. Clinical guideline for the evaluation, management and long-term care of obstructive sleep apnea in adults. *J Clin Sleep Med.* 2009;5: 263-76.

7. Johns MW. A new method for measuring daytime sleepiness: the Epworth sleepiness scale. *Sleep.* 1991;14:540-45.
8. Pouliot Z, Peters M, Neufeld H, et al. Using self-reported questionnaire data to prioritize OSA patients for polysomnography. *Sleep.* 1997;20:232-36.
9. Osman EZ, Osborne J, Hill PD, et al. The Epworth Sleepiness Scale: can it be used for sleep apnoea screening among snorers? *Clin Otolaryngol Allied Sci.* 1999;24:239-41.
10. Netzer NC, Stoohs RA, Netzer CM, et al. Using the Berlin Questionnaire to identify patients at risk for the sleep apnea syndrome. *Ann Intern Med.* 1999;131:485-91.
11. Weinreich G, Plein K, Teschler T, et al. Ist der Berlin-Fragebogen ein geeignetes Instrument der schlafmedizinischen Diagnostik in der pneumologischen Rehabilitation? *Pneumologie.* 2006;60:737-42
12. Ahmadi N, Chung SA, Gibbs A, et al. The Berlin questionnaire for sleep apnea in a sleep clinic population: relationship to polysomnographic measurement of respiratory disturbance. *Sleep Breath.* 2008;12:39-45.
13. Sharma SK, Vasudev C, Sinha S, et al. Validation of the modified Berlin questionnaire to identify patients at risk for the obstructive sleep apnoea syndrome. *Indian J Med Res.* 2006;124:281-90.
14. Friedman M, Tanyeri H, La Rosa M, et al. Clinical predictors of obstructive sleep apnea. *Laryngoscope.* 1999;109:1901-7.
15. Viner S, Szalai JP, Hoffstein V. Are history and physical examination a good screening test for sleep apnea? *Ann Intern Med.* 1991;115:356-59.
16. Hoffstein V, Szalai JP. Predictive value of clinical features in diagnosing obstructive sleep apnea. *Sleep.* 1993;16:118-22.
17. Dreher A, de la Chaux R, Klemens C, et al. Correlation between otorhinolaryngologic evaluation and severity of obstructive sleep apnea syndrome in snorers. *Arch Otolaryngol Head Neck Surg.* 2005;131:95-8.
18. Nuckton TJ, Glidden DV, Browner WS, et al. Physical examination: Mallampati score as an independent predictor of obstructive sleep apnea. *Sleep.* 2006;29:903-8.
19. Pouliot Z, Peters M, Neufeld H, et al. Using self-reported questionnaire data to prioritize OSA patients for polysomnography. *Sleep.* 1997;20:232-36.

CHAPTER 4

Diagnostic Approach to Sleep Disordered Breathing

Nagarajan Ramakrishnan, Anup Bansal

INTRODUCTION

Sleep problems are common among all age groups and increasingly recognized by the public. The most common presenting symptom remains difficulty in sleeping (insomnia) followed closely in number by those presenting with excessive sleepiness (hypersomnolence). Insufficient quantity or altered quality of sleep due to any reason may lead to hypersomnolence. Obstructive sleep apnea (OSA) with a prevalence of 2–4% in adult population[1,2] as reported in community based epidemiological studies in India remains a frequent cause of daytime hypersomnolence. It is estimated that a significant proportion of patients with OSA remain undiagnosed and untreated. This could result in memory impairment, accidents while at work or driving, psychosocial and medical complications, and overall impaired quality of life. Early diagnosis and appropriate treatment would have a positive impact on preventing complications and improving quality of life. This chapter provides an overview on diagnostic approach to sleep disordered breathing.

DIAGNOSIS

Diagnostic approach to sleep apnea is based on evaluation of symptoms obtained by detailed sleep history, clinical examination, and findings of sleep testing.

History and Physical Examination

Detailed sleep history should be obtained in patients presenting with suspected sleep apnea. Nocturnal symptoms often include loud snoring (usually reported by bed partners and denied by the patient), choking, witnessed apneas, nocturia, and dryness of the mouth. This in association with daytime symptoms such as not feeling refreshed upon wakening, morning headache, and excessive daytime sleepiness (EDS) may strongly suggest the possibility of sleep apnea. Interestingly, patients often do not accept that they are sleepy and use surrogate terminology such as frequent yawning, fatigue, and a feeling of exhaustion. It is also important to elicit subtle symptoms such as irritability, memory impairment, and lack of libido which are often not voluntarily disclosed.

It would be important to particularly screen those with the following clinical associations who are at high risk for OSA.[3]

- Obesity [body mass index (BMI) > 35 kg/m^2]
- Hypothyroid
- Type 2 diabetes
- Congestive heart failure
- Atrial fibrillation
- Refractory hypertension
- Stroke
- Pulmonary hypertension
- Preoperative for bariatric surgery.

The Berlin questionnaire[4] (Box 1) was developed as a screening test to evaluate patients for possible OSA. It includes a list of questions mainly based on sleep related symptoms. Responses to this questionnaire were grouped into different categories based on snoring, daytime sleepiness, hypertension, and BMI. High risk patients are those who respond positively to at least two to three categories and this helps to predict OSA [defined as apnea hypopnea index (AHI) > 5] with a sensitivity of 86% and specificity of 77%.

Positive findings of initial screening should lead to more focused questions relating to medication history, family history of snoring, and physical examination. In physical examination, specific attention should be paid to waist and neck circumference, upper airway anatomy, presence of macroglossia, tonsillar hypertrophy, elongated uvula, and also craniofacial changes such as retrognathia and mandibular hypoplasia. The nares should be examined to exclude polyp, rhinitis, or deviated nasal septum. Increased neck circumference (> 18 inches in male and > 16 inches in female) and BMI of more than 30 kg/m^2 are strong predictors of sleep apnea hypopnea syndrome (SAHS).

Box 1: Berlin questionnaire

Has your weight changed?
Increased/Decreased/No change
Do you snore?
Yes/No/Do not know
Snoring loudness
Loud as breathing/Loud as talking/Louder than talking/Very loud
Snoring frequency
Almost every day/3–4 times per week/1–2 times per week/1–2 times per month/Never
Does your snoring bother other people?
Yes/No
How often have you been told that your breathing has been paused?
Almost every day/3–4 times per week/1–2 times per week/1–2 times per month/Never
Are you tired after sleeping?
Almost every day/3–4 times per week/1–2 times per week/1–2 times per month/Never
Are you tired during wake time?
Almost every day/3–4 times per week/1-2 times per week/1–2 times per month/Never
Have you ever fallen asleep while driving?
Yes/No
Do you have high blood pressure?
Yes/No/Do not know

Table 1: Epworth sleepiness scale[5]

Situation		Chance of dozing			
1.	Sitting and reading	0	1	2	3
2.	Watching television	0	1	2	3
3.	Sitting inactive in a public place	0	1	2	3
4.	As a passenger in a car for an hour without a break	0	1	2	3
5.	Lying down to rest in the afternoon when circumstances permit	0	1	2	3
6.	Sitting quietly after a lunch without alcohol	0	1	2	3
7.	Sitting and talking to someone	0	1	2	3
8.	In a car, while stopped for a minute in traffic	0	1	2	3

0 = would never doze, 1 = slight chance of dozing, 2 = moderate chance of dozing, 3 = high chances of dozing.

Subjective Assessment

Epworth sleepiness scale (ESS)[5] (Table 1) is one of the commonly used subjective methods for assessing symptoms of EDS. This metric system consists of short questionnaire of eight social circumstances when the individual assesses the probability of falling asleep on a four point scale (0–3). A score of 0–8 is considered to be normal, 9–12 suggests mild sleepiness, 13–16 moderate, and more than 16 is considered to be severe sleepiness. Modified and translated versions of the ESS have been adopted in various parts of the world.

Other scales available to assess sleepiness are:

1. *Stanford sleepiness scale*:[6] A subjective, introspective assessment of current state of alertness on a scale of 1 (feeling wide awake) to 7 (sleep onset likely to happen soon).
2. *Karolinska sleepiness scale*: A measure of subjective level of sleepiness at a particular time of the day which best reflects the psychophysical state in the last 10 minutes prior to the assessment.
3. *Visual-analog scale*: A simplified method that could be used across categories of patients with varying literacy level where the degree of alertness-sleepiness is reflected on a pictorial scale.
4. *Fatigue severity scale*: This provides a subjective assessment of daytime fatigue intensity on various functional and behavioral aspects of life. Each item is rated from 1 to 7 and higher the score greater the level of fatigue.[7]

Systemic Examination

Detailed systemic examination[8] mainly cardiopulmonary is important to detect any cardiac or lung disease that may predispose patients to sleep related breathing disorders. Baseline arterial blood gas analysis and pulmonary function test helps in differentiating obstructive sleep apnea from obesity hypoventilation syndrome and overlap syndrome. It is also essential to diagnose underlying obstructive or restrictive lung disease as it would influence the decision on the type of positive pressure therapy. Cardiac examination should focus on signs of cardiac failure as Cheyne-Stokes respirations and central sleep apnea may be the associated findings with it.[9] Neurologic examination would help to diagnose central nervous system problems and neuromuscular disorders, which may contribute to sleep related breathing disorder.

Following detailed clinical history and examination, suspected patients should undergo objective testing to confirm the diagnosis and severity of obstructive sleep apnea. Patients should be explained the need for the evaluation and also the steps and procedures involved. It would be particularly important for the sleep lab to provide a comfortable environment for sleep and the technician should take the time to allay all fears and concerns of the patients.

Objective Tests

Sleep study is needed for an accurate diagnosis of sleep apnea (both obstructive and central sleep apneas). Polysomnography (PSG) in the sleep lab remains the gold standard objective test for the diagnosis and assessment of severity of OSA, although there is increasing acceptance of portable studies. The severity of sleep apnea is estimated based on the AHI which reflects the average number of apneas and hypopneas per hour during sleep (Table 2). In addition, respiratory effort related arousals (RERAs) can be evaluated in a full polysomnogram which helps to calculate the respiratory disturbance index (RDI). Recent evidence suggests that severity of oxygen desaturation assessed by oxygen desaturation index (ODI) is an important factor in assessment of severity of OSA.

On the basis of number of recorded channels and data analyzed, sleep studies have been classified into four levels (Table 3). As per American Academy for Sleep Medicine (AASM)[10] in-lab PSG and modified portable PSG are both acceptable objective methods recommended for diagnosis of OSA.

Table 2: Classification of severity of obstructive sleep apnea

Apnea hypopnea index	Classification of severity
<5	Normal
5–15	Mild OSA
16–30	Moderate OSA
>30	Severe OSA

OSA, obstructive sleep apnea.

Table 3: Levels of sleep study[10]

Level-1	Gold standard
	Attended full PSG
	Intervention is possible
Level-2	Unattended full PSG
	Same parameters as like level 1
	Intervention not possible
Level-3	Cardio respiratory sleep study
	4 bioparameters
	Airflow, SpO_2, respiratory effort, ECG
Level-4	1 or 2 bioparameters
	Airflow and SpO_2

PSG, polysomnography; ECG, electrocardiogram.

Polysomnography[11]

Polysomnography consists of the continuous and simultaneous recordings of several physiologic variables during sleep. This includes electroencephalogram (EEG), electrooculogram (EOG), electromyogram (EMG) of chin [to diagnose reduced muscle tone during rapid eye movements (REM) sleep] and legs [to evaluate periodic limb movements (PLM)], electrocardiogram (ECG), nasal airflow, snoring microphone, respiratory effort channels, and pulse oximetry. PSG is helpful both for diagnosis and titration of positive airway pressure therapy as it is important to evaluate optimal pressures during REM sleep when the pressure requirement may be higher than during non-REM sleep.

Electroencephalogram: The international 10–20 system is used for the placement of EEG electrodes. Each electrode is provided with a letter representing a region of brain Frontal (F), Central (C), Occipital (O), Mastoid (M) and numeric subscripts represent the side of placement side (odd numbers represent left side and even numbers right side) of electrode. The designation "Z" is used for electrodes placed in the midline. The landmarks are the nasion, inion, and preauricular point. According to AASM F_4M_1, C_4M_1, O_2M_1 represents a recommended electrode placement in polysomnography.

On the basis of frequency and voltage the resultant waves can be classified into delta (4 Hz), theta (4–7Hz), α (8–13 Hz), and β (>13Hz). Delta waves have high amplitude (>75 μV) and alpha waves is generally less than 50 μV in adults. Alpha activity is more prominent in occipital leads and delta in central and frontal leads.

Electrooculogram: It records the potential difference between the cornea (positively charged) and retina (negatively charged). A positive voltage (downward deflection) is recorded when the eye moves towards an electrode and negative voltage (upward deflection) when it moves away from the electrode. The AASM recommended E_1M_2 and E_2M_2 for the placement of EOG electrodes. E_1 is placed 1 cm below the left outer canthus and E_2 at 1 cm above the right outer canthus. With this electrode placement usually two types of eye movements are recorded namely slow rolling at sleep onset and REM during REM sleep. Slow rolling eye movements often occur with drowsiness and stage 1 sleep.

Electromyogram: Usually three EMG leads are placed in the mental and submental areas. It is an essential element for identifying stage of sleep as reduction or absence of muscle tone is an important feature of REM sleep. The reduction in EMG amplitude during REM sleep represents generalized muscle atonia. Additional electrode over the masseter muscle is used to detect bruxism. The activity of anterior tibialis muscle is also routinely monitored to diagnose PLM based on specific criteria such as duration (0.5–10 sec), amplitude (>8 μV above baseline), sequence (four or more movements), and onset [consecutive leg movements (LMs) >5 and <90 sec].

Airflow: Oronasal thermal sensor is used for identifying apneas but nasal air pressure transducers are more sensitive to identify hypopneas as per AASM guidelines. Obstructive event appear as a flattening signal while central are associated with reduced but rounded signals in the inspiratory flow. A reduction in airflow of 30% or more from baselines is essential for diagnosing hypopneas.

Respiratory effort: There is no universally accepted method for measuring respiratory effort but AASM recommends esophageal manometry and inductance plethysmography sensors. It is important to look at simultaneous recordings of airflow and respiratory effort to diagnose obstructive (respiratory effort without airflow), central (absence of respiratory effort and airflow) and mixed apneas (initial absence of respiratory effort, with subsequent efforts although there is no significant airflow). While it is generally accepted that a drop in airflow by 30% is essential for diagnosing hypopneas, there have been significant controversies and variations in definition of oxygen desaturations. AASM continues to recommend scoring hypopneas in adults when there is more than 3% oxygen desaturation from baseline and/or the event is associated with an arousal. However, AASM has clarified that it is acceptable for accredited sleep centers to score hypopneas in adults when there is a more than 4% oxygen desaturation from pre-event baseline.

SLEEP STAGE SCORING

Sleep is divided into two phases: (1) nonrapid eye movement (NREM) and (2) REM. NREM sleep is further divided into three stages: stage 1 (N1) representing light sleep which usually occurs during transition from wakefulness to sleep; stage 2 (N2) representing the most predominant stage of sleep; and stage 3 often referred as slow wave sleep, delta sleep, or deep sleep. Polysomnographic data are evaluated and scored as 30 second periods or epochs. Each epoch is labeled as single sleep stage that occupies the majority of time within that epoch. Following EEG activities and frequencies encountered in PSG are beta: more than 16 Hz, alpha: 8–12Hz, theta: 3–7 Hz, delta: less than 2 Hz. Sleep spindle and K complexes are characteristic findings of stage N2. Sleep spindle is brief oscillations of 12–14 Hz lasting for 0.5 s to 1.5 s with amplitude of less than 50 μV. K complex is a high amplitude diphasic waveform with slow negative (upward) deflection followed by positive (downward) component. Table 4 shows various sleep stages with their characteristic findings.

Table 4: Stages of sleep

	Stages of sleep (Normal)	Electroencephalogram characteristics
1.	Stage W	• >50% of epoch has α wave—best seen over occipital region • If α waves are absent—conjugate vertical eye blinks, conjugate slow movements followed by rapid movement in opposite direction or voluntary rapid eye movements • High chin EMG tone
2.	Stage N1 (5%)	• <50% of α activity • >50% epoch contains low voltage, mixed frequency waves (4–7 Hz) • Vertex sharp waves of duration of <0.5 sec over the central region
3.	Stage N2 (45–55 %)	• Presence of sleep spindles and K complexes
4.	Stage N3 (20–25%)	• More than 20% of slow wave activity (0.5–2 Hz and 75 µV) • Best seen over the frontal region
5.	Stage REM (20–25%)	• Low amplitude, mixed frequency EEG waves • Rapid eye movement • Low chin EMG tone

EEG, electroencephalogram; REM, rapid eye movements; EMG, electromyogram.

There are some polysomnographic parameters which are commonly used in characterizing the quality, composition, and quantity of sleep. These are:
1. Time in bed (TIB): The total time of recording of data from "light out" to "light on".
2. Total sleep time (TST): The sum of all the time (in minutes) spent in various stages of sleep.
4. Sleep efficiency: The total sleep time divided by the time in bed, multiplied by 100 (expressed as %).
5. Sleep latency: Time from "light out" to the 1st epoch of sleep. Normal is less than 15 minutes.
6. REM latency: Time from sleep onset to first epoch of REM sleep. Normal is 60–120 minutes.
7. Lights out: Time when sleep recording started.
8. Lights on: Time when sleep recording ended.

Split Night Polysomnography

Split night study combining diagnostic study and continuous positive airway pressure (CPAP) titration may be initiated by the sleep technician based on established sleep lab protocols. Commonly accepted criteria are AHI more than or equal to 40 with significant oxygen desaturations during the initial two hours of the study. It would be important to ensure that adequate time is available (preferably at least 4 hours) for the CPAP titration as titration in supine position and REM sleep would be important to accurately assess the pressure required for nocturnal CPAP therapy. Although split night PSG saves time and is thought to be a cost effective option, it is important to educate the patient about CPAP during the study and also avoid suboptimal titration due to lack of time or absence of REM sleep in the titration period.

Portable Sleep Monitoring (Level 3 Studies)

Portable sleep monitoring is recommended for patients with high index of suspicion for sleep apnea on the basis of comprehensive sleep evaluation.[12] Commonly accepted indications are: (1) patients with severe clinical symptoms of SAHS; (2) follow-up studies to evaluate treatment response; and (3) patients who are unable to undergo in-lab sleep studies for any reason. Such portable studies should record minimum four parameters of respiratory effort, airflow, heart rate and oxygen saturation.[13] An experienced sleep technician or other trained healthcare personel must hook up the study and also educate the patient about the correct application of sensors. Level 3 PSG usually underestimates the severity of sleep apnea because total recording time is used for the calculation of respiratory disturbances index (RDI) rather than total sleep time.

Other Diagnostic Tests

Multiple Sleep Latency Test and Maintenance of Wakefulness Test

The multiple sleep latency test (MSLT)[14] is designed to evaluate propensity to sleep and is indicated when patient has problem of excessive sleepiness despite optimal treatment for OSA or when the severity of daytime hypersomnolence is out of proportion to severity of sleep disordered breathing. It helps in evaluation for possible diagnosis of narcolepsy in hyper somnolent patients. Maintenance of wakefulness test (MWT) which is designed to evaluate ability to stay awake is useful in following up patients with OSA after treatment.

Cephalometry

Cephalometry[15] is a plain lateral radiograph of the head and neck. It is used to examine the upper airway and craniofacial structures. Some of the common measures include distance from maxilla to cranial base (SNA), mandible to cranial base (SNB), posterior airway space (PAS), soft palate length (PNS), and distance of hyoid from inferior mandible (MPH). It is cost effective and useful in evaluating the efficacy of oral appliances or upper airway surgery, if required for treatment.

Actigraphy

Actigraphy is the continuous recording of the body (often wrist) movements using a device which is worn, to detect and record the movements. This information can be stored for days, weeks, months, or years.[16] Actigraphy is not an alternative to polysomnography but a tool to record for long periods and hence more reliable then sleep logs, which are a patients' recall of their sleep pattern.[17] However, inactivity on actigraphy may not necessarily be interpreted as sleep. While actigraphy is helpful in evaluating sleep patterns, it is not of significant value in diagnosis of sleep disordered breathing.

CONCLUSION

Obstructive sleep apnea is a common sleep disorder that often remains under diagnosed and untreated. Screening patients at high risk with appropriate history and subjective questionnaires will help to identify and treat the condition early to prevent long-term complications. Prudent use of appropriate diagnostic tests such as polysomnogram (in-lab or portable as appropriate) and supplementary tests such as MSLT would help in accurate diagnosis and assessment of severity (Flowchart 1).[18] While split night studies are appropriate for those with severe

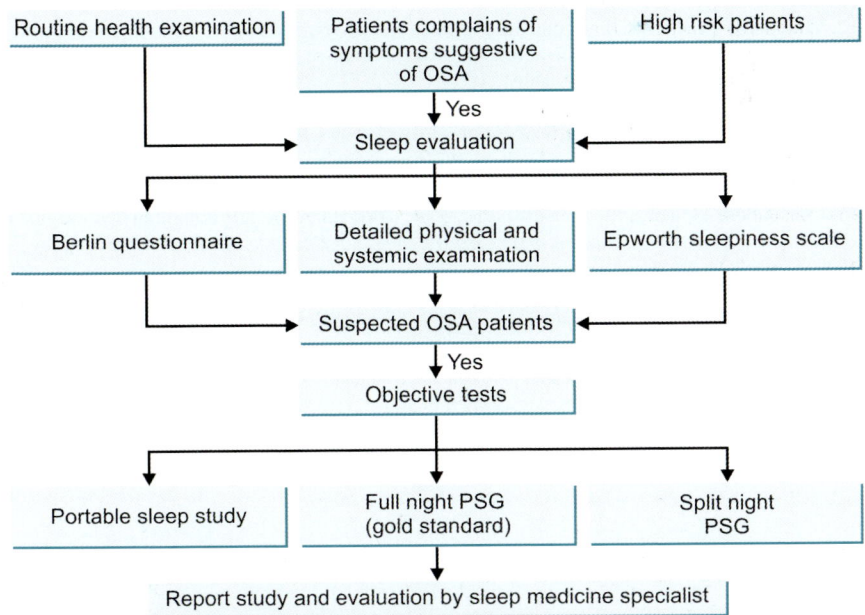

OSA, obstructive sleep apnea; PSG, polysomnography.
Flowchart 1: Evaluation of patients with suspected OSA.[18]

OSA and AHI more than or equal to 40 in the first 2 hours of study, caution must be exercised to ensure that adequate time is available for positive airway pressure including periods of supine position and REM sleep.

REFERENCES

1. Reddy EV, Kadhivaran T, Mishra HK, et al. Prevalence and risk factors of obstructive sleep apnea among middle-aged urban Indians: A community based study. *Sleep Med.* 2009;10:913-8.
2. Mysliwiec V, Henderson JH, Strollo PJ. Epidemiology, consequences and evaluation of excessive daytime sleepiness. In: Lee-Chiong TL, Sateia MJ, Carskadon MA, (Eds). Sleep Medicine. Philadelphia: Hanley & Belfus; 2002. pp. 187-92.
3. Friedman M, Tanyeri H, La Rosa M, et al. Clinical predictors of obstructive sleep apnea. *Laryngoscope.* 1999;109:1901-7.
4. Netzer NC, Stoohs RA, Netzer CM, et al. Using the Berlin Questionnaire to identify patients at risk for the sleep apnea syndrome. *Ann Intern Med.* 1999;131:485-91.
5. Johns MW. A new method for measuring daytime sleepiness: the Epworth sleepiness scale. *Sleep.* 1991;14:540-5.
6. Glenville M, Broughton R. Reliability of the Stanford sleepiness scale compared to short duration performance tests and the Wilkinson auditory vigilance task. *Adv Biosci.* 1978;21:235-44.
7. Hossain JL, Ahmad P, Reinish LW, et al .Subjective fatigue and subjective sleepiness: two independent consequences of sleep disorders? *J Sleep Res.* 2005;14:245-53.
8. Kushida CA, Littner MR, Morgenthaler T, et al. Practice parameters for the indications for polysomnography and related procedures: an update for 2005. *Sleep.* 2005;28:499-521.
9. Sin DD, Fitzgerald F, Parker JD, et al. Risk factors for central and obstructive sleep apnea in 450 men and women with congestive heart failure. *Am J Respir Crit Care Med.* 1999;160:1101-6.
10. American Academy of Sleep Medicine. Standards for Accreditation. Westchester: American Academy of Sleep Medicine; 2007.
11. Iber C, Ancoli-Israel S, Chesson A, et al. For the American Academy of Sleep Medicine. The AASM manual for the scoring of sleep and associated events: rules, terminology and technical specifications. Westchester, IL: American Academy of Sleep Medicine 2007.
12. Standards practice Committee of the American Sleep Disorders Association: Practice parameters for the use of portable recording in the assessment of obstructive sleep apnea: ASDA standards of practice. *Sleep.* 1994;17:372-77.
13. Ferber R, Milliman R, Coppola M, et al. Portable recording in assessment of obstructive sleep apnea: ASDA Standards of Practice. *Sleep.* 1991;14:378-92.
14. Littner MR, Kushida C, Wise M, et al. Practice parameters for clinical use of the multiple sleep latency test and the maintenance of wakefulness test. *Sleep.* 2005;28:113-21.
15. Sakakibara H, Tong M, Matsushita K, et al. Cephalometric abnormalities in non-obese and obese patients with obstructive sleep apnea. *Eur Respir J.* 1999;13:403-10.
16. Tryon WW. Activity measurement in psychology and medicine. New York: Plenum Press, 1991
17. Ancoli-Israel S, Cole R, Alessi C, et al. The role of actigraphy in the study of sleep and circadian rhythms. American Academy of Sleep Medicine Review Paper. *Sleep.* 2003;26(3):342-92.
18. Epstein Lj, Kristo D, Strollo Pj, et al. Clinical guideline for the evaluation, management and long term care of obstructive sleep apnea in adults. J Clin Sleep Med. 2009;5(3):263-76.

CHAPTER 5

Snoring and Upper Airways Resistance Syndrome

Raja Dhar, Debdeep Sen

INTRODUCTION

Sleep medicine has undergone a revolution since the first description of abnormal airflow through the upper airway during sleep in patients with Pickwickian Syndrome in 1965.[1] In 1982, Guilleminault and co-workers[2] found a subgroup of sleepy patients who had increased sleep fragmentation [characterized by short electroencephalographic (EEG) arousal] secondary to increased respiratory effort as measured by an esophageal monitor, without apneas, hypopneas, or oxygen desaturation which was called the respiratory effort-related arousals (RERA) and thus initiated the concept of upper airway respiratory syndrome (UARS).[2] This brought into focus a hitherto ignored section of population who were left undiagnosed and untreated despite severe problems. In the past, it has been thought that UARS and obstructive sleep apnea (OSA) are two different entities with the distinguishing feature being the gradation of severity (OSA being a more severe form) but the International Classification of Sleep Disorders (ICSD-II) published in 2005 recommends that UARS be included as a part of OSA.[3] However, RERAs are described as a distinct entity and require a special mention.

DEFINITION AND PREVALANCE

Snoring is defined as the repetitive sound produced by the vibrations of the upper airways during sleep. RERA is defined as a series of breaths occurring over at least 10 seconds associated with ever-increasing respiratory effort against a narrowed upper airway that terminates with an arousal before criteria for an apnea or hypopnea are met. And UARS is defined as occurrence of excessive daytime sleepiness unexplained by another cause and associated with more than 50% RERAs.

The exact prevalence of UARS is unknown. But considering that 71% of men and 11% of women suffering from UARS are snorers[4] and that 41% of the general population aged between 26 years and 50 years are reported to be snorers[5] implies that that the numbers could be enormous.

PATHOPHYSIOLOGY

The nasal passage nasopharynx, oropharynx, hypopharynx, and supraglottic larynx constitute the upper airway in humans. Investigations in children and adults have revealed that this upper airway could undergo a partial and transient reduction in size which could lead to an increase in respiratory effort and respiratory rate without accompanying apnea and hypopnea and oxygen desaturation.[6-8] This increased upper airway resistance (IUAR)[9] can be measured by various means including esophageal manometry, measurement of airflow with a tight fitting mask, or calculation of increased resistance using a pneumotachograph. Research for depicting IUAR is based on increasing negative inspiratory PES as measured by an esophageal catheter, with decreased oronasal air flow in the absence of frank apnea or oxygen desaturation. Guilleminault et al described the phenomenon of IUAR[9] in a group of adult patients based on increased air way resistance accompanied by EEG arousal the symptoms of which would be improved with nasal continuous positive airway pressure (CPAP). The adults described in their paper were individuals who had excessive daytime somnolence (EDS). Ordinarily these individuals would have been classified as idiopathic hypersomnia prior to their path breaking paper.

It has been suggested that OSA is a polyneuropathy resulted from repetitive trauma and prolonged stretching of the pharyngeal structures during an apnea. OSA also results in malfunction of receptors which become hyporesponsive or unresponsive. The UARS is on the other hand present in individuals who have intact sensory responses but malfunctioning mechanoreceptors located in the pharyngeal area.[10] Hence, negative intrathoracic and airway pressure with resultant minimal flow limitations stimulate the sensory pathway and hence arousal (with no obvious hypopneas or apneas). This is what leads to sleep fragmentation and day time symptoms in patients with UARS.[11]

CLINICAL FEATURES

Increased daytime somnolence and fatigue are intrinsic to the definition to UARS and hence are the commonest symptoms.[9] Unlike OSA, this condition has no gender preference.[9] The patients here are generally slim [body mass index (BMI) are less than equal to 25 kg/m² and relatively young) age 37.5 ± 7 years.[9,12,13] They have a smaller circumference neck circumference (38 ± 3.5 cm).[13] This is all in distinction to patients with OSA. Such patients usually have a distinct craniofacial characteristic that includes long face with short and narrow chin and reduced mouth opening.[4]

Chronic insomnia seems to be a more prominent feature of UARS in comparison to OSA. The patients in this condition have more of day time fatigue in comparison to sleepiness (Table 1). They often complain of sleep onset and

Table 1: Comparison of clinical variables				
Variable	UARS		OSAS	
	Mean ± SD	Range	Mean ± SD	Range
Body mass index, kg/m²	28.2 ± 4.1	18–33	29.0 ± 3.7	19–33
Neck circumference (cm)	38.2 ± 3.5	31–45	41.5 ± 4.2	32–49
Age (years)	44.1 ± 13.2	14–81	50.3 ± 13.8	14–76
Epworth sleepiness scale scores	11.0 ± 6.1	0–24	10.5 ± 5.0	0–24
Subjects with wisdom teeth extraction (%)	74.2	(n = 95)	73.3	(n = 129)

UARS, upper airway respiratory syndrome; OSAS, obstructive sleep apnea syndrome; SD, standard denvation.

Table 2: Symptoms indicated in questionnaires and confirmed on interview

	UARS	OSAS
Male: female ratio	1:1	2:1
Sleep onset	Insomnia	Short sleep latency
Snoring	Common	Almost all patients
Apnea	None	Common
Daytime symptoms	Tiredness/fatigue	Sleepiness
Body habitus	Mostly slim or thin	Mostly obese
Somatic functional complaints	Common: fibromyalgia, chronic pain syndrome	Rare
Orthostatic symptoms	Common: cold hands/feet, fainting, dizziness	Rare
Blood pressure	Low	Normal to high
Neck circumference	Normal	Increased

UARS, upper airway respiratory syndrome; OSAS, obstructive sleep apnea syndrome.

sleep maintenance insomnia,[14] which is thought to be result of the conditioning as a consequence of frequent sleep disruptions. There are other presentations which include parasomnias like sleep walking and sleep terror, muscle ache, psychiatric manifestations like anxiety and depression.[15,16] Because of its atypical presentation, UARS is often confused with syndromes like fibromyalgia, chronic fatigue syndrome, or other psychosomatic conditions. Symptoms may include headaches, irritable bowel syndrome, dry mouth, drooling sore throat headaches, sweating cold extremities, and postural dizziness. This tendency to faint is presented about 25% of patients, more commonly teenagers and young adults, and may be explained by the finding of low blood pressure (systolic blood pressure of less than 100 mmHg) associated with UARS (Table 2). There is, however, a different subgroup of patients of UARS who might have hypertension as seen in patients with OSA.

DIAGNOSIS

A general examination would reveal craniofacial abnormalities especially retrognathia. Polysomnography reveals AHI of less than 5, oxygen saturation more than 92%, and presence of respiratory related respiratory arousal (RERAS) and other non apnea-hypopnea respiratory events.[17,18] PES measurement remains the gold standard for detecting respiratory abnormalities. However, other techniques like respiratory plethysmography, pneumotachograph, nasal cannula/pressure transducer, and variations in pulse transit time have been tried to measure subtle respiratory alterations. Three abnormal forms of PES recording have been described.

1. Esophageal pressure crescendo: Increase in negative peak inspiratory pressure in each breath which then terminates with an alpha wave EEG arousal or a first of delta wave. Oxygen saturation does not drop here.
2. The sustained continuous respiratory effort: The tracing shows stable persistent negative peak inspiratory pressure more than that for baseline and non obstructed breaths. This lasts longer than four breaths.

3. Esophageal pressure reversal: Abrupt drop in respiratory effort indicated by less negative peak inspiratory pressure after a sequence of increased respiratory efforts independent of EEG pattern.

Esophageal pressure measurement has, however, not become popular because it is considered "invasive". Hence despite significant scientific validation, good tolerability and low complications rates, the use of this modality has not become widespread except in centers which have a wide research umbrella.

CONSEQUENCES OF UPPER AIRWAY RESPIRATORY SYNDROME

1. Daytime somnolence: Arousal lasts only a few seconds due to IUAR during sleep and results in sleep fragmentation and increased daytime sleepiness.[11]
2. Effect on blood pressure: Several studies have established a causal association between OSA and hypertension.[19-21] A similar association has also been described in UARS by Guilleminault et al.[22] using 48 hours continuous blood pressure monitoring the blood pressure was measured before and after treatment with nasal CPAP. A significant increase in blood pressure was noted with the arousal. A small minority of the subjects underwent echocardiography during sleep which showed a left ward shift of the intraventricular septum with pulsus paradoxus at the time that peak end inspiratory pressure was more negative than minus 35 cm of water. Similar changes have been noted by Lofazo et al. However, autonomic response to arousal is also thought to be a strong contributor to blood pressure variations. The exact mechanism is likely to be a combination of both arousal and hemodynamic factors. The presence of orthostatic hypotension (as discussed previously) was also documented in some subjects.

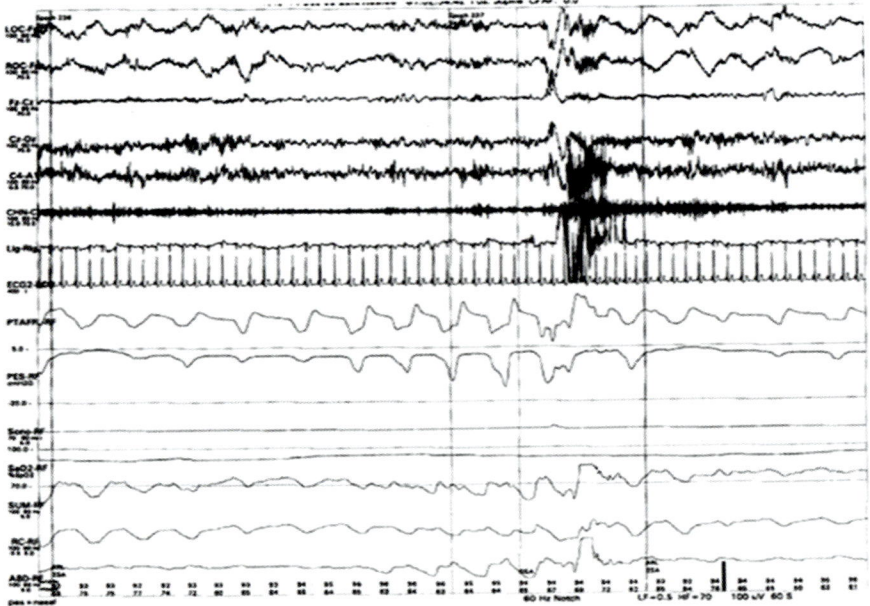

Figure 1: Epoch shows an increasing respiratory effort (as indicated by a progressive negative pressure on the Pes - Pes crescendo) along with flow limitation leading to an arousal.

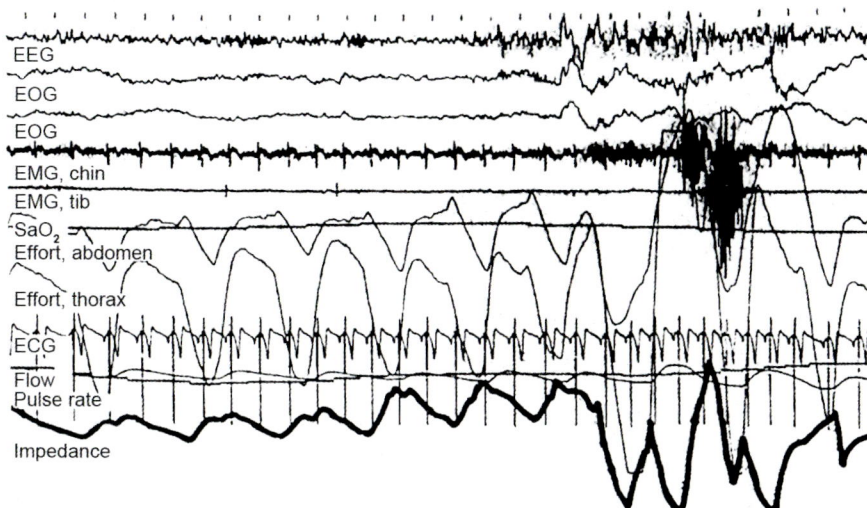

Figure 2: Conventional registration of oronasal flow, thoracic and abdominal effort in comparison with impedance, measured by the forced oscillationtechnique. The impedance (bold tracing) increases without obvious changes in flow and effort until a respiratory arousal occurs. Without impedance measurement, the arousal cannot be explained.

TREATMENT

1. Nasal continuous positive airway pressure: Nasal CPAP continues to be the most frequently used treatment modality in this condition. It seems to work by preventing inspiratory flow limitations and hence decreasing the frequency of arousal. This improved day time fatigue and sleepiness. This has also been used as a reputed trial to prove the diagnosis of UARS. Unfortunately, nasal CPAP seems to be poorly tolerated on a long term basis which has forced researchers to look at other treatment modalities.
2. Turbinectomy: Radiofrequency ablation of the inferior nasal turbinates in post menopausal women with UARS and chronic insomnia seem to work at least as well as CPAP at 6 months post intervention.[23]
3. Oral appliances: This seems to work satisfactorily in a majority of patients with UARS. Oral appliances combined with turbinate surgery and/or palatal surgical procedures seem to work well.[24]
   A combination of septoplasty and radiofrequency reduction of nasal inferior turbinates also seems successful in treating UARS related to pure nasal problems.[25,26]
4. More invasive surgeries: Uvuloflap, lateral pharyngoplasty,[27,28] and distraction osteogenesis have been found helpful in the management of UARS.
5. Orthodontic procedures: Rapid maxillary distraction are more commonly used in children and teenagers (but not directly applicable to adult who need mid line incision of maxilla and mandible for placement of jaw distractors). Combined surgical of orthodontic treatment is less invasive than the traditional jaw advancement surgery. However, patients need to have braces for a long time after jaw expansion for orthodontic procedures.[26]

6. Cognitive behavioral therapy: Recent studies have demonstrated that adding cognitive behavioral therapy to CPAP treatment is beneficial for patients with chronic insomnia or psychosomatic symptoms secondary to UARS.[24,25]

CONCLUSION

At present there is an ongoing debate whether UARS is an independent entity or a subset of OSA. However, this condition still remains quite difficult to diagnose and recent studies show that these patients are often left untreated or poorly treated. With the obesity epidemic throughout the world OSA gets highlighted but UARS is often the forgotten step sister. With better understanding of this condition it is suggested that benign snoring should be questioned and further evaluated because it might be an early pointer to the existence of UARS. RERAs are distinct respiratory events resulting in micro-arousals and should be included in the calculation of respiratory distress index (RDI). Further treatment modalities need to be explored for better management of this condition.

REFERENCES

1. Gastaut H, Tassinari CA, Duron B. Polygraphic study of the episodic diurnal and nocturnal (hypnic and respiratory) manifestations of the Pickwick syndrome. *Brain Res.* 1965;2:167-86.
2. Guilleminault C, Winkle R, Koroblin R, et al. Children and nocturnal snoring: evaluation of effects of sleep related respiratory resistive load and daytime functioning. *Eur J Pediatr.* 1982;139:165-71.
3. International Classification of Sleep Disorders: Diagnostic and Coding Manual. 2nd ed. Westchester, American Academy of Sleep Medicine, 2005.
4. Guilleminault C, Black JE, Palombini L. High (or abnormal) upper airway resistance (in French). *Rev Mal Respir.* 1999;16:173-80.
5. Strohl KP, Redline S. Recognition of obstructive sleep apnea. *Am J Respir Crit Care Med.* 1996;154:279-89.
6. Guilleminault C, Stoohs R. The upper airway resistance syndrome. *Sleep Res.* 1991; 20:250.
7. Guilleminault C, Stoohs R, Clerk A, et al. Excessive daytime somnolence in women with abnormal respiratory efforts during sleep. *Sleep.* 1993;16(suppl):137– 138.
8. Guilleminault C, Winkle R, Korobkin R, et al. Children and nocturnal snoring: Evaluation of the effects of sleep related respiratory resistive load and daytime functioning. *Eur J Pediatr.* 1982;139:165-71.
9. Guilleminault C, Stoohs R, Clerk A, et al. A cause of excessive daytime sleep iness: The upper airway resistance syndrome. *Chest.* 1993;104:781-7.
10. Guilleminault C, Li K, Chen NH, et al. Two-point palatal discrimination in patients with upper airway resistance syndrome, obstructive sleep apnea syndrome, and normal control subjects. *Chest.* 2002;122:866-70.
11. Sleep Disorders Atlas Task Force: EEG arousals: Scoring rules and examples–a preliminary report from the Sleep Disorders Atlas Task Force of the American Sleep Disorders Association. *Sleep.* 1992;15:174-84.
12. Guilleminault C, Stoohs R, Duncan S. Snoring I. Daytime sleepiness in regular heavy snorers. *Chest.* 1991;99:40-8.
13. Woodson BT. Upper airway resistance syndrome after uvulopalatopharyngoplasty for obstructive sleep apnea syndrome. *Otolaryngol Head Neck Surg.* 1996;114:457-61.
14. Guilleminault C, Palombini L, Poyares D, et al. Chronic insomnia, post menopausal women, and SDB, part 2: comparison of non drug treatment trials in normal breathing and UARS post menopausal women complaining of insomnia. *J Psychosom Res.* 2002;53:617-23.
15. Afifi L, Guilleminault C, Colrain I. Sleep and respiratory stimulus specific dampening of cortical responsiveness in OSAS. *Respir Physiol Neurobiol.* 2003;136:221-34.

16. Guilleminault C, Li K, Chen NH, et al. Two-point palatal discrimination in patients with upper airway resistance syndrome, obstructive sleep apnea syndrome, and normal control subjects. *Chest.* 2002;122:866-70.
17. Epstein MD, Chicoine SA, Hanumara RC. Detection of upper airway resistance syndrome using a nasal cannula/pressure transducer. *Chest.* 2000;117:1073-7.
18. Epstein MD, Chicoine SA, Hanumara RC. Detection of upper airway resistance syndrome using a nasal canula/pressure transducer. *Chest.* 2000;117:1073-77.
19. Guilleminault C, Anstella R. Sleep-disordered breathing and hypertension: Past lesson, future directions. *Sleep.* 1997;20:806-11.
20. Hoffstein V, Mateika S, Rubinstein I, et al. Determinants of blood pressure in snorers. *Lancet.* 1988;ii:992-4.
21. Carlson JT, Hedner JA, Ejnell H, et al. High prevalence of hypertension in sleep apnea patients independent of obesity. *Am J Respir Crit Care Med.* 1994;150:72-7.
22. Guilleminault C, Stoohs R, Young-Do K, et al. Upper airway sleep-disordered breathing in women. *Ann Intern Med.* 1995;122:493-501.
23. Guilleminault C, Palombini L, Poyares D, et al. Chronic insomnia, post menopausal women, and SDB, part 2: comparison of non drug treatment trials in normal breathing and UARS post menopausal women complaining of insomnia. *J Psychosom Res.* 2002;53:617-23.
24. Krakow B, Melendrez D, Lee SA, et al. Refractory insomnia and sleep disordered breathing: a pilot study. *Sleep Breath.* 2004;8:15-29. [32]
25. Yoshida K. Oral device therapy for the upper airway resistance syndrome patient. *J Prodthet Dent.* 2002;87:427-30.
26. Powell N, Riley R, Guilleminault C, et al. A reversible uvulopalatal flap for snoring and sleep apnea syndrome. *Sleep.* 1996;19:593-9.
27. Pirelli P, Saponara M, Guilleminault C. Rapid maxillary expansion in children with obstructive sleep apnea syndrome. *Sleep.* 2004;27:761-6.
28. Guilleminault C, Li KK. Maxillomandibular expansion for the treatment of sleep-disordered breathing: preliminary result. *Laryngoscope.* 2004;114:893-6.

CHAPTER 6

Obstructive Sleep Apnea

Vivek Nangia, Shivani Swami

INTRODUCTION

Obstructive sleep apnea (OSA) is a major health problem which has been described for decades but has not got its due recognition. Most of the research and understanding of the disorder has taken place in the last 4–5 decades, more so, after the invention of continuous positive airway pressure (CPAP) device in 1981.[1] The spectrum of OSA ranges from mild to severe and encompasses apneas, hypopneas, and upper airway resistance syndrome. It is multifactorial in origin and has far-fetched deleterious consequences on the various organ systems of the body. It is simple to diagnose but demands extensive counseling to convince the patient to comply with the therapeutic modality.

PATHOPHYSIOLOGY

Snoring signifies the intermediate collapsibility of upper airways. It is expected to be pathologically advancing towards an OSA hypopnea syndrome (OSAHS) if this collapsibility results in significant diminution of airflow. Airflow depends upon the size, compliance, and shape of the upper airway. The patency of the upper airways is accomplished by complex interactions among anatomic structures, neuromuscular tone, ventilatory control mechanisms, level of consciousness, upper airway reflexes, peripheral nervous system mechanisms, body position, vascular tone, surface tension forces, lung volume effects, and expiratory collapse.[2] Skeletal morphology, soft tissue abnormality and obesity influence the upper airway configuration. Two structural abnormalities, micrognathia and retrognathia, commonly cause impingement of the airways due to displacement of the tongue, soft palate, and soft tissues backwards towards the oropharynx.[3] The hyoid bone if displaced inferiorly commonly results in the inferior displacement of the tongue, thus, reducing the pharyngeal lumen.[4] Larger volumes of the adenoids, tonsils, tongue and soft palate, and thickening of the lateral pharyngeal walls play a major role in the narrowing the upper airways during sleep.[5] Obesity contributes by increasing the fat distribution around the neck and airway and by altering the metabolism and ventilation via leptin and other cytokines.[6] During normal awake respiration, the collapsing tendency of the negative inspiratory pressure within the upper airway lumen is balanced by the outward force of pharyngeal dilator muscle activity under central nervous system control. During sleep, reduction of tonic pharyngeal muscle activity and loss of compensatory reflex dilator mechanisms, results in insufficient ability to maintain airway stability in the context of an anatomically or functionally vulnerable pharynx.[7] Clinically significant upper airway narrowing most commonly occurs behind the uvula and soft palate (velopharynx), behind the tongue, or at both sites. With obstruction comes increasing ventilatory effort and possible arousal. Insufficient ventilation due to advanced obstruction, results in hypopneas or apneas and resultant hypercapnia and hypoxia.

By definition, a reduction in airflow of more than 30% is called hypopnea while complete cessation of airflow is called apnea. Both the events, last for at least 10 seconds, are associated with at least 4% drop in oxygen saturation and are terminated by an arousal.[8] This results in fragmentation of sleep, frequent arousals in the night, bradytachycardias, frequent drops in oxygen saturation, despite the presence of an increasing respiratory effort. Many apneas and hypopneas are terminated in the absence of detectable arousals, and recent work suggests that arousals may actually contribute to the severity of OSAHS by promoting airflow overshoot, thereby increasing respiratory control instability.[9]

EPIDEMIOLOGY

Country specific data regarding the prevalence of OSA is now available. Various studies have revealed it to be 2–3 times more common in adult males, with a prevalence of 3–7%, as compared to female adults in general population, in whom the prevalence is 2–5%.[10] Various population based studies from India have revealed the prevalence of OSA and OSAHS to range from 2.4% to 13.4%, being threefold higher in men as compared to women.[11] The exact reason for the gender difference is not known but hormonal differences may be responsible for it. The prevalence is comparable to that in the Western world thus implying that it is not a disease of affluence only. It occurs more commonly in overweight or obese individuals. OSA can affect all age groups but occurs more commonly in the elderly population, in men between the fifth and the seventh decades and in females around the perimenopausal and postmenopausal age group.

RISK FACTORS

Amongst the various attributable risk factors, greater than ideal body weight or obesity is clearly the strongest one. OSAHS occurs in approximately 30% of patients with a body mass index (BMI) more than 30 and 50% of patients with a BMI more than 40. A 1 standard deviation increase in BMI was associated with a 4.5-fold increased risk for OSAHS.[12] Obese individuals have nearly four times higher risk of having OSAHS as compared to non obese individuals independent of age and gender.

Familial inheritance of OSA was recognized way back in 1978 when it was first demonstrated in the study of a single family with high prevalence of OSA.[13] Subsequently, The Cleveland Family Study has clearly shown that there was an increased relative risk of OSA in first-degree relatives of patients with OSA and that this was not affected by controlling the BMI, as a covariate. Thus implying, that familial aggregation cannot be explained only on the basis of obesity.[14]

Craniofacial dysmorphism is another important risk factor. Retrognathia, micrognathia, cleft palate, glossoptosis, retropositioned maxilla and inferiorly positioned hyoid bone are some of the structural factors associated with increased risk of OSA.

The airway inflammation and damage caused by smoking cigarette, results in changes in the structure and function of upper airway, thus leading to increased collapsibility during sleep. The Wisconsin Sleep Cohort Study, showed that current smokers had a much greater risk of moderate or worse degree of OSA (odds ratio, 4.44) compared with never smokers.[15]

Alcohol, increases upper airway resistance by relaxing upper airway dilator muscles and thus narrowing the lumen of upper airways. Therefore, alcohol intake can prolong apnea duration, suppress arousals, increase frequency of occlusive episodes and worsen the severity of hypoxaemia,[16] however, the exact underlying mechanisms are not well understood.

Nasal congestion, use of sedatives and hypnotics are the other risk factors.

CLINICAL PRESENTATION

Such patients, classically, present with loud snoring, disturbed sleep, choking during sleep, waking up non refreshed and excessive daytime sleepiness (Box 1).

CONSEQUENCES

There is increasing evidence to suggest that a disturbed sleep is not the only consequence of OSAHS. Through the inflammatory cascade, endothelial dysfunction, increased coagulability, oxidative stresses, and sympathetic activation, it adversely impacts body's metabolic system and the various organs of the body especially cardiovascular, central nervous system, and the kidneys.

Box 1: Nonrefreshed and excessive daytime sleep

Breathing disturbances during sleep
- Habitual, socially-disruptive snoring
- Witnessed apneas
- Gasping or choking

Difficulties maintaining sleep
- Snort arousals
- Dyspnea spells
- Restlessness
- Nocturia
- Diaphoresis
- Gastroesophageal reflux

Daytime dysfunction
- Nonrestorative sleep
- Excessive daytime sleepiness
- Impaired concentration, cognition, or memory
- Motor vehicle accidents
- Headaches upon arising
- Mood liability
- Weakened libido

Inflammatory Changes[17]

Evidence is also accumulating that OSA can be associated with upper airway inflammation. Exhaled nasal pentane and nitric oxide have been found to be increased after sleep only in patients with OSA. Increased levels of 8-isoprostane (another indicator of oxidative stress) and interleukin (IL)-6 in breath condensate have also been reported. These changes correlated with measured apnea-hypopnea index (AHI).

Systemic markers of inflammatory cascade have also been investigated. Neutrophil superoxide, reactive oxygen species intercellular adhesion molecule 1, IL-8, and monocyte chemoattractant protein 1, are some of the biomarkers studied and found to be elevated. Studies have confirmed that the levels of these markers settle down to normal levels with regular usage of CPAP therapy. It is tempting to speculate that the apparently proinflammatory effect of OSA could account for the associations of this disorder with cardiovascular disease and asthma severity

Pulmonary[17]

Fifteen percent of the OSA patients have been seen to have mildly elevated pulmonary artery pressures. Clinically evident right heart failure occurs only in the presence of daytime hypoxia or coexistent pulmonary disease. In patients of bronchial asthma, the severity and the frequency of nocturnal exacerbations increase in the presence of concomitant OSA. Effective treatment of OSA in such patients is associated with improvement in asthma control and symptoms. Approximately, 10% of patients with OSA also have a coexisting chronic obstructive pulmonary disease (COPD). Such patients experience a greater degree of nocturnal desaturation especially during the rapid eye movement (REM) sleep. This may occur due to REM sleep-associated hypoventilation, sleep-associated ventilation perfusion mismatch and decreased functional residual capacity.

Metabolic

The classical metabolic syndrome which includes insulin resistance, android-central obesity, hypertension, and dyslipidemia is frequently associated with OSAHS and is then referred to as Syndrome Z. Two large prospective studies, one from Sweden and another from the US have shown that regular snoring is associated with a 2- to 7-fold higher risk for type II diabetes over a 10-year period.[18]

Cardiovascular

Obstructive sleep apnea hypopnea syndrome has been implicated in the pathogenesis of ischemic heart disease, left ventricular failure, nocturnal arrhythmias, and atherosclerosis. Enhanced sympathetic tone is considered to be responsible for the association between hypertension and OSAHS. The guidelines of the seventh Joint National Committee on Hypertension have identified OSA as a treatable cause of hypertension and recommend that all patients with refractory hypertension must be evaluated for OSAHS.[19] Nocturnal ST-segment changes consistent with myocardial ischemia are evident even in patients with OSA who do not have clinically significant coronary artery disease. OSA may contribute to nocturnal angina, and ST-segment depression during sleep and this appears to be directly related to the severity of oxygen desaturation.[20] Studies conducted over 7 years have shown that patients with OSA were five times more likely to have cardiovascular disease than those without OSA, even after controlling for age, BMI, and blood pressure. More than 50% of the patients with incompletely treated OSA had cardiovascular events, compared to 10% of those appropriately treated. Patients with untreated severe OSA had a 2.9 folds higher risk of fatal and 3.2 folds higher risk of nonfatal cardiovascular events as compared to healthy subjects.[21] Hypertension, left ventricular diastolic dysfunction, and atrial fibrillation (AF) are the pathogenetic mechanisms for the development of heart failure. OSAHS is tenfold more common in patients with heart failure than general population. Several studies have suggested an association between OSAHS and AF. Thirty to fifty percent of the patients suffering from lone AF have a co-existing OSAHS. Untreated sleep apnea in patients successfully cardioverted to normal sinus rhythm was accompanied by an 80% likelihood of recurrence of AF within 1 year, which is twice as high as the recurrence rate in patients in whom sleep apnea was appropriately treated. OSA has been proposed as a possible contributor to aortic dilation and dissection. Anecdotal and unpublished observations have also suggested that severe OSA may be associated with sudden cardiac death during sleep. A study conducted in Minnesota, examining the time distribution of deaths among residents who had undergone polysomnography and subsequently suffered a sudden cardiac death, showed that amongst the residents dying between 10:00 pm and 6:00 am, 54% of them had an underlying untreated OSA.[22]

Cerebrovascular

The relationship between OSAS and cerebrovascular disease is bidirectional. Habitual snoring increases the risk of cerebrovascular disease with odds ratios (95% CI) ranging from 2.1 to 3.3. Nocturnal apneas and hypopneas may be a predisposing factor for atherosclerosis and may precipitate plaque formation. Carotid intimal-medial thickness, which is considered as a surrogate for stroke risk, is reportedly increased in patients with severe OSA. The risk of stroke in patients with OSAHS is directly proportional to its severity.[23]

Erectile Dysfunction

Erectile dysfunction has also been linked to OSA. While, as many as 33% patients of OSA have been reported to have an erectile dysfunction or decreased libido, 20% of patients with erectile dysfunction have been noted to have OSA.[22]

Renal Disease

Severe hypoxic events in OSA have also been shown to lead to kidney damage. The lowest oxygen saturation level reached at night modestly but significantly predicted chronic kidney disease as indicated by a below-normal estimated glomerular filtration rate (eGFR). OSA has been linked to proteinuria, which is a manifestation of renal disease and a risk factor for chronic kidney disease progression to end-stage renal disease. OSA is exceedingly common among individuals with end-stage renal disease, affecting an estimated 50% of patients.[24]

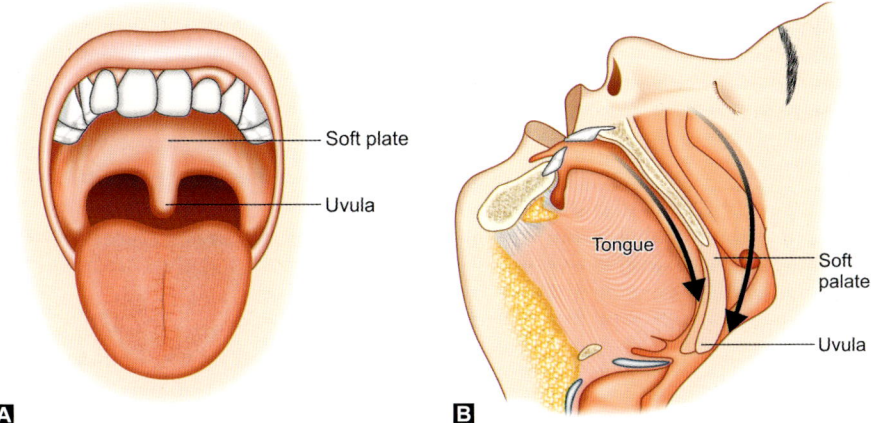

Figure 1: Illustration of the upper airway.[22]

Neurobehavioral and Social

The excessive daytime sleepiness, impaired vigilance, mood disturbances, and cognitive dysfunction that are commonly seen in patient with OSAHS can result in poor quality of life, poor performance at work, increased risk for motor vehicle accidents and occupational injuries, and decreased quality of life. The odds ratio for involvement in automotive collisions for drivers who have OSAHS versus those who do not is 2.5.[25]

Perioperative risk may be higher in OSAHS patients because of difficult endotracheal intubation, upper airway edema from intubation, forced supine sleep positioning, and anesthetic agents/narcotic analgesics. Anesthetic agents and narcotic analgesics increase upper airway collapsibility, impair protective arousal mechanisms, and decrease central respiratory drive. Substantial studies have shown that patients suffering from OSAHS experienced complications (39% vs. 18% in controls) and longer hospital stays (6.8 ± 2.8 days vs. 5.1 ± 4.1 days).[25]

DIAGNOSIS

The search for a diagnosis should begin with a detailed physical examination with special emphasis on the facial structure (retrognathia and micrognathia), body mass index and neck circumference. A BMI more than 30 and neck circumference (shirt collar size) more than 43 cm (17 inches) correlates well with snoring and OSA. A thorough nose and oropharyngeal examination to look for overcrowding of the upper airways is a must. Patients with Mallampati grades 3 and 4 are more likely to have OSA.

Epworth sleepiness scale is used as a validated, reproducible, and sensitive tool for the assessment and quantification of daytime sleepiness. Patient is asked about his or her likelihood of falling asleep in various common situations like: sitting and reading, watching television, sitting inactive in a public place (e.g., meeting), as a passenger in a car for an hour without a break, lying down to rest in the afternoon, sitting and talking to someone, sitting quietly after lunch without alcohol, in a car, while stopped for a few minutes in the traffic, etc.

and is then given a score for each situation and totaled. A score of more than 7 strongly correlates with the presence of OSA.

Polysomnography or a full night sleep study is the gold standard test for the diagnosis of OSA. It is a laboratory-based, technician-attended recording of various parameters during sleep. Sleep architecture is assessed by electroencephalography (EEG), electro-oculography (EOG), and electromyography (EMG). Airflow is assessed by oronasal temperature-sensitive sensors or nasal pressure detectors. Respiratory effort is assessed by strain gauges, piezo sensors, diaphragmatic EMG, or thoracoabdominal inductance plethysmography. Oxyhemoglobin saturation is assessed by pulse oximetry. Cardiac activity is assessed by electrocardiography (ECG). Leg EMG may be added to detect periodic limb movements of sleep and esophageal pressure monitoring may supplement standard respiratory monitoring.[26] OSAHS is then graded by the AHI, which is the polysomnographically-derived number of apneas and hypopneas per hour of sleep. By consensus, OSAHS is diagnosed in patients who have an AHI greater than or equal to five along with daytime dysfunction or who have an AHI greater than or equal to 15. It is classified as mild if AHI is 5–14, moderate if 15–30, and severe if AHI is greater than 30.[20] A limited channel "home" sleep study may be done in patients with a very high pre test probability of OSA.[23]

TREATMENT

The treatment of OSA includes a multidisciplinary approach involving behavioral, medical and surgical options. Weight loss, risk factor modifications like quitting smoking and alcohol and avoiding to sleep in supine position have to be discussed with the patient. The relationship between weight loss and apneas is apparently curvilinear. A critical amount of weight loss must often occur before

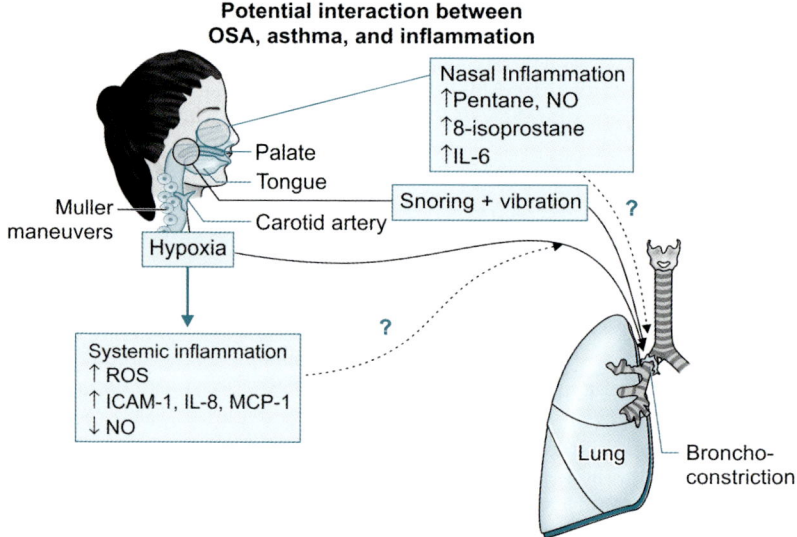

NO, nitric oxide; IL, interleukin; ROS, reactive oxygen species; ICAM-1, intercellular adhesion molecule 1; MCP-1, Monocyte chemoattractant protein 1.

Figure 2: Potential interactions among obstructive sleep apnea, nasal inflammation systemic inflammation, and a possible link to asthma severity.

a significant reduction in AHI is seen. Weight loss alone does not cure OSA in the majority of patients. However, it would always need to be combined with the primary treatment.[27]

Positive airway pressure (PAP) therapy, commonly using the CPAP device is the first line therapy for moderate to severe OSA. Effective CPAP therapy reduces nocturnal respiratory disturbances and improves nocturnal oxygenation, sleep architecture, daytime sleepiness, neurocognitive performance, driving performance, and perceived health status. Regular usage of CPAP therapy during sleep has also been shown to favorably impact the cardiovascular, cerebrovascular, renal, and metabolic consequences. Bilevel PAP device (commonly known as BiPAP), which allows independent adjustment of inspiratory and expiratory pressures, can be use on patients who cannot tolerate CPAP, because of persistent massive nasal mask air leak or discomfort exhaling against positive pressure, or have concomitant nocturnal breathing disorders, such as restrictive thoracic disorders, COPD, or nocturnal hypoventilation (Obesity Hypoventilation Syndrome).

Oral appliances which reduce the upper airway collapsibility may be used during sleep in patients with mild to moderate OSA who are either not candidates or refuse for PAP therapy. Mandibular repositioning appliances and tongue-retaining devices have been used to hold the mandible in an advanced position and the tongue in a forward position. They are successful in bringing the mandible forward by 5–6 mm.[1]

Surgical treatment of OSA includes a wide variety of procedures targeting relief of obstruction at different levels of the airway. It is directed toward site-specific obstruction in the upper airway. The three major anatomic regions of obstruction for OSA are (1) nose; (2) palate (oropharynx); and (3) the base of the tongue (hypopharynx). They involve either extirpation of soft tissue, secondary soft tissue repositioning through primary skeletal mobilization, or bypass of the

Table 1: Prevalence of obstructive sleep apnea in different ethnic groups[10]

Reference	Study population	Age (years)	Prevalence
Young et al. 1993	American men and women	30–60	Men: 4*–25[#]
			Women: 2*–19[#]
Bixler et al. 1998	American men	20–100	17[#]
Bixler et al. 2001	American men and women	20–100	Men: 3.9*
			Women: 1.2*
Duran et al. 2001	Spanish men and women	30–70	Men: 14*–26[#]
			Women: 1.2*
Ip et al. 2001	Chinese men	30–60	4.1*–8.8[#]
Ip et al. 2004	Chinese women	30–60	2.1*–3.7[#]
Kim et al. 2004	Korean men and women	40–69	Men: 4.5*–27[#]
			Women: 3.2*–16[#]
Udwadia et al. 2004	Indian men	25–65	7.5*–19.5*
Sharma et al. 2006	Indian men and women	30–60	Men: 4.9*–19.7[#]
			Women: 2.1*–7.4[#]

*Obstructive sleep apnea syndrome is defined as apnea-hypopnea index ≥5 with excessive daytime sleepiness; #Obstructive sleep apnoea is defined as apnea-hypopnoea index >15. All these prevalence studies were assessed with standard polysomnography.

pharyngeal airway. The most common surgical intervention to be performed is the uvulopalatopharyngoglossoplasty (UPPP), which enlarges the retropalatal airway through tonsillectomy (if present); trimming and reorientation of the posterior and anterior tonsillar pillars; and excision of the uvula and the posterior portion of the palate. Surgical procedure may be considered as a secondary treatment for inadequate treatment outcome from PAP treatment and oral appliances. Tracheostomy may be used as a life saving procedure to bypass the pharyngeal airway in OSA patients with morbid obesity; severe facial skeletal deformity (mandibular deficiency) with excessive daytime somnolence; hypoxemia (SaO_2 <70%); or significant cardiac arrhythmias.[23]

Adjunctive therapies of OSA include bariatric surgery which is indicated in patients with BMI more than 40 or more than 35 with comorbidities. No pharmacologic agent exists which can fully prevent or overcome upper airway obstruction, sufficient enough to justify itself as a primary therapy in the management of OSA. Topical nasal steroid sprays have been found to improve AHI in children and in adults with perennial allergic rhinitis, modafinil are armodafinil are recommended to be used for residual excessive daytime sleepiness despite CPAP and oxygen therapy.[28]

CONCLUSION

Obstructive sleep disorder is a common but often undiagnosed condition in the general population. The classical symptoms of OSA are loud snoring, disturbed sleep, choking during sleep, waking up unrefreshed, early morning headaches and excessive daytime sleepiness. It is commonly seen in obese males and if left untreated can result in deleterious consequences impacting cardiovascular, cerebrovascular, neurocognitive, and social as also metabolic systems. A thorough physical examination looking for crowded upper airways, BMI more than 30, neck circumference more than 17 inches clubbed together with Epworth sleepiness scale more than 7 can point towards the diagnosis. Overnight polysomnography is the gold standard test for its diagnosis. The cornerstone of treatment remains nasal CPAP. Effective treatment provides significant relief and prevents the various systemic complications.

REFERENCES

1. Sullivan CE, Issa FG, Berthon-Jones M, et al. Reversal of obstructive sleep apnoea by continuous positive airway pressure applied through the nares. Lancet. 1981;1:862-5.
2. Woodson BT, Franco R. Physiology of sleep disordered breathing. Otolaryngol Clin North Am. 2007;40(4):691-711.
3. Watanabe T, Isono S, Tanaka A, et al. Contribution of body habitus and craniofacial characteristics to segmental closing pressures of the passive pharynx in patients with sleep-disordered breathing. Am J Respir Crit Care Med. 2002;165:260-5.
4. Young JW, McDonald JP. An investigation into the relationship between the severity of obstructive sleep apnoea/hypopnoea syndrome and the vertical position of the hyoid bone. Surgeon. 2004;2:145-51.
5. Stauffer JL, Buick MK, Bixler EO, et al. Morphology of the uvula in obstructive sleep apnea. Am Rev Respir Dis. 1989;140:724-8.
6. Kryger M, Quesney LF, Holder D, et al. The sleep deprivation syndrome of the obese patient—a problem of periodic nocturnal upper airway obstruction. Am J Med. 1974;56:530-9.

7. Fogel RB, Malhotra A, White DP. Sleep 2: pathophysiology of obstructive sleep apnoea/hypopnoea syndrome. *Thorax*. 2004;59:159-63.
8. Meoli AL, Casey KR, Clark RW, et al. Hypopnea in sleep-disordered breathing in adults. *Sleep*. 2001;24:469-70.
9. Younes M. Role of arousals in the pathogenesis of obstructive sleep apnea. *Am J Respir Crit Care Med*. 2004;169:623-33.
10. Lam CM, Sharma SK, Lam B. Obstructive sleep apnoea: Definitions, epidemiology & natural history. *Indian J Med Res*. 2010;131:165-170.
11. Sharma SK, Ahluwalia G. Epidemiology of adult obstructive sleep apnoea syndrome in India. *In J Med Res*. 2010;131:171-5.
12. Young T, Palta M, Dempsey J, et al. The occurrence of sleep-disordered breathing among middle-aged adults. *N Engl J Med*. 1993;328:1230-5.
13. Strohl KP, Saunders NA, Feldman NT, et al. Obstructive sleep apnea in family members. *N Engl J Med*. 1978;299:969-73.
14. Redline S, Tishler PV, Tosteson TD, et al. The familial aggregation of obstructive sleep apnea. *Am J Respir Crit Care Med*. 1995;151:682-7.
15. Wetter DW, Young TB, Bidwell TR, et al. Smoking as a risk factor for sleep-disordered breathing. *Arch Intern Med*. 1994;154:2219-24.
16. Mitler MM, Dawson A, Henriksen SJ, et al. Bedtime ethanol increases resistance of upper airways and produces sleep apneas in asymptomatic snorers. *Alcohol Clin Exp Res*. 1998;12:801-5.
17. Ballard RD, Quershi A. Obstructive sleep apnea. *J Allergy Clin Immunol*. 2003;112(4):643-51.
18. Vgontzas AN, Bixler EO, Chrousos GP. Sleep apnea is a manifestation of the metabolic syndrome. *Sleep Med Rev*. 2005;9:211-24.
19. Chobanian AV, Bakris GL, Black HR, et al. The seventh report of the Joint National Committee on Prevention, Detection, Evaluation, and Treatment of High Blood Pressure: the JNC 7 report. *JAMA*. 2003;289:2560-72.
20. Hanly P, Sasson Z, Zuberi N, et al. ST-segment depression during sleep in obstructive sleep apnea. *Am J Cardiol*. 1993;71:1341-5.
21. Marin JM, Carrizo SJ, Vicente E, et al. Long-term cardiovascular outcomes in men with obstructive sleep apnoea hypopnoea with or without treatment with continuous positive airway pressure: an observational study. *Lancet*. 2005;365:1046-53.
22. Lopez-Jimenez F, Sert Kuniyoshi FH, Gami A, et al. Obstructive sleep apnea: implications of cardiac and vascular disease. *Chest*. 2008;133:793-804.
23. Guilleminault C, Abad VC. Obstructive sleep apnea syndromes. *Med Clin North Am*. 2004;88(3):611-30.
24. Adeseun GA, Rosas SE. The impact of obstructive sleep apnea on chronic kidney disease. *Curr Hypertens Rep*. 2010;12(5):378-83.
25. Olson EJ, Park JG, Morgenthaler TI. Obstructive sleep apnea-hypopnea syndrome. *Prim Care*. 2005;32(2):329-59.
26. Sleep-related breathing disorders in adults: recommendations for syndrome definition and measurement techniques in clinical research. The report of an American Academy of Sleep Medicine Task Force. *Sleep*. 1999;22:667-89.
27. Morgenthaler TI, Kapen S, Lee-Choing T, et al. Practice parameters for the medical therapy of OSA. *Sleep*. 2006;(29):1031-35.
28. Abad VC. Pharmacologic therapy for obstructive sleep apnea. *Sleep Med Clin*. 2013;527-42.

CHAPTER 7

Central Sleep Apnea

Manas K Sen

INTRODUCTION

Central sleep apnea (CSA) is the cessation of breathing due to absence of respiratory effort during sleep. CSA syndrome (CSAS) is recognized by a diminution or absence of respiratory effort associated with symptoms of daytime sleepiness, frequent nocturnal awakenings or both.[1]

DEFINITION

Central sleep apnea is a polysomnographic terminology and, therefore, it would be prudent to review some of the operational polysomnographic terms. Apnea is the absence of airflow at nose or mouth for 10 seconds.[2,3] Whereas an obstructive apnea is characterized by the absence of tidal volume with continued respiratory effort as monitored by thoracoabdominal bands, a central apnea is the absence of tidal volume with a complete absence of respiratory effort (Figures 1 and 2).[2,4] Although central apnea index (CAI) of more than or equal to 5 per hour is abnormal, it is difficult to identify the minimum number of CSA events needed to cause a distinct disorder or syndrome (insomnia, excessive daytime sleepiness, impaired quality of life etc.).[5,6]

Also, in contrast to obstructive apnea-hypopnea index, the number of hypopneas is not included in CAI. CSA syndrome is an acceptable diagnosis in case the apnea-hypopnea index (AHI) is more than or equal to five events per hour with more than 50% of the respiratory events classified as central rather than obstructive.[7,8] In many sleep apnea patients, central apneas can lead to

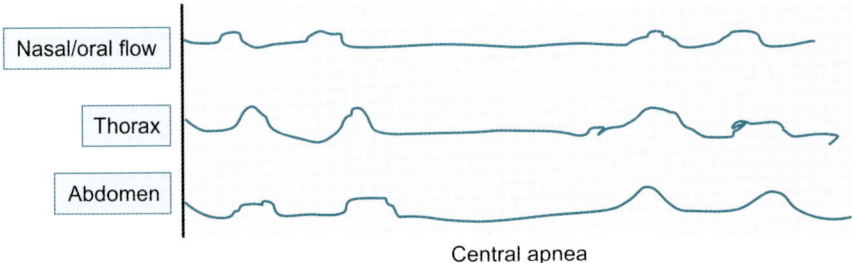

Figure 1: Central sleep apnea

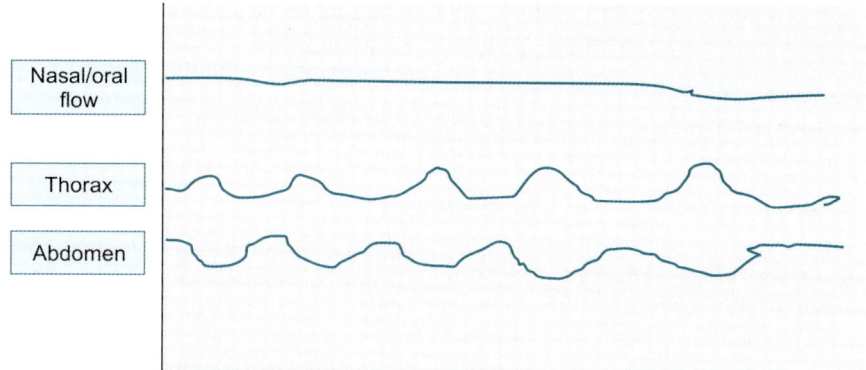

Figure 2: Obstructive sleep apnea.

obstructive respiratory events and vice-versa; in others, there may be an overlap, or mixed apnea syndrome.[8-10] Although obstructive hypopnea has the widest variety of definitions, the most practical one identifies it as a reduction in airflow of 30% from baseline for more than or equal to 10 seconds with an oxygen desaturation of more than or equal to 4%. In the recently revised American Academy of Sleep Medicine (AASM) Scoring Manual, an obstructive hypopnea has been redefined to incorporate paradoxical movements, snoring, and inspiratory flattening relative to baseline.[11] A central hypopnea is characterized by absence of these indicators.[12] As evolution takes place in the "definitions of sleep apnea" and the "metrics used to define respiratory events", recent efforts have attempted to utilize esophageal manometry to design an algorithm to distinguish central from obstructive apneas.[13]

CLASSIFICATION

According to the International Classification of Sleep Disorders (ICSD)-3 there are eight different forms of CSA.[14]
1. Primary central sleep apnea.
2. Central sleep apnea due to Cheyne-Stokes breathing pattern.
3. Central sleep apnea due to medical conditions not Cheyne-Stokes.
4. Central sleep apnea due to high altitude periodic breathing.
5. Central sleep apnea due to drug or substance.
6. Primary sleep apnea of infancy.
7. Primary central sleep apnea of prematurity.
8. Treatment-emergent central sleep apnea.

Based on pathophysiologic mechanisms, CSA can be classified into two broad categories.
A. Central sleep apnea due to post-hypocapnia hyperventilation as seen in CSA associated with congestive heart failure, high altitude sickness and primary CSA.
B. Central sleep apnea due to hypoventilation as seen in CSA associated with compromised neuromuscular ventilatory control, central nervous system (CNS) disease (encephalitis) and chest wall disease (kyphoscoliosis).

When CSA occurs due to no attributable cause, it is known as primary CSA.

In a patient with OSA, central apneas frequently coexist, with more than 50% apneas being obstructive in nature. Such entities are termed as "complex apnea". Quite often, it may so occur that central apneas develop in patients with OSA upon initial continuous positive airway pressure (CPAP) exposure. These are often also labeled as "treatment emergent central apneas".

Epidemiology of Central Sleep Apnea

Central sleep apnea is more prevalent in older adults compared to middle aged individuals.[15-18] In a study of elderly men, obstructive apnea was observed to be present in 35% whereas central apnea in 7.5% of the subjects.[19] Cheyne-Stokes breathing pattern (CSBP) or Cheyne-Stokes respiration (CSR) is identified by central apnea followed by hyperventilation in a crescendo-decrescendo pattern. It may occur in 30–40% patients with congestive heart failure (CHF).[20,21] In patients of systolic CHF, CSA is commoner than OSA (40% vs. 11%).[21] CSA predicts a higher morbidity and mortality in CHF patients. In randomly selected men >60 years old who were inpatients on a medical ward and followed up for 17.5 years, there were significantly greater mortality rates in patients who had both CHF and CSA than those with just CSA or just OSA.[22] CSA occurring in individuals with cardiac, renal and neurological disorders without any CSR pattern is then termed as CSAS due to medical conditions not Cheyne-Stokes.

Mechanisms of Causation of Central Sleep Apnea

The principal pattern generator of respiratory rhythm (inspiration) is said to be the Pre-Botzinger Complex (PBC) group of neurons located in the brainstem; some role is also played by the retro-trapezoid nucleus (RTN) as expiratory rhythm generator.[23,24] Central chemoreceptors in the medulla respond to changes in $PaCO_2$; peripheral chemoreceptors in the carotid body respond to changes in $PaCO_2$ as well as PaO_2—both influencing the respiratory center. Other factors influencing the respiratory center include Golgi tendon organs and muscle spindles from chest wall and respiratory muscles; emotional influences during wakefulness and stretch receptors in the lungs. The augmented ventilatory drive to breathe that prevails during wakefulness is lost during sleep (Figure 3).[25-27] Thus breathing during sleep is predominantly under the metabolic control factors mentioned above, and becomes increasingly sensitive to small changes in $PaCO_2$.[28] At onset of sleep, normally ventilation decreases and $PaCO_2$ increases mildly. The $PaCO_2$ level

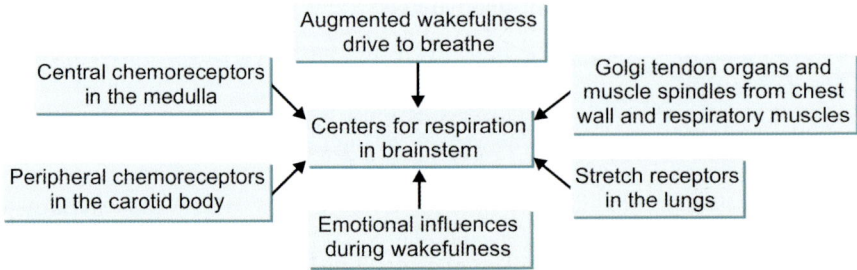

Figure 3: Factors influencing control of breathing.

below which rhythmical breathing stops and central apnea ensues is known as apneic threshold. Rhythmical breathing is maintained as long as the prevailing $PaCO_2$ (eupneic $PaCO_2$) is above the apneic threshold.[28] Hyperventilation (due to arousal or any other reason) may decrease the eupneic $PaCO_2$ below the arousal threshold, thus precipitating a central apnea. Subsequently, $PaCO_2$ increases as a result of central apnea, till the apneic threshold is exceeded, when breathing resumes. The difference between eupneic $PaCO_2$ and the apnea threshold (also known as $PaCO_2$ reserve) is thus crucial in the pathogenesis of CSA, which in disease states results from unmasking of the apneic threshold during sleep.[28,29] At sleep onset, in healthy subjects, respiratory control is unstable, upper airway resistance increases due to a reduction in the tone of upper airway dilators, and ventilatory drive and chemosensitivity reduce.[30,33] During sleep, the ventilatory response to chemical stimuli as well as compensation to respiratory load are reduced.[34-37]

This feedback loop of ventilatory control is referred to as "loop gain" which is the ratio of the magnitude of the corrective action (response) to the magnitude of disturbance (stimulus) = corrective action/disturbance or ventilatory response.[8,38] There are two types of loop gain, namely, controller gain (hypoxic and hypercapnic ventilatory chemo-responsiveness of the system plus responses) and plant gain (efficiency of CO_2 excretion). A third variety of loop gain, namely, mixing gain reflects circulatory delay and binding of hemoglobin to oxygen and carbon dioxide, and is important in the genesis of CSA and heart failure.[8,39,40] A high loop gain, characterized by over-enthusiastic corrective action to a relatively small disturbance can precipitate periodic breathing with central apneas.

Conditions Associated with Central Sleep Apnea

The various conditions associated with CSA are outlined in table 1.

Type of CSA	Condition
Table 1: Conditions associated with central sleep apnea	
Physiologic	
Non-hypercapnic	Systolic heart failure
	Cerebrovascular accident
	High altitude
	Idiopathic
	Idiopathic pulmonary arterial hypertension
Hypercapnic	Congenital central hypoventilation syndrome
	Idiopathic (primary) alveolar hypoventilation syndrome
	Brain stem pathology
	Opioid Induced CSA
	Neuromuscular disorders
CSA associated with endocrine disorders	Acromegaly
	Hypothyroidism
CSA associated with OSA	Treatment emergent sleep apnea or complex sleep apnea

CSA, central sleep apnea; OSA, obstructive sleep apnea

Physiologic Central Sleep Apnea

As mentioned earlier, CSA may occur in normal subjects at onset of sleep, after a sigh or an arousal and sometimes during phasic rapid eye movement (REM) during sleep.[28,41]

Non-hypercapnic Central Sleep Apnea

Conditions like systolic heart failure, idiopathic pulmonary arterial hypertension, high altitude, and cerebrovascular accidents are often associated with CSA. The $PaCO_2$ in awake steady state is usually low normal or below normal range.

Systolic heart failure: In an analysis of 1,250 patients with systolic heart failure, 52% had moderate to severe sleep apnea, 31% had CSA, and 21% had OSA.[28,42-46] There are several mechanisms that could precipitate CSA in patients with heart failure.[40]

- Increased venous return and pulmonary capillary wedge pressure during sleep as a result of diastolic ventricular dysfunction may prevent a normal rise in $PaCO_2$. Prevailing $PaCO_2$, thus, remains close to an exposed apnea threshold thus predisposing to CSA
- Pulmonary congestion increases the CO_2 chemosensitivity below eupnea and decreases $PaCO_2$ reserve. There is a high ventilatory response, mainly to hypercapnia, but also to hypoxia (high controller gain) favoring ventilatory instability
- Restrictive lung volumes and alveolocapillary membrane dysfunction increases the plant gain
- Transit between lung and chemoreceptors is slower due to prolongation of circulation time
- Central sleep apnea occurs in heart failure with periodic breathing (PB), which is characterized by long crescendo-decrescendo ventilation arms. It results from prolongation in circulation time between pulmonary capillary blood and the respiratory center.

High altitude: Hypoxemia at high altitude increases chemosensitivity below apneic threshold and also reduces the $PaCO_2$ reserve. Administration of supplemental oxygen and small amounts of CO_2 as well as acetazolamide decreases periodic breathing.[28,47,48]

Cerebrovascular accident: Central sleep apnea can be caused by acute, chronic, and ischemic strokes and may decrease with time.[28,49] A pattern similar to Hunter-Cheyne-Stokes breathing has been observed.[25,58]

Idiopathic CSA: This is a diagnosis arrived at by exclusion of all other causes and is rare. Such patients have a low $PaCO_2$ and increased hypercapnic ventilatory response during wakeful state.[28]

Idiopathic pulmonary arterial hypertension: This condition is often associated with CSA which may result from a diminution in stroke volume and prolongation of arterial circulation time.[28]

Hypercapnic Central Sleep Apnea

In this group of conditions, the daytime $PaCO_2$ is either raised or is close to the upper limit of normal. Hypoventilation leads to this hypercapnia, which is magnified during sleep due to the loss of wakefulness drive to breathe. The plant gain in such patients is increased. As a result, with regaining of wakefulness drive to breathe, the $PaCO_2$ falls to disproportionately low levels, and may precipitate central apnea in case the apneic threshold is also increased, which in such patients is common.[5,25,28] In certain conditions, due to the involvement of respiratory centers, absences of the wakefulness drive to breathe results in central apneas. There are several such "won't breathe" situations that need to be mentioned.

Congenital central hypoventilation syndrome: Previously known as Ondine's Curse, a rare autosomal dominant genetic disorder resulting from a mutation in the *PHOX2B* gene, this usually presents in the neonatal period. The automatic/metabolic pathway is at fault, ventilatory responses and sensing of dyspnea in response to hypoxia and hypercapnia and processing of respiratory afferent information is diminished.[8,28,51,52]

Idiopathic (primary) alveolar hypoventilation syndrome: This disorder manifests in adult men and may have a genetic basis. There may be no demonstrable neuromuscular, thoracic, pulmonary or CNS pathology.[28]

Brain stem pathology: Brain stem conditions resulting from edema, infarct, compression, ischemia, tumor, encephalitis, neurodegenerative disease, and Chiari malformation can lead to a "won't breathe" like situation as outlined earlier.[53-60]

Opioid Induced CSA: Chronic pain is commonly managed with opioids on a long-term basis. Although daytime hypoventilation is mild, sleep apnea is widely prevalent among chronic opioid users.[24,61-65] A study polysomnographically documented that 75% of such patients had AHI more than or equal to 5/hour, 50% had AHI more than or equal to 15/hour, and 36% AHI more than or equal to 30/hour.[62] It has been suggested that opioids inhibit the inspiratory rhythm generator neurons in the PBC, that was referred to earlier, resulting in central apneas.[28] Nocturnal hypoxemia due to central apneas, besides other reasons, has been demonstrated in chronic opioid users.[66] There is a heightened ventilatory response to hypoxia and a blunted hypercapnic response in these patients. The opioid agonist is said to directly depress the central respiratory controller leading to a central apnea. This, in turn, results in worsening of an already prevailing low grade hypoxia.[8] Such events initiate an over-enthusiastic peripheral chemoreceptor response which resolves the hypoxia and then subsides, leading to a decrease in $PaCO_2$. The response of central chemoreceptors to changes in $PaCO_2$ is blunted in such patients, although they remain susceptible to the depressant effects of opiates, thus precipitating the cycle of events.[8]

Neuromuscular disorders: These are situations which resemble a "can't breathe" scenario. Patients with cervical cord pathology (disc disease), motor neuron disease, post-polio syndrome, neuromuscular junction pathology (myasthenia gravis), and myopathies (kyphoscoliosis) are included in this group.

Central Sleep Apnea Associated with Endocrine Disorders

Acromegaly and hypothyroidism are both associated with sleep apnea. Obstructive apneas occur in excess of CSA in both situations. In acromegaly, human growth hormone, insulin-like growth factor-1 and hypercapnic ventilatory response have all been hypothesized to attribute to the occurrence of CSA.[8,28,68-70]

CSA Associated with OSA (Complex Sleep Apnea/Treatment Emergent Sleep Apnea)

As referred to above (see section on classification of CSA), some patients of severe obstructive sleep apnea, those with systolic heart failure, atrial fibrillation, chronic opioid use, and neuromuscular disorders often have excess central apneas or develop CSA during commencement of CPAP therapy and are often termed as "treatment emergent" CSA.[28,71,72] Those who continue to have OSA and CSA on CPAP are often termed as "complex sleep apnea".[28]

Diagnosis of Central Sleep Apnea

The standard of diagnosis of sleep apnea is nocturnal in-laboratory polysomnography.[15,73] Distinction between obstructive and central apneas can be made by assessment of pleural pressure changes as reflected by esophageal manometry.[74] However, respiratory inductance plethysmography (RIP) or strain gauges and pulse transit time (PTT) (the time taken by the pulse signal to reach the periphery) can also measure respiratory effort accurately and non-invasively.

Treatment of Central Sleep Apnea

The sheet anchor of treatment of CSA is positive airway pressure (PAP) therapy. However, acetazolamide, oxygen therapy, and carbon dioxide gas supplementation have also been utilized. The practice parameters for treatment of CSAS have been lucidly outlined in the recommendations of the Standards of Practice Committee of the American Academy of Sleep Medicine in 2012.[1]

With regard to CSAS related to congestive heart failure, the following modalities have been recommended as standard of care.
- Continuous positive airway pressure therapy targeted to normalize the AHI for initial treatment
- Nocturnal oxygen therapy
- Adaptive servoventilation (ASV) targeted to normalize the AHI.

The following modalities have been listed as optional:
- Bilevel positive airway pressure (BPAP) therapy in spontaneous-timed (ST) mode targeted to normalize the AHI in CSAS with CHF only if there is no response to adequate trials of CPAP, ASV, and oxygen therapies
- Positive airway therapy (PAP), acetazolamide, zolpidem and triazolam (in case there is no risk for respiratory depression)
- Continuous positive airway pressure, supplemental oxygen, bicarbonate buffer use during dialysis, and nocturnal dialysis in case of CSAS related to end stage renal disease.

Optimization of pharmacotherapy is of seminal importance in patients of CSAS with CHF. Important nonpharmacological treatment modalities include cardiac resynchronization therapy, atrial overdrive pacing, and cardiac transplant. The CANPAP Trial suggested that CPAP therapy had no direct effect on cardiac function or survival in case sleep-disordered breathing was not controlled adequately.[1,75] However, in a *post hoc* analysis of the trial, a positive effect on both left ventricular ejection fraction (LVEF) and transplant free survival is noted if CSAS is adequately treated.[76]

Adaptive servoventilation is a pressure preset, volume or flow cycled, closed loop mechanical ventilation mode that provides breath by breath adjustment of inspiratory pressure support with a back-up rate to normalize breathing patterns relative to a pre-determined target.[1,77] Consistent improvement in AHI and LVEF has been demonstrated, though no survival or long-term data is available. The cost of this device is more than CPAP and its data is consistent and is "at least comparable if not better than data supporting CPAP use".[1]

Oxygen therapy in CSA with CHF acts by reduction in CO_2 chemoreflex sensitivity.[78] Although there is no evidence demonstrating any outcome advantage of oxygen therapy over CPAP therapy, it is easily administered and can be prescribed to those not compliant to CPAP therapy in patients of CSA with CHF.[1]

It has been opined that bilevel positive airway pressure (BPAP) can be used in those patients who require high positive airway pressure (PAP) level or as a pressure support ventilatory method to augment alveolar ventilation.[1]

Raising the eucapnic $PaCO_2$ during sleep to above the apneic threshold may minimize the risk of central apneas in some patients.[8] Addition of CO_2 or increasing the dead space via a mask may be beneficial in idiopathic CSA.[79] However, CO_2 induced sympathetic stimulation may be detrimental in patients with CSA-CHF.[8,80] A mathematical model found some advantage with dynamic administration of CO_2 adjusting the dose and duration in real time.[81]

Positional therapy (seated, upright, right sided) has been reported to reduce cardiac work.[40,82,83] The role of exercise therapy and newer PAP therapies, as therapeutic options for CSA, are being explored.[84,85] The SERVE-HF and ADVENT-HF (Effect of ASV on Survival and Hospital Admissions in Heart failure) are new trials that look into the role of PAP therapy in CSA-CHF.[1,86,87]

CONCLUSION

Central sleep apnea manifests in a heterogeneous group of disorders. Important pathogenetic mechanisms have been discussed. Options of the multiple therapeutic modalities have also been highlighted with a view to underscore the significance of early diagnosis and its prompt treatment.

REFERENCES

1. Aurora RN, Choudhuri S, Ramar K, et al. The treatment of central apnea syndrome in adults: Practice Parameters with an evidence based literature review and meta-analyses. *Sleep.* 2012;35(1):17-40.
2. Connolly TA, Sharafkhaneh A. Sleep-related breathing disorder and heart disease-central sleep apnea. *Sleep Med Clin.* 2007;2:107-17.
3. Kryger MH. Monitoring respiratory and cardiac function. In: Kryger MH, Roth T, Dement WC, editors. Principles and practice of sleep medicine. Philadelphia: WB Saunders; 2000. pp.1217-30.
4. Berry RB. Sleep medicine pearls. 2nd ed. Philadelphia: Hanley & Belfus Inc; 2003.
5. Javaheri S. Central sleep apnea. In: Lee-Chiong T, editors. Sleep Medicine essentials, Hoboken: Wiley-Blackwell; 2009. pp. 81-9.
6. Javaheri S, Dempsey JA. Central sleep apnea. *Compr Physiol.* 2013;3:141-63.
7. Sin DD, Fitzgerald F, Parker JD, et al. Risk factors for central and obstructive sleep apnea in 450 men and women with congestive heart failure. *Am J Respir Crit Care Med.* 1999;160(4):1101-6.
8. McSharry DG, Eckert DJ, Malhotra A. Central sleep apnea. *Eur Respir Mon.* 2010;50:381-95.
9. Badr MS, Toiber F, et al. Pharyngeal narrowing/occlusion during central sleep apnea. *J Appl Physiol.* 1995;78:1806-15.

10. Sankri-Tarbichi AG, Rowley JA, Badr MS. Expiratory pharyngeal narrowing during central hypocapnic hypopnea. *Am J Respire Crit Care Med.* 2009;179:313-9.
11. Berry RB, Budhiraja R, Gottlieb DJ, et al. Rules for scoring of sleep associated events. Deliberations of the sleep apnea definitions task force of American Academy of Sleep Medicine. *J Clin Sleep Med.* 2012;8:597-619.
12. Iber C. Are we ready to define central hypopneas? *Sleep.* 2013;36(3):305-6.
13. Randerath WJTM, Preignitz C, Steiglitz S, et al. Evaluation of a non-invasive algorithm for differentiation of obstructive and central hypopneas. *Sleep.* 2013;36:363-8.
14. American Academy of Sleep Medicine (2014). The international classification of sleep disorders. 3rd ed. Diagnostic and coding manual. Darien, IL: American Academy of Sleep Medicine; 2014.
15. Chowdhuri S, Badr MS. Central sleep apnea. *Indian J Med Res.* 2010;131:150-64.
16. Bixler EO, Vgontzas AN, Lin HM, et al. Prevalence of sleep-disordered breathing in women: effects of gender. *Am J Respir Crit Care Med.* 2001; 163:608-13.
17. Mason WJ, Ancoli-Israel S, Kripke DF. Apnea revisited: a longitudinal follow up. *Sleep.* 1989;12:423-9.
18. Bliwise DL, Bliwise NG, Partinen M, et al. Sleep apnea and mortality in an aged cohort. *Am J Public Health.* 1988;78:544-7.
19. Mehra R, Stone KL, Blackwell T, Israel SA, et al. Prevalence and correlates of sleep-disordered breathing in older men: Osteoporotic Fractures in Men Sleep Study. Osteoporotic Fractures in Men Study. *J Am Geriatr Soc.* 2007;55:1356-64.
20. Bitter T, Faber L, Hering D, Langer C, Horstkotte D, Oldenburg O. Sleep disordered breathing in heart failure with normal left ventricular ejection fraction. *Eur Heart J.* 2009; 11:602-8.
21. Javaheri S, Parker TJ, Liming JD, Corbett WS, Nishiyama H, Wexler L, Roselle GA. Sleep apnea in 81 ambulatory male patients with stable heart failure: types and their prevalence, consequences, and presentations. *Circulation.* 1998;97:2154-9.
22. Ancoli-Israel S, Duhamel ER, Stepnowski C, et al. The relationship between congestive heart failure, sleep apnea, and mortality in older men. *Chest.* 2003;124:1400-5.
23. Boden AG, Harris MC, Parkes MJ. Apneic threshold for CO2 in the anaesthetized rat: fundamental properties under steady state conditions. *J Appl Physiol.* 1998;85:898-907.
24. Feldman J, Del Negro C. Looking for inspiration: New perspectives on respiratory rhythm. *Nat Rev.* 2006;7:232-42.
25. Orem J. The nature of wakefulness stimulus for breathing. *Prog Clin Biol Res.* 1990;345:23-30.
26. Kay A, Trinder J, Bowes G, et al. Changes in airway resistance during sleep onset. *J Appl Physiol.* 1994;76:1600-7.
27. Worsnop C, Kay A, Pierce R, et al. Activity of respiratory pump and upper airway muscles during sleep onset. *J Appl Physiol.* 1998;85:908-20.
28. Javaheri S. Central sleep apnea. *Clin Chest Med.* 2010;31:235-48.
29. Chowdhuri S, Shanidze I, Pierchala L, et al. Effect of episodic hypoxia on the susceptibility to hypocapnic central apnea during NREM sleep. *J Appl Physiol.* 2010;108:368-77.
30. Trinder J, Whitworth F, Kay A, et al. Respiratory instability during sleep onset. *J Appl Physiol.* 1992;73:2462-9.
31. Dunai J, Wilkinson M, Trinder J. Interaction of chemical and state effects on ventilation during sleep onset. *J Appl Physiol.* 1996;81:2235-43.
32. Harms CA, Zeng YJ, Smith CA, et al. Negative pressure induced deformation of the upper airway causes central apnea in awake and sleeping dogs. *J Appl Physiol.* 1996;80:1528-39.
33. Davis AM, Koenig JC, Thack BT. Upper airway chemoreflex responses to saline and water in preterm infants. *J Appl Physiol.* 1988;64:1412-20.
34. Douglas NJ, White DP, Weil JV, et al. Hypoxic ventilatory response decreases during sleep in normal men. *Am Rev Respir Dis.* 1982;125:286-9.
35. Skatrud JB, Dempsey JA, Badr S, et al. Effect of respiratory muscle activity during NREM sleep. *J Appl Physiol.* 1988;65:1676-85.
36. White DP, Douglas NJ, Picket CK, et al. Hypoxic ventilatory response during sleep in premenopausal women. *J Appl Physiol.* 1982;126:530-3.
37. Weigand L, Zwillich CW, White DP. Sleep and the ventilatory response to resistive loading in normal men. *J Appl Physiol.* 1988;64:1186-95.

38. Khoo MC, Kronauer RE, Strohl KP, et al. Factors inducing periodic breathing in humans: a general model. *J Appl Physiol.* 1982;53:644-59.
39. Stanchina MI, Ellison K, Malhotra A, et al. The impact of cardiac resynchronization therapy on obstructive sleep apnea in heart failure patients: a pilot study. *Chest.* 2007;132:433-9.
40. Naughton MT, Andreas S. Sleep apnea in chronic heart failure. *Eur Respir Mono.* 2010;50:396-420.
41. Orem J, Kubin L. Respiratory physiology: central neural control. In: Kryger MH, Roth T, Dement WC, editors. Principles and Practice of Sleep medicine. 3rd ed. Philadelphia: WB Saunders; 2000. pp. 295-208.
42. Javaheri S. Sleep disorders in 100 male patients with systolic heart failure. A prospective study. *Int J Cardiol.* 2006;106:21-8.
43. Vazir A, Hastings PC, Dayer M, et al. A high prevalence of sleep disordered breathing in men with mild symptomatic chronic heart failure due to left ventricular systolic dysfunction. *Eur J Heart Failure.* 2007;9:243-50.
44. Oldenburg O, Lamp B, Faber L, et al. Sleep disordered breathing in symptomatic heart failure: a contemporary study of prevalence in and characteristics of 700 patients. *Eur J Heart Fail.* 2007;9:251-7.
45. MacDonald M, Fang J, Pittman SD, et al. The current prevalence of sleep disordered breathing in congestive heart failure in patients treated with beta-blockers. *J Clin Sleep Med.* 2008;4:38-42.
46. Wang H, Parker JD, Newton GE, et al. Effect of obstructive sleep apnea on mortality in patients with heart failure. *J Am Coll Cardiol.* 2007;49:1625-31.
47. Nakayama H, Smith CA, Rodman JR, et al. Effect of ventilatory drive on CO2 sensitivity below eupnea during sleep. *Am J Respir Crit Care Med.* 2002;165:1251-8.
48. White DP, Gleeson K, Pickett CK, et al. Altitude acclimatization influence on periodic breathing and chemo-responsiveness during sleep. *J Appl Physiol.* 1987;63:401-12.
49. Parra O, Arboix A, Bechich S, et al. Time course of sleep related breathing disorders in first-ever stroke or transient ischemic attack. *Am J Respir Crit care Med.* 2000;161:375-80.
50. Natchmann A, Siebler M, Rose G, et al. Cheyne Stokes respiration in ischemic stroke. *Neurology.* 1995;45:820-1.
51. Idiopathic congenital central hypoventilation syndrome. *Am J Respir Crit Care Med.* 1999;160:368-73.
52. Huang J, Marcus CL, Bandla P, et al. Cortical processing of respiratory occlusion stimuli in children with central hypoventilation syndrome. *Am J Respir Crit Care Med.* 2008;178:757-64.
53. White DP, Miller F, Erickson RW. Sleep apnea and nocturnal hypoventilation after western equine encephalitis. *Am Rev Respir Dis.* 1983;137:132-3.
54. Devereaux MW, Keane JR, Davis RL. Automatic respiratory failure associated with infarction of the medulla: report of two cases with pathologic study of one. *Arch Neurol.* 1973;29:46-52.
55. Levin BE, Margolis G. Acute failure of automatic respirations secondary to unilateral brainstem infarct. *Ann Neurol.* 1977;1:583-6.
56. Kraus J, Heckmann JG, Druschky A, et al. Ondine's curse in association with diabetes insipidus following transient vertebrobasilar ischemia. *Clin Neurol Neurosurg.* 1999;101:196-8.
57. Yglesias A, Narbona J, Vanaclocha V, et al. Chiari Type-1 malformation, glossopharyngeal neuralgia and central sleep apnea in a child. *Dev Med Child Neurol.* 1996;38:1126-30.
58. Manning HL, Leiter JC. Respiratory control and respiratory sensation in a patient with a ganglioglioma within the dorsocaudal brainstem. *Am J Respir Crit Care Med.* 2000;161:2100-6.
59. Schulz R, Fegbeutel C, Althoff A, et al. Central sleep apnea and unilateral diaphragmatic paralysis associated with vertebral artery compression of the medulla oblongata. *J Neurol.* 2003;250(4):503-5.
60. Cummiskey J, Guilleminault C, Davis R, et al. Automatic respiratory failure: sleep studies and Leigh's disease. *Neurology.* 1987;37:1876-8.
61. Teichtahl H, Prodromidis A, Miller B, et al. Sleep disordered breathing in stable methahdone programme patients: a pilot study. *Addiction.* 2001;96:395-403.
62. Webster LR, Choi Y, Desai H, et al. Sleep disordered breathing and chronic opioid thearpy. *Pain Med.* 2008;9:425-32.

63. Fareny RJ, Walker JM, Cloward RS. Sleep disordered breathing associated with long-term opioid therapy. *Chest.* 2003;123:632-9.
64. Walker M Farney RJ, Rhondeau SM, et al. Chronic opioid use a risk factor for the development of central sleep apnea and ataxic breathing. *J Clin Sleep Med.* 2007;3:455-61.
65. Wang D, Teichtahl H, Drummer O, et al. Central sleep apnea in stable methadone maintenance treatment patients. *Chest.* 2005;128:1348-56.
66. Mogri M, Desai H, Webster L, et al. Hypoxemia in patients on chronic opiate therapy with and without sleep apnea. *Sleep Breath.* 2009;13:49-57.
67. Teichtahl H, Wang D, Cunnington D, et al. Ventilatory responses to hypoxia and hypercapnia in stable methadone maintenance treatment patients. *Chest.* 2005;128:1339-47.
68. Grunstein RR, Ho KY, Sullivan CE. Effect of octreotide and somatostatin analog, on sleep apnea in patients with acromegaly. *Ann Intern Med.* 1994; 121:478-87.
69. Grunstein RR, Ho KY, Sullivan CE. Acromegaly and sleep apnea. *Ann Intern Med.* 1991;115;527-32.
70. Grunstein RR, Ho KY, Berthon-Jones M, et al. Central sleep apnea is associated with increased ventilatory response to carbon dioxide and hypersecretion of growth hormone in patients with acromegaly. *Am J Respir Crit Care Med.* 1994;150:496-502.
77. Javaheri S, Malik A, Smith J, et al. Adaptive pressure support ventilation: a novel treatment for sleep apnea associated with use of opioids. *J Clin Sleep Med.* 2008;4:305-10.
71. Endo Y, Suzuki M, Inoue Y, et al. Prevalence of complex sleep apnea amongst Japanese patients with sleep apnea syndrome. *Tohoku J Exp Med.* 2008;215:349-54.
72. Yaegashi H, Fujimoto K, Abe H, et al. Characteristics of Japanese patients with complex sleep apnea syndrome: a retrospective comparison with obstructive sleep apnea syndrome. *Intern Med.* 2009;48:427-32.
73. Farre R, Montserrat JM, Navajas D. Noninvasive monitoring of respiratory mechanics during sleep. *Eur Respir J.* 2004; 24:1052-60.
74. Boudewyns A, Willeman M, Wagemans M, et al. Assessment of respiratory effort by means of strain guage and esophageal pressure swings: A comparative study. *Sleep.* 1997;20:168-70.
75. Bradley T, Logan A, Kimoff R, et al. CANPAP Investigators. Continuous positive airway pressure for central sleep apnea in heart failure. *New Engl J Med.* 2005;353:2025-33.
76. Artz M, Floras J, Logan A, et al. The CANPAP Investigators. et al. Suppression of central sleep apnea by continuous positive airway pressure and transplant-free survival in heart failure: a post-hoc analysis of the Canadian positive airway pressure therapy of patients with central sleep apnea and heart failure trial (CANPAP). *Circulation.* 2007;115:3173-80.
78. Xie A, Skatrud J, Pulco D, et al. Influence of arterial O2 on the susceptibility to post hyperventilation apnea during sleep. *J Appl Physiol.* 2006;100:171-7.
79. Xie A, Rankin F, Rutherford R, et al. Effects of inhaled CO2 and added dead space on idiopathic central sleep apnea. *J Appl Physiol.* 1997;82:918-26.
80. Andreas S, Weidel K, Hagenah G, et al. Treatment of Cheyne-Stokes respiration with nasal oxygen and carbon dioxide. *Eur Respir J.* 1998; 12:414-9.
81. Mebrate Y, Willson K, Manisty CH, et al. Dynamic CO2 therapy in periodic breathing: a modeling study to determine optimal timing and dosage regimes. *J Appl Physiol.* 2009;107:696-706.
82. Joho S, Oda Y, Hirai T, et al. Impact of sleeping position on central sleep apnea/Cheyne Stokes respiration in patients with heart failure. *Sleep Med.* 2010;11:143-8.
83. Soll BA, Yeo KK, Davis JW, et al. The effect of posture on Cheyne-Stokes respirations and hemodynamics in patients with heart failure. *Sleep.* 2009;32:1499-506.
84. Ueno LM, Drager LF, Rodrigues AC, et al. Effects of exercise training in patients with chronic heart failure and sleep apnea. *Sleep.* 2009;32:637-47.
85. Randerath WJ, Galetke W, Kenter M, et al. Combined adaptive servo ventilation and automatic positive airway pressure (anti-cyclic modulated ventilation) in co-existing obstructive and central sleep apnea syndrome and periodic breathing. *Sleep Med.* 2009;10:898-903.
86. SERVE-HF. Treatment of sleep disordered breathing by adaptive servo-ventilation in HF patients. [online] Available from http:/www.servehf.com. [Accessed May 2014].
87. ADVENT-HF. Effect of Adaptive Servo Ventilation (ASV) on Survival and Hospital Admissions in Heart Failure. [online] Available from: http://www.clinicaltrials.gov/show/NCT 0112886. [Accessed May 2014].

CHAPTER 8

Obesity Hypoventilation Syndrome and Complex Sleep Apnea

Vivek Nangia, Shivani Swami

INTRODUCTION

Obesity hypoventilation syndrome (OHS), also known as Pickwickian syndrome,[1] was initially described in the Pickwick papers by Charles Dickens in 1867, in which the fat and red-faced boy Joe was consuming a lot of food and would fall asleep constantly in daytime. However, the first case report in the medical literature, appeared only in 1955, in which a patient with obesity, hypersomnolence and alveolar hypoventilation was described.[2] As the name suggests, it refers to an association between obesity and daytime chronic hypoventilation. With the ongoing global epidemic of extreme obesity, the prevalence of OHS is also on the rise. The syndrome arises from a complex interaction between sleep-disordered breathing (SDB), diminished respiratory drive, and obesity-related respiratory impairment, and is associated with significant morbidity and mortality.

DEFINITION AND PREVALENCE

Obesity hypoventilation syndrome is defined as obesity [body mass index (BMI) ≥ 30 kg/m^2] and chronic alveolar hypoventilation [arterial carbon dioxide tension (PaCO$_2$) >45 mmHg] during wakefulness, which occurs in the absence of other diseases that could account for awake hypoventilation, such as lung or neuromuscular disease (Table 1). Whether presence of obstructive sleep apnea

Table 1: Definition of obesity hypoventilation syndrome[7]	
Required conditions	**Description**
Obesity	BMI $\geq$30 kg/m^2
Chronic hypoventilation	Awake daytime hypereapnia (PaCO$_2$ $\geq$45 mmHg)
Sleep-disordered breathing	OSA (AHI $\geq$5 with or without sleep hypoventilation) present in 90% of cases; sleep hypoventilation (AHI <5) present in 10% of caes
Exclusion of other causes of hypercapnia	Severe obstructive airways disease; severe interstitial lung disease; severe chest wall disorders (e.g., kyphoscoliosis): severe hypothyroidism; neuromuscular disease; and congenital central hypoventilation syndrome

BMI, body mass index; OSA, obstructive sleep apnea; AHI, apnea-hypopnea index.

(OSA) is a part of the definition or not, is debatable. However, approximately 90% of patients with OHS also have SDB which consists of OSA.[3] Due to this association, the term *hypercapnic OSA* has been interchangeably used with OHS. In the remaining 10%, flow limitation causing obstructive hypoventilation, through to hypoventilation in all sleep stages is seen.[4]

The incidence of OHS increases significantly with the increase in obesity. The prevalence is reported to range from around 10–20% in outpatients presenting to sleep clinics[3] to almost 50% of hospitalized patients with a BMI greater than 50 kg/sqm.[5] Overall, 0.3–0.4% of the population may have OHS.[6] The prevalence of OHS tends to be higher in men with no clear racial or ethnic predominance. However, it may be reasonable to presume that it would be higher in the United States especially the African-Americans, amongst whom obesity is almost an epidemic. Nearly, 20% of OSA patients may have an associated OHS.[7]

PATHOPHYSIOLOGY

The important factors involved in the pathogenesis of OHS include increased work of breathing, respiratory muscle impairment, a depressed central ventilatory drive, and diminished effects of neurohumoral modulators (e.g., leptin) due to decreased levels or resistance, some degree of ventilation perfusion mismatch and sleep disordered breathing (Figure 1).

Work of breathing is increased by threefolds in patients with OHS as compared to eucapnic morbidly obese patients and non-obese control subjects. This occurs due to a greater than 50% reduction in chest wall compliance and a threefold increase in lung resistance. The increase in lung resistance results from closure of the small airways and the engorgement of pulmonary capillaries due to increased blood volume.[8] As a result, morbidly obese patients dedicate 15% of their oxygen consumption to the work of breathing compared to 3% in non-obese individuals.[9] While patients with OSA have an increased upper airway resistance only in supine position, patients with OHS have a higher upper airway resistance both in the sitting and supine position.[10] This also contributes to the increased work of breathing.

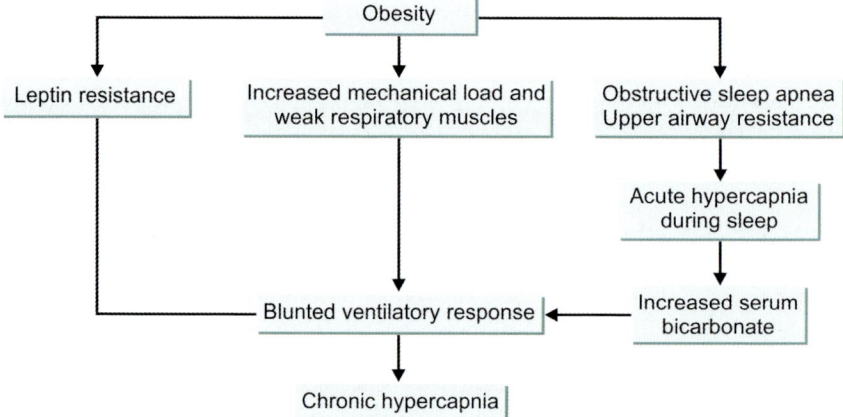

Figure 1: Potential pathphysiological mechanisms of obesity hypoventilation syndrome.[7]

Respiratory Muscle Function

A modest reduction in respiratory muscle strength and endurance occurs in OHS. The severity of OHS is directly proportional to this reduction. The maximal inspiratory and expiratory pressures are normal in eucapnic morbidly obese patients but are reduced in patients with OHS.[11] Whether diaphragmatic weakness has a role to play or not is still not clear.

Central Ventilatory Drive

The ability to increase the respiration in response to hypoxia and/or hypercapnea is diminished or blunted in patients with OHS while it is well maintained in obese individuals without OHS. Thus, implying that this may be an adaptation, rather than a primary defect.[12] The slope of the ventilatory response to hypercapnia is less than 1 L/min/mmHg in patients with obesity hypoventilation, 2 L/min/mmHg in eucapnic obese subjects, and 3 L/min/mmHg in healthy subjects. The response of the timing components in the breathing pattern to hypercapnia (i.e., duration of respiratory cycle, inspiratory time, and duty cycle ratio) is similar among the three subject groups.[13] The mechanisms proposed for this blunted response include obesity, genetic predisposition, SDB, and leptin resistance. In some patients, this response starts to improve within 2 weeks after the treatment for OHS is initiated and touches normal by the sixth week.[14]

Neurohumoral modulator (Leptin) is a circulating protein produced by the adipose tissue (adipokine) that interacts with hypothalamic receptors to inhibit eating. Experiments with the mice have shown that the mice deficient in leptin develop obesity and exhibit features of OHS like impaired respiratory mechanics, depressed ventilatory responsiveness and awake hypercapnea. The total lung capacity (TLC) and the lung compliance of these mice are half of that in wild-type mice. The proportion of the diaphragmatic myosin heavy chain type I is increased, and the proportion of the type II myosin chain is decreased, conferring resistance to fatigue. The long-term replacement of leptin in these mice prevents or attenuates these changes in the breathing pattern, lung mechanics, and myosin level.

Patients with OSA have high serum leptin levels that are mostly associated with obesity and are unrelated to OSA. In humans, deficiency of leptin is rare even in extremely obese individuals. In fact, in one study, the patients with OHS, the levels of leptin were seen to be higher than eucapnic subjects with OSA. If this leptin was biologically active then there would be reduced eating and subsequently weight loss. However, this does not happen, thus suggesting a state of "leptin resistance". Higher leptin levels are associated with both a reduced respiratory drive and a reduced response to hypercapnea in severely obese individuals. It also impacts the mechanical properties of lungs and the chest wall. Since, there is a state of leptin resistance; treatment with leptin does not help the patient.[15] In another study, patients with OHS without a concomitant OSA were reported to have lower leptin levels as compared to matched obese subjects without OSA. Serum leptin levels were seen to increase with effective therapy for OHS without significantly changing the BMI. This was also associated with improvement in chemosensitivity.[16]

Ventilation Perfusion (V/Q) Mismatching

A diminished lung compliance, difficulty in moving the ribcage and diaphragm, and premature closure of some alveoli prior to the end of expiration in obese individuals results in poor ventilation of the lower lobes of their lungs. On the other hand there is an increased blood flow to the lower lobes thus resulting in a state of V/Q mismatching and hypoxemia in obese patients.[8]

Sleep-Disordered Breathing

Obstructive sleep apnea is one of the major contributors to the pathogenesis of OHS. This is evident by the fact that treatment of OSA [with either positive airway pressure (PAP) therapy or tracheostomy] eliminates OHS in many patients[17] and that OSA is present in 85–92% patients who have OHS.[18]

The main patterns of sleep disordered breathing seen in patients with OHS include obstructive apneas and hypopneas as well as obstructive and central hypoventilation. Such patients would usually have a lower baseline oxygen saturation. In them, even with apnea-hypopnea index (AHI) of less than 5, minute ventilation reduces by 25% during non-rapid eye movement (NREM) sleep and by 40% during rapid eye movement (REM) sleep. As a result, with each apnea and hypopnea, there is slight rise in $PaCO_2$, which a patient of OHS is unable to normalize. In order to maintain the pH, kidneys reduce the bicarbonate excretion, resulting in an increase in bicarbonate levels, which then results in blunting of the ventilatory response to rising pCO_2 levels. This vicious cycle of rising pCO_2, compensatory rise in bicarbonate levels to maintain the pH and a suppressed ventilator response result in daytime hypercarbia, which is a hallmark feature of OHS.[7]

CLINICAL FEATURES

Obesity hypoventilation syndrome usually occurs in the extremely obese male patients (twice more common than females), in their middle ages.[7] The patients characteristically present with two groups of symptoms: (1) those attributable to OSA and (2) those to chronic hypoxia. Fatigue, morning headaches, excessive daytime sleepiness, loud habitual snoring and nocturnal choking episodes, and cognitive difficulties are the common complaints which are similar to those seen in patients with OSA. Patients suffering from chronic hypoxia present with peripheral edema, secondary pulmonary hypertension and polycythemia. Dyspnea and lower oxygen saturation measured by pulse oximetry are distinguishing features which are present more often in OHS than in OSA patients. Some patients may present with acute decompensation characterized by severe hypoxia, uncompensated hypercarbia, corpulmonale, massive edema and altered mental status. Hypertension, heart failure, type II diabetes mellitus, and asthma are the common comorbidities.

DIAGNOSIS

Arterial Blood Gases

A typical awake state arterial blood gas report will show presence of hypercapnia ($PaCO_2$ > 45 mmHg), hypoxemia (PaO_2 < 70 mmHg) with elevated bicarbonate

Obesity Hypoventilation Syndrome and Complex Sleep Apnea

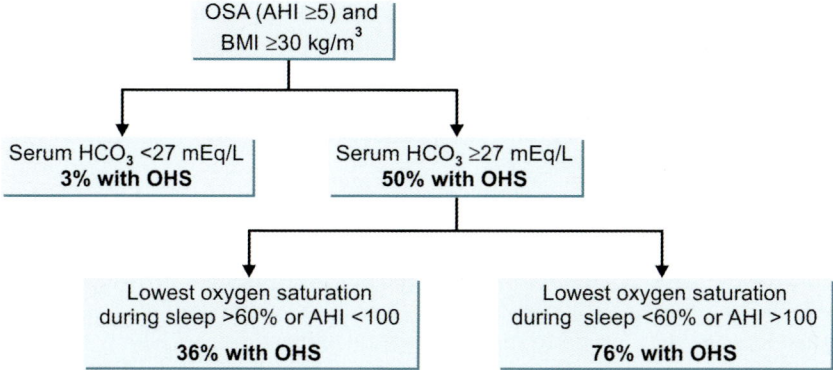

OSA, obstructive sleep apnea; AHI, apnea-hypopnea index; BMI, body mass index; OHS, obesity hypoventilation syndrome.

Figure 2: Clinical prediction of obesity hypoventilation syndrome based on serum bicarbonate and severity of obstructive sleep apnea.[37]

levels ($HCO_3 > 27$ meq/L). Serum bicarbonate levels along with severity of OSA have been used as clinical predictors of OHS in patients with morbid obesity and OSA (Figure 2). Elevated hematocrit may be present and indicate a state of chronic hypoxia[7].

Pulmonary Function Tests

A pulmonary function tests (PFT) is performed primarily to rule out the presence of obstructive lung disease. OHS patients will have a PFT that is characteristic of obesity. A low forced vital capacity (FVC), a low forced expiratory volume in one second (FEV_1), a normal FEV_1/FVC ratio, and a low expiratory reserve volume (ERV) with diminished TLC in some patients are the characteristic features.[19]

Chest Radiograph

It would usually show small volume lungs with both diaphragms elevated due to obese abdomen. The cardiac shadow may be enlarged due to right ventricular hypertrophy and in late stages may show evidence of congestive heart failure.

Cardiac Studies

The ECG and echocardiogram may show right heart strain, right atrial and right ventricular hypertrophy, while the cardiac catheterization frequently reveals pulmonary hypertension.[20]

Polysomnography

An overnight polysomnography will be essential in making the diagnosis of OHS. Most patients will have an abnormal number of apneas and hypopneas per hour of sleep (i.e., a high AHI) due to coexisting OSA. They usually have a more profound oxyhemoglobin desaturation during sleep than patients with OSA alone. Transcutaneous monitoring of CO_2 is of value in documenting the degree to which CO_2 is retained especially during REM sleep. An increase in pCO_2 by 10 mmHg or an oxygen desaturation not explained by apnea or hypopnea, are often seen on polysomnography. Although, nocturnal transcutaneous monitoring of CO_2 is a useful technique in detecting prodromal OHS in obese patients, yet, clinical trials have not shown any benefit of it, neither in the diagnosis nor management of such patients.[15]

Specific Tests

Serum electrolytes (including magnesium and phosphorus), thyroid functions, computerized tomography of thorax with pulmonary angiography or ventilation-perfusion scan may be performed to exclude other diseases which can cause alveolar hypoventilation. These diseases include hypothyroidism, diaphragmatic paralysis, chronic obstructive pulmonary disease (COPD), restrictive diseases (e.g., neuromuscular weakness, interstitial lung disease, chest wall disease), and chronic pulmonary embolism.

TREATMENT

The goals of treatment for a patient of OHS include normalization of $PaCO_2$ during wakefulness and sleep, relief of hypersomnia and altered mentation, and prevention of complications like polycythemia and pulmonary hypertension. The three chief modalities of treatment are weight loss, PAP therapy, and to some extent pharmacotherapy. Oxygen supplementation may be required in a substantial number while tracheostomy may be considered in refractory or life threatening situations.

Positive Airway Pressure Therapy

The first line of treatment for OHS is nocturnal noninvasive PAP device. It should be offered to all irrespective of whether there is a coexistent OSA or not and should not be delayed while the patient is trying to lose weight. Two types of devices can be used: bilevel positive airway pressure (BPAP) or continuous positive airway pressure (CPAP). The choice of the most optimal device remains uncertain, however, given that majority of the patients of OHS have a concomitant OSA, use of CPAP device seems to be reasonable[21] while patients with purely OHS are managed best with BPAP. There are no long-term follow-up studies to establish whether outcomes of CPAP would be different from those with BPAP. Also, that a patient initiated on CPAP can be switched to BPAP if oxygen desaturation persists below 90% despite resolution of apneas, hypopneas, and flow limitation while those initiated on BPAP can be switched over to CPAP once hypercarbia is corrected. BPAP does have certain advantages. It provides active ventilation rather than just splinting of the upper airways, provides rest to the respiratory muscles, achieves a lower mean airway pressure which is more comfortable to the patient, and helps correct the hypercarbia faster.

Consistent use of PAP therapy as defined by the duration of daily use, irrespective of the mode used (BPAP or CPAP), results in decline in nocturnal as well as daytime hypercarbia and daytime sleepiness.[22] $PaCO_2$ decreases by 1.8 mmHg and PaO_2 increases by 3 mmHg per hour of daily use. Patients who use it for longer than 4.5 hours per night, experience an even better restoration of $PaCO_2$ and PaO_2 levels.[23] It also improves quality of life.

In an acutely ill patient presenting with acute hypercarbic respiratory failure, BPAP is the modality of choice with volume cycle positive pressure ventilation (VCPPV) reserved for those who fail to improve. Average volume-assured pressure support (AVAPS) is a hybrid mode, with features of standard BPAP and VCPPV, and is reasonable alternative to BPAP when rapid correction of hypercarbia is needed.

The pressures in CPAP are titrated in the conventional manner, upwards till all episodes of apneas, hypopneas, flow limitation are eliminated and oxygen saturation stabilized. During the titration of BPAP pressures, expiratory positive airway pressure (EPAP) is adjusted to eliminate the obstructive events while inspiratory positive airway pressure (IPAP) is increased over EPAP to improve alveolar hypoventilation. A minimum of 4 cm H_2O gap is mandatory to be kept between the EPAP and the IPAP.

Supplemental Oxygen

Almost 20–50% patients may require supplemental nocturnal oxygen in addition to PAP therapy while a small proportion may require it during the day too. However, in most patients, both daytime and nocturnal oxygen supplementation can be withdrawn over a period of months if the patient is adherent with PAP therapy.[23]

Weight Loss

Initial studies have shown that loss of weight whether by lifestyle modification or surgically is associated with better lung functions, central respiratory drive, and daytime hypercarbia.[24] A reduction in BMI from 56 kg/m² to 36 kg/m² has been shown to result in a drop in AHI from 72 to 19.[25] Thus reflecting that even after significant weight loss, the SDB only improves but is not fully cured. Bariatric surgery, especially the Roux-en-Y procedure is the most effective approach to achieving a substantial weight loss.[26] In order to reduce the perioperative morbidity and mortality, it is believed that PAP therapy must be provided in the pre-operative period and then again in the immediate postoperative period without any fears of an anastamotic leakage or disruption.[27]

Tracheostomy

This is rarely necessary and indicated only for patients with life-threatening complications or those totally intolerant to PAP therapy. It helps in overcoming the upper airway obstruction during sleep but the daytime hypoventilation may persist.[28] Continued sleep disordered breathing after tracheotomy may be attributed to obstruction of the tracheotomy stoma by fatty tissue[29] or the appearance of central apneic events.

Pharmacotherapy

Amongst the various respiratory stimulants, while Theophylline has not been studied for this purpose, acetazolamide and medroxyprogesterone[30] and acetazolamide[31] have been shown to improve awake hypercarbia and hypoxemia.

However, neither of them impact the SDB and thus are considered a therapy of last resort for patients with persistent hypercarbia despite PAP therapy.

MORBIDITY AND MORTALITY

Obesity hypoventilation syndrome is associated with a significantly poorer quality of life, higher healthcare expenses and a greater risk of pulmonary hypertension as compared to patients with OSA alone.[32] Such patients have a higher rate of ICU admission (6% vs. 40%) and a greater need for mechanical ventilation (0% vs. 6%) when compared to patients with eucapnic obesity.[33]

Mortality is also significantly higher in patients with OHS as compared to eucapnic obese individuals with similar degree of obesity (23% vs. 9%).[33] It is even higher in patients who refuse treatment. According to a small, retrospective study, 46% patients who refused long-term PAP therapy died during an average 50 months follow-up period[34] while those complying with treatment have been reported to have a 2-year and 4-year mortality rate of less than 10%.[35] Another large prospective study of patients complying with treatment has reported 1-, 2-, 3-, and 5-year survival rates of 98%, 93%, 88%, and 77%, respectively.

CONCLUSION

Obesity hypoventilation syndrome, a state of chronic daytime hypoventilation associated with obesity, despite being associated with a high morbidity and mortality, is grossly under-recognized. It has a complex pathophysiological mechanism resulting in symptoms similar to those of OSA and chronic hypoxia. An individual with SDB and BMI more than or equal to 30 kg/m^2 with serum bicarbonates more than or equal to 27 mEq/L must be evaluated further with a polysomnography. PAP therapy is the first line therapy and if combined with weight loss significantly impacts the survival rates.

COMPLEX SLEEP APNEA

INTRODUCTION

Complex sleep apnea (CSA), also called "treatment-emergent central sleep apnea", refers to the emergence or increase of central apneas and hypopneas, in a patient of OSA during the application of continuous positive airway pressure (CPAP) therapy or BPAP without a backup respiratory rate.[38-42] The term was coined only, as late as 2006 even though the pattern has been described in the past. Some authors have held the opinion that it is not a distinct entity but instead, comprises a vaguely defined group of entities with varying etiologies.[42] These are generally innocuous and self-limiting.

Epidemiology and Natural History

Complex sleep apnea may be detected in up to 18% of patients of OSA who undergo positive airway pressure therapy.[39,41,43-46] More often than not, these apneas are transitory and resolve spontaneously by 8 weeks of PAP therapy.[47] For some reason, it is more common in males. Forty to fifty percent of patients with systolic heart failure with periodic breathing and CSA have CPAP-resistant

CSA.[48] Patients with severe OSA, patients with both obstructive and central apneic events during initial polysomnography are more likely to develop CSA after application of CPAP.[49-52] Other factors commonly associated are NREM sleep, high altitude, oral breathing, opioid narcotics, and supine position sleep.[41,46,47,53-55]

PATHOGENESIS

Use of PAP therapy in patients of OSA invariably results in the elimination of disordered breathing (i.e., obstructive apneas and hypopneas). However, in some patients, central apneas emerge after the initiation of PAP therapy. The mechanism behind it, however, remains elusive.[56] Several hypothesis have emerged, in this respect:
1. Changes in the CO_2 excretion with the relief of upper airway obstruction, on using the PAP therapy. If these changes yield a value below the CO_2 apnea threshold, it could explain the occurrence of central apneas. The CO_2 apnea threshold may change over weeks hence, the central apneas may resolve.[57,58]
2. Overtitration with CPAP is thought to also lead to central apneas, even though the mechanism remains unexplained. Inhibition of central respiratory drive due to the activation of lung stretch receptors, may be responsible.[47]
3. Once CPAP therapy is initiated, it may initially lead to increased sleep disturbances, and the repeated transitions from sleep to wake to sleep, may contribute to central apneas.[59]

Clinical Presentation

Patients of OSA using CPAP may either remain asymptomatic or may present with persisting excessive daytime sleepiness, poor sleep quality, frequent arousals, fatigue, morning headaches, poor concentration. These symptoms may persist due to disrupted sleep, even though snoring may be absent. Diagnosis can only be made on titration polysomnography. On application of PAP therapy, the following criteria must be met.[60]
- Apnea hypopnea index more than or equal to 5 events per hour
- Central apneas and hypopneas, more than 50% of the AHI
- Central AHI more than or equal to 5
- Symptoms of disturbed sleep or excessive daytime sleepiness.

The following conditions will need to be excluded before reaching a diagnosis of CSA:[47]
- Inadequate titration, overtitration, substantial mask leak, residual sleepiness on CPAP, change in CPAP requirements due to gain in body weight, sleep transition apneas upon CPAP initiation, narcotic induced central apneas, and other causes of sleepiness

TREATMENT

Treatment options include switching to adaptive servoventilation (ASV) or BPAP with a back up rate or continue CPAP therapy.

Adaptive servoventilation provides a varying amount of inspiratory pressure over a low level of continuous pressure, along with a backup rate.[61-64] The changes in peak flow determine the inspiratory pressure provided. Hence, when the peak flow is lower than average, it induces an increased inspiratory pressure and *vice versa*. The backup rate can either be manually or automatically set.[65,66] It can be used to treat not only CSA, but also CSA associated with Cheyne-Stokes respiration and central sleep apneas.[65]

In more than half the patients, CSA may disappear with continued use of CPAP only thus simply continuing the use of CPAP is a reasonable option.[41]

CONCLUSION

Patients of OSA, who continue to be symptomatic despite PAP therapy, must be evaluated for CSA. An overnight polysomnography with on going PAP device will yield the diagnosis. CSA may disappear on its own with continued use of CPAP or may require a switch to ASV or BPAP with a backup respiratory rate.

REFERENCES

1. Bickelmann AG, Burwell CS, Robin ED, et al. Extreme obesity associated with alveolar hypoventilation; a Pickwickian syndrome. *Am J Med.* 1956;21:811.
2. Auchincloss JH Jr, Cook E, Renzetti AD. Clinical and physiological aspects of a case of obesity, polycythemia and alveolar hypoventilation. *J Clin Invest.* 1955;34:1537-45.
3. Mokhlesi, B, Tulaimat, A, Faibussowitsch, I, et al Obesity hypoventilation syndrome: prevalence and predictors in patients with obstructive sleep apnea. *Sleep Breath.* 2007;11:117-24.
4. Berger KI, Ayappa I, Chatr-Amontri B, et al. Obesity hypoventilation syndrome as a spectrum of respiratory disturbances during sleep. *Chest.* 2001;120:1231-8.
5. Nowbar S, Burkart KM, Gonzales R, et al. Obesity-associated hypoventilation in hospitalized patients: prevalence, effects, and outcome. *Am J Med.* 2004;116:1-7.
6. Kaw R, Hernandez AV, Walker E, et al. Determinants of hypercapnia in obese patients with obstructive sleep apnea: a systematic review and metaanalysis of cohort studies. *Chest.* 2009;136:787-96.
7. Mokhlesi, B, Tulaimat A. Recent advances in Obesity Hypoventilation syndrome. *CHEST.* 2007;132:1322-36
8. Rochester DF, Arora NS. Respiratory failure from obesity. In: Medical Complications of obesity, Mancini M, Lewis B, Contaldo F, editors. Academic Press; London: 1980. p. 183.
9. Lopata M, Onal E. Mass loading, sleep apnea, and the pathogenesis of obesity hypoventilation. *Am Rev Respir Dis.* 1982;126:640-5.
10. Lin CC, Wu KM, Chou CS, et al. Oral airway resistance during wakefulness in eucapnic and hypercapnic sleep apnea syndrome. *Respir Physiol Neurobiol.* 2004;139:215-24.
11. Kelly TM, Jensen RL, Elliott CG, et al Maximum respiratory pressures in morbidly obese subjects. *Respiration.* 1988;54:73-7.
12. Zwillich CW, Sutton FD, Pierson DJ, et al. Decreased hypoxic ventilatory drive in the obesity-hypoventilation syndrome. *Am J Med.* 1975;59:343.
13. Sampson MG, Grassino K. Neuromechanical properties in obese patients during carbon dioxide rebreathing. *Am J Med.* 1983;75:81-90.
14. Han F, Chen E, Wei H, et al. Treatment effects on carbon dioxide retention in patients with obstructive sleep apnea-hypopnea syndrome. *Chest.* 2001;119:1814-9.
15. Piper AJ, Grunstein RR. Obesity Hypoventilation syndrome. *Am J Respircrit Care Med.* 2011;183:292-8.
16. Redolfi S, Corda L, La Piana G, et al. Long-term non-invasive ventilation increases chemosensitivity and leptin in obesity-hypoventilation syndrome. *Respir Med.* 2007;101:1191-5.
17. Chaouat A, Weitzenblum E, Krieger J, et al. Association of chronic obstructive pulmonary disease and sleep apnea syndrome. *Am J Respir Crit Care Med.* 1995;151:82-6.

18. Bednarek M, Plywaczewski R, Jonczak L, et al. There is no relationship between chronic obstructive pulmonary disease and obstructive sleep apnea syndrome: a population study. *Respiration*. 2005;72:142-9.
19. Heinemann F, Budweiser S, Dobroschke J, et al. Non-invasive positive pressure ventilation improves lung volumes in the obesity hypoventilation syndrome. *Respir Med*. 2007;101:1229.
20. Kessler R, Chaouat A, Schinkewitch P, et al. The obesity-hypoventilation syndrome revisited: a prospective study of 34 consecutive cases. *Chest*. 2001;120:369.
21. Rapoport DM, Sorkin B, Garay SM, et al. Reversal of the "Pickwickian syndrome" by long-term use of nocturnal nasal-airway pressure. *N Engl J Med*. 1982;307:931-3.
22. Waldhorn RE. Nocturnal nasal intermittent positive pressure ventilation with bi-level positive airway pressure (BiPAP) in respiratory failure. *Chest*. 1992;101:516.
23. Mokhlesi B, Tulaimat A, Evans AT, et al. Impact of adherence with positive airway pressure therapy on hypercapnia in obstructive sleep apnea. *J Clin Sleep Med*. 2006;2:57-62.
24. Rochester DF, Enson Y. Current concepts in the pathogenesis of the obesity-hypoventilation syndrome. Mechanical and circulatory factors. *Am J Med*. 1974;57:402-20.
25. Verse T. Bariatric surgery for obstructive sleep apnea. *Chest*. 2005;128:485-7.
26. Foster GD Principles and practices in the management of obesity. *Am J RespirCrit Care Med*. 2003;168:274-80.
27. Ebeo CT, Benotti PN, Byrd RP Jr, et al. The effect of bi-level positive airway pressure on postoperative pulmonary function following gastric surgery for obesity. *Respir Med*. 2002;96:672-6.
28. Rapoport DM, Garay SM, Epstein H, et al. Hypercapnia in the obstructive sleep apnea syndrome. A reevaluation of the "Pickwickian syndrome". *Chest*. 1986;89:627-35.
29. El Solh AA, Jaafar W. A comparative study of the complications of surgical tracheostomy in morbidly obese critically ill patients. *Crit Care*. 2007;11:R3.
30. Lyons HA, Huang CT. Therapeutic use of progesterone in alveolar hypoventilation associated with obesity. *Am J Med*. 1968;44:881.
31. Rapoport DM, Garay SM, Epstein H, et al. Hypercapnia in the obstructive sleep apnea syndrome. A reevaluation of the "Pickwickian syndrome". *Chest*. 1986;89:627.
32. Hida W, Okabe S, Tatsumi K, et al Nasal continuous positive airway pressure improves quality of life in obesity hypoventilation syndrome. *Sleep Breath*. 2003;7:3-12.
33. Nowbar S, Burkart KM, Gonzales R, et al. Obesity-associated hypoventilation in hospitalized patients: prevalence, effects, and outcome. *Am J Med*. 2004;116:1-7.
34. Perez de Llano LA, Golpe R, Ortiz Piquer M, et al. Short-term and long-term effects of nasal intermittent positive pressure ventilation in patients with obesity-hypoventilation syndrome. *Chest*. 2005;128:587-94.
35. Heinemann F, Budweiser S, Dobroschke J, et al Non-invasive positive pressure ventilation improves lung volumes in the obesity hypoventilation syndrome. *Respir Med*. 2007;101:1229-35.
36. Priou P, Hamel JF, Person C, et al. Long-term outcome of noninvasive positive pressure ventilation for obesity hypoventilation syndrome. *Chest*. 2010;138:84.
37. Mokhlesi B. Obesity Hypoventilation Syndrome: A State-of-the-Art Review. *Respir Care*. 2010;55(10):1347-62.
38. Gay PC. Complex sleep apnea: it really is a disease. *J Clin Sleep Med*. 2008;4:403.
39. Morgenthaler TI, Kagramanov V, Hanak V, et al: Complex sleep apnea syndrome: is it a unique clinical syndrome? *Sleep*. 2006;29:1203-9.
40. Malhotra A, Bertisch A, Wellman A. complex Sleep Apnea: it is a disease. *J Clin Sleep Med*. 2008;4:406
41. Javaheri S, Smith J, Chung E, et al. The prevalence and natural history of complex sleep apnea. *J Clin Sleep Med*. 2009;5:205-11.
42. Gilmartin GS, Daly RW, Thomas RJ, et al. Recognition and management of complex sleep disordered breathing. *Curr Opin Pulm Med*. 2005;11:485-93.
43. Marrone O, Stallone A, Salvaggio A, et al. Occurrence of breathing disorders during CPAP administration in obstructive sleep apnea syndrome. *Eur Respir J*. 1991;4:660-6.

44. Lehman S, Antic NA, Thompson C, et al. Central sleep apnea on commencement of continuous positive airway pressure in patients with a primary diagnosis of obstructive sleep apnea-hypopnea. *J Clin Sleep Med.* 2007;3:462-6.
45. Westhoff M, Arzt M, Litterst P. Prevalence and treatment of central sleep apnea emerging after initiation of continuous positive airway pressure in patients with obstructive sleep apnea without evidence of heart failure. *Sleep Breath.* 2012;16:71-8.
46. Younes M1, Ostrowski M, Thompson W, et al. Chemical control stability in patients with obstructive sleep apnea. *Am J Respir Crit Care Med.* 2001;163:1181-90.
47. Malhotra A1, Bertisch S, Wellman A. Complex Sleep Apnea: It Isn't Really a disease. *J Clin Sleep Med.* 2008;4:406-8.
48. Javaheri S. Effects of continuous positive airway pressure on sleep apnea and ventricular irritability in patients with heart failure. *Circulation.* 2000;101:392-7.
49. Morgenthaler TI1, Kagramanov V, Hanak V, et al. Complex sleep apnea syndrome: is it aunique clinical syndrome? *Sleep.* 2006;29:1203-9.
50. Lehman S, Antic NA, Thompson C, et al. Central Sleep Apnea on commencement of continuous positive airway pressure in patients with a primary diagnosis of obstructive sleep apnea-hypopnea. *J Clin Sleep Med.* 2007;3:462-6.
51. Younes M, Ostrowski M, Thompson W, et al. Chemical control stability in patients with obstructive sleep apnea. *Am J Respir Crit Care Med.* 2001;163:1181-90.
52. Thomas RJ, Terzano MG, Parrino L, et al. Obstructive sleep disordered breathing with a dominant cyclic alternating pattern- a recognizable polysomnographic variant with practical clinical implications. *Sleep.* 2004;27:229-34.
53. Allam JS, Olson EJ, Gay PC, et al. Efficacy of adaptive servoventilation in treatment of complex and central sleep apnea syndromes. *Chest.* 2007;132:1839-46.
54. Nussbaumer-Ochsner Y, Schuepfer N, Ulrich S, et al. Exacerbation of sleep apnea by frequent central events in patients with obstructive sleep apnea syndrome at altitude: a randomized trial. *Thorax.* 2010;65:429-35.
55. Ambrogio C, Lowman X, Kuo M, et al. Sleep and non invasive ventilation in patients with chronic respiratory insufficiency. *Intensive Care Med.* 2009;35:306-13.
56. Eckert DJ, Jordan AS, Merchia P, et al. Central Sleep Apnea: pathophysiology and treatment. *Chest.* 2007;131:595-607.
57. Skatrud JB, Dempsey JA, Badr S, et al. Effect of airway impedance on CO2 retention and respiratory muscle activity during NREM sleep. *J Appl Physio.* 1988;65:1676-85.
58. Dempsey JA. Crossing the apneic threshold: causes and consequences. *Exp Physiol.* 2005;90:13-24.
59. Jordan AS, McEvoy RD, Edwards JK, et al. The influence of gender and upper airway resistance on the ventilator response to arousal in obstructive sleep apnea in humans. *J Physiol.* 2004;558:993-1004.
60. Local Coverage Determination for Respiratory Assist Devices. Available from: https://www.noridianmedicare.com/dme/coverage/docs/lcds/current_lcds/respiratory_assist_devices.htm.
61. Morgenthaler TI, Gay PC, Gordon N, et al. Adaptive servo ventilation versus noninvasive positive airway pressure ventilation for central, mixed and complex sleep apnea syndromes. *Sleep.* 2007;30:468-75.
62. Teschler H, Döhring J, Wang YM, et al. Adaptive pressure support servo ventilation: a novel treatment for Cheyne Stokes respiration in heart failure. *Am J Respir Crit Care Med.* 2001;164:614-9.
63. Arzt M, Wensel R, Montalvan S, et al. Effects of dynamic bilevel positive airway pressure support on central sleep apnea in men with heart failure. *Chest.* 2008;134:61
64. Pepperell JC, , Maskell NA, Jones DR, et al. A randomized controlled trial of adaptive ventilation for Cheyne Stokes breathing in heart failure. *Am J Respir Crit Care Med.* 2003;168:1109-14.
65. Antonescu-Turcu A, Parthasarathy S. CPAP and bilevel PAP therapy: New and established roles. *Respir Care.* 2010;55:1216.
66. Javaheri S, Goetting MG, Khayat R, et al: The performance of two automatic servo ventilation devices in the treatment of central sleep apnea. *Sleep.* 2011;34:1693-8.

CHAPTER 9

Cardiac Effects of Sleep Related Breathing Disorders

Manish Bansal, Kapil D Mohindra

INTRODUCTION

For long, sleep related breathing disorders (SRBDs) have largely been overlooked by the health care providers, disregarded often as merely a form of habitual snoring or excessive daytime sleepiness. However, over the past couple of decades, there has been a growing recognition of their significance as an important health problem and as a source of considerable morbidity and mortality.

Sleep related breathing disorders are not isolated disorders of sleep or breathing but are characterized by multisystem disturbances. Involvement of the cardiovascular (CV) system is amongst the most common and the most serious complications of SRBDs. Many epidemiologic and clinical studies, conducted in cross-sectional and longitudinal pattern, have shown that SRBDs increase the relative risk and progression of CV disease, and both these diseases tend to coexist as comorbid conditions. Prevalence of hypertension (HTN), diabetes mellitus (DM), coronary artery disease (CAD), heart failure (HF), and stroke have all been shown to be higher in patients with SRBDs.[1-11] Furthermore, amelioration of many of the adverse CV effects by correction of the underlying breathing disorder, through either weight reduction or continuous positive airway pressure (CPAP), provides further evidence linking these two entities.

CARDIOVASCULAR INVOLVEMENT IN OBSTRUCTIVE SLEEP APNEA

Pathophysiology

Obstructive sleep apnea (OSA) is characterized by disordered breathing resulting from partial or complete obstruction of the airway during sleep leading to hypopneic or apneic spells. The resultant intermittent nocturnal hypoxia and CO_2 retention initiate a cascade of pathophysiological mechanisms involving activation of autonomic, neurohormonal and metabolic pathways which, in turn, lead to endothelial dysfunction, inflammation, increased oxidative stress and metabolic dysregulation. These pathophysiological events eventually lead to the development of CV diseases such as HTN, CAD, HF, and arrhythmias (Figure 1).

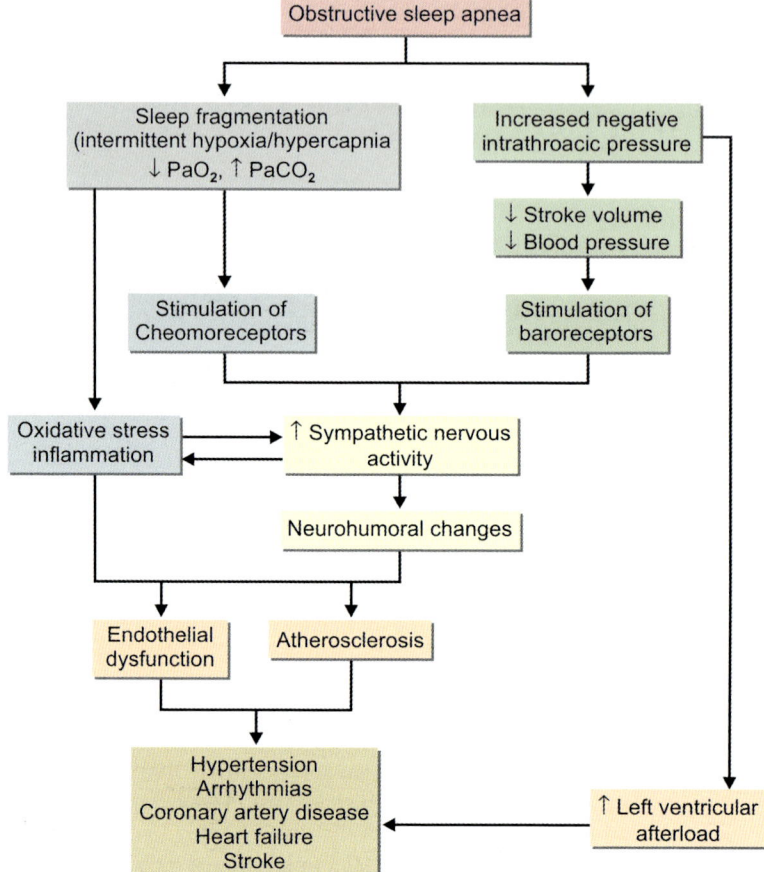

Figure 1: Pathophysiology of cardiovascular effects in obstructive sleep apnea.

Mechanical Effects

In patients with OSA, high intrathoracic pressure against the occluded upper airway results in increased left ventricular (LV) transmural pressure, and thus, the LV afterload. At the same time, right ventricle (RV) preload is also increased due to augmented venous return in response to increased negative intrathoracic pressure. As a consequence, the interventricular septum gets displaced towards left side during diastole, impeding LV filling.[12] The combined effect of increased LV afterload and reduced LV preload results in lower stroke volume and cardiac output.[13,14] In addition, intermittent hypoxia and increased LV afterload may also induce oxygen supply-demand mismatch which may provoke myocardial ischemia, impair myocardial contractility, and precipitate diastolic dysfunction.[15,16]

Autonomic Effects

In patients with OSA, in response to intermittent hypoxia and CO_2 retention, peripheral and central chemoreceptors are stimulated, inducing high level of tonic sympathetic activation.[17,18] Apneic spells, by eliminating reflex sympathetic inhibition arising from pulmonary stretch receptors, further augment sympathetic nervous activity (SNA).[18] At the same time, reduced vagal activity during arousal also increases SNA, resulting in postapneic surges in blood pressure (BP) and heart rate.[19]

Sympathetic tone is shown to be high in patients with OSA during wakefulness, and it further increases during sleep. As compared to the controls, the patients with OSA have a higher baseline heart rate, reduced heart rate variability and increased BP variability, all manifestations of increased SNA. Numerous studies have shown these abnormalities to be associated with an increased risk of development of future HTN and of target organ damage.[20-23]

Inflammation and Oxidative Stress

Intermittent hypoxia lowers arterial oxygen tension which serves as a stimulus for polymorph activation. Once activated, these polymorphs release highly reactive oxygen species that lead to endothelial damage and atherogenesis through the release of inflammatory markers such as tumor necrosis factor-α, interlukein-6, interlukein-8, C-reactive protein, adhesion molecules, etc. These inflammatory markers not only cause direct endothelial injury but also suppress production of nitric oxide by inhibiting nitric oxide synthase.[24-26] Several studies have demonstrated increased levels of inflammatory markers in patients with OSA, which fall with CPAP therapy.[27-30]

Endothelial Dysfunction

Endothelial dysfunction is common in patients with OSA and, being an early marker of atherogenesis, may be present even in absence of overt CVD.[31,32] As discussed above, hypoxia, increased SNA and oxidative stress induce release of inflammatory markers and vasoactive substances such as endothelin,[33] whereas the synthesis of nitric oxide is suppressed.[34,35] Altogether, these abnormalities result in endothelial dysfunction. Endothelin levels have been shown to be increased in untreated patients with OSA and fall with adequate therapy with CPAP.[36]

Thrombosis

Increased nocturnal SNA in response to hypoxia results in elevated catecholamine levels, which results in augmented platelet activity and other potential markers of thrombosis.[37,38] Several other factors such as fibrinogen, hematocrit, etc. have also been found to be elevated in patients with OSA.[29,39,40]

Burden of Cardiovascular Disease in Patients with Obstructive Sleep Apnea

Numerous studies have shown increased prevalence of a wide range of CV disorders in patients with OSA. The risk may be higher in relatively young subjects (<50 years of age) in whom OSA may have a more serious CV effect.[41] Previous studies have shown that there is higher prevalence of HTN[42] and atrial fibrillation (AF)[43] and greater risk of mortality[44] in young subjects with OSA.

Several persuasive data now suggest an association independent of obesity, between OSA and CV disorders such as HTN, CAD, HF, and arrhythmias. For example, in the Sleep Heart Health Study (SHHS), several CV outcomes including myocardial infarction and stroke were found to be associated with sleep disordered breathing.[7] However, establishing a definite causal role of OSA has remained difficult because of the presence of multiple confounding factors and also because most of these conditions are chronic in nature, have long latent periods, and are multifactorial in origin.

Hypertension

Hypertension is among the most prevalent CV disorders in patients with OSA and is an important risk factor for the development of CAD, HF, and stroke.[11] Almost half of all patients with OSA have HTN.[45] The converse is also true with as many as 30% of all hypertensives having OSA, though OSA often remains undiagnosed in these patients.[46-49] Wisconsin Sleep Cohort study suggested OSA to be an independent risk factor for HTN by showing dose-dependent relationship between OSA and HTN. The association was independent of age, sex, body mass index (BMI), smoking and antihypertensive medications.[11] Similarly, a strong association between OSA and HTN was shown in patients less than 65 years of age in SHHS study also.[8] The prevalence of OSA in patients with drug-resistant HTN is even higher and is reported to be in excess of 80%.[50] Increased aldosterone levels have been postulated as one of the mechanisms responsible for resistant HTN in patients with OSA.[51-53] Reduction in BP with CPAP therapy further supports causative role of OSA in HTN.[54] In view of these observations, the Joint National Committee guidelines on evaluation and management of HTN listed OSA as one of the few identifiable causes of secondary HTN.[55] In fact, a large percentage of patients who are classified as "essential HTN" may actually be having undiagnosed and untreated OSA leading to secondary HTN.

An important feature of HTN in OSA is the absence of normal nocturnal fall in BP and heart rate.[56] This "nondipping" pattern of BP is associated with increased risk of development of LV hypertrophy and HF[57] and is a cause of increased CV morbidity and mortality.[58]

Arrhythmias

A wide range of arrhythmias are common in patients with OSA, including AF, ventricular ectopics, nonsustained ventricular tachycardia (NSVT), sinus arrest, and atrioventricular (AV) blocks. It is estimated that almost up to 50% patients with OSA have some form of arrhythmia.

Most of the arrhythmias in OSA occur during sleep, particularly during the episodes of apnea/hypopnea. As per the SSHS study, there was a 17-fold increase in the odds of AF and NSVT occurring after apnea/hypopnea episodes as compared to normal breathing during sleep.[59-62] The nocturnal incidence of arrhythmias in OSA also affects the timing of sudden cardiac death in these patients. Unlike the patients without OSA, in whom most of the sudden deaths occur between 6 am and 11 am, the incidence of sudden death in OSA is highest between 10 pm and 6 am.[63]

Atrial fibrillation is the most common tachyarrhythmia encountered in patients with OSA. This is partly due to the fact that AF and OSA share many risk factors such as male sex, HTN, CAD, and HF.[64] Not only AF is more common in

OSA, it also responds poorly to the conventional treatment. A large multicentric study of 3,000 patients with OSA undergoing AF ablation showed a relatively inferior procedural success and increased procedure-related complications. However, the patients who were on CPAP had lower AF recurrences.[65] The lower AF recurrence with CPAP has also been reported in patients undergoing cardioversion for AF.[66] Ventricular arrhythmias are another common form of tachyarrhythmias in patients with OSA and are seen in almost 66% of these patients as compared to only 0–12% patients without OSA.[67,68]

Much like tachyarrhythmias, bradyarrhythmias are also commonly observed in patients with OSA and can occur even in absence of conduction system disease. Apnea/hypopnea episodes heighten vagal tone which can induce bradyarrhythmias such as sinus bradycardia, sinus arrest and AV blocks.[67,69,70] Although bradyarrhythmias may have a cardioprotective effect by reducing myocardial oxygen demand and prolonging diastole, extreme and persistent bradycardia may be deleterious and may result in impaired myocardial perfusion and myocardial ischemia. Fortunately, most of these patients have normal electrophysiological studies[71] and respond well to CPAP alone,[70] without the need for permanent pacemaker implantation.

Heart Failure

The prevalence of OSA in patients with HF is reported to be 11–37%.[72-74] Conversely, more than 50% of the patients with OSA are known to have diastolic dysfunction. The incidence of HF increases with increasing severity of OSA,[72] as is the risk of associated mortality. It has been shown that, independent of the confounding factors, HF patients with untreated OSA [apnea-hypopnea index (AHI) >15] have much higher mortality as compared to those with an AHI less than 15.[72]

Heart failure may also contribute to the development and worsening of OSA. Nocturnal fluid displacement in patients with HF, particularly in supine position, increases neck circumference as a result of edema of the upper airway. This may cause the upper airway to narrow and collapse due to increased airway resistance.[75] Poor respiratory drive in HF patients may also cause the upper airway to collapse and could further potentiate the development of OSA.[76,77]

Coronary Artery Disease

Based on several studies, prevalence of OSA in CAD patients appears to be up to twofold higher as compared to those without CAD.[78-81] Cross-sectional data from SHHS study over 8 years' follow-up showed higher odds ratio for CAD, HF and stroke in those with AHI greater than 15.[82] Similar findings have been reported in other prospective observational studies also.[83,84]

The presence of OSA in patients with CAD is associated with worse clinical outcomes. Not only the CV mortality is higher,[85] the outcome of revascularization is also relatively poorer with comparatively small increase in left ventricular ejection fraction (LVEF) post revascularization.[86]

The effect of OSA on development and progression of subclinical atherosclerosis has also been assessed in several studies. The patients with OSA have been shown to have increased carotid intima-media thickness (CIMT)[87-89] and arterial stiffness[88] as compared to those without OSA. Moreover, these abnormalities tend to resolve with adequate treatment of OSA.[89] In a study involving young patients with OSA, CPAP therapy was administered for 4 months and its effect on markers of inflammation and atherosclerosis was studied. CPAP significantly reduced inflammatory markers and CIMT in the studied population.[89]

Cardiovascular Diagnostic Evaluation in Patients with Obstructive Sleep Apnea

Given the association between OSA and CV disease, a patient with OSA can either present to a cardiologist or to a pulmonologist (or a sleep physician). When such a patient presents to a cardiologist, the cardiologist has a unique opportunity to not only diagnose the CV disease but also to recognize the underlying sleep disorder and to involve sleep physician colleagues in the management of the patient. Unfortunately, the diagnosis of OSA often gets overlooked, resulting not only in incomplete resolution of the patient's symptoms but also exposing the patient to unwarranted potential risk of long-term complications. It is, therefore, very important for all nonrespiratory physicians to have a high degree of alertness and a high index of suspicion so as to not miss OSA. It should be a routine practice to look for symptoms suggestive of OSA in all patients with one or more of the following:

- Obesity (BMI > 35 kg/m^2)
- Heart failure
- Refractory HTN
- Atrial fibrillation
- Nocturnal arrhythmias
- Pulmonary HTN.

In all such patients, a comprehensive sleep history should be obtained. An inquiry should be made about snoring, any witnessed apnea or gasping/choking at night, unexplained excessive daytime sleepiness, morning headaches, decreased concentration, and general irritability. If there is any suggestion of OSA, the patient should be referred for a detailed polysomnography to confirm or refute the diagnosis of OSA.

Not infrequently though, the patients with signs and symptoms suggestive of OSA may also approach a pulmonologist directly. In such circumstances and in all other patients diagnosed to have OSA, a comprehensive cardiac assessment is essential to detect any pre-existing CV disease, to define future risk of CV events and to devise an optimum treatment strategy (Table 1).

A detailed clinical examination is required which should include BP measurement, anthropometric assessment, and a search for any clinical evidence of target organ damage. The biochemical investigations should include fasting blood glucose, glycosylated hemoglobin, fasting lipid profile, renal function test, and thyroid function test among others. All patients should also have an ECG and echocardiogram done. Echocardiogram will help uncover many of the deleterious cardiac effects of OSA such as LV hypertrophy, LV systolic or diastolic dysfunction, pulmonary HTN, or atrial enlargement. Patients with refractory or labile HTN, should also have a 24-hour ambulatory BP monitoring performed whereas those with arrhythmias will require a 24-hour ambulatory ECG recording. If the patient complains of angina, a cardiac stress test or even coronary angiogram may be required.

Table 1: Approach to cardiovascular evaluation in patients with sleep related breathing disorders

Diagnostic tool	Indication
Required in all patients	
• Detailed clinical examination	
• Fasting blood glucose	
• Glycosylated hemoglobin	
• Fasting lipid profile	
• Blood urea, serum creatinine	
• Serum electrolytes	
• Thyroid function test	
• Chest X-ray	
• Electrocardiogram (ECG)	
• Echocardiogram	
Optional tests	
• 24-hour ambulatory blood pressure monitoring	• Patients with labile hypertension or refractory hypertension
• 24-hour ambulatory ECG monitoring	• Patients with undiagnosed arrhythmias or those requiring more detailed analysis of arrhythmias
• Cardiac stress test	• Patients presenting with symptoms suggestive of angina
• Carotid intima-media thickness measurement	• OSA patients without overt atherosclerotic vascular disease
• Arterial stiffness assessment	• OSA patients with hypertension
• Coronary angiography	• Patients with significant angina or abnormal cardiac stress test or evidence of LV systolic dysfunction

LV, left ventricular; OSA, obstructive sleep apnea.

Most patients with OSA usually do not have any overt evidence of atherosclerotic vascular disease at the time of initial presentation. However, given their clinical profile, they may still be at substantial risk of developing CV disease in future. In such patients, assessment of subclinical atherosclerosis may be of help. By providing a more accurate estimate of future CV risk, it allows more appropriate adjustment of treatment intensity according to the patients' "true" CV risk. Over the past 2–3 decades, numerous noninvasive tools for detection of subclinical atherosclerosis have become available for clinical use. Of these, CIMT appears to be the most suited because of its simplicity, wider availability, relatively low cost and lack of any radiation or contrast-related hazards.[90] Although not mandatory, CIMT measurement may be recommended in all patients with OSA who do not have overt vascular disease at the time of initial presentation. Assessment of arterial stiffness is another useful tool, particularly in patients with HTN, in whom it can help in guiding antihypertensive treatment.[91]

Management of Cardiovascular Disease in Obstructive Sleep Apnea

As discussed above, CV diseases are common in patients with OSA and OSA may aggravate preexisting CV conditions. In addition, OSA may also impair the efficacy of conventional therapy for CV diseases, thus making it important to diagnose and treat OSA effectively.

Continuous positive airway pressure is the treatment of choice for all types of OSA and as discussed below, CPAP itself can reverse many of the adverse CV effects of OSA. Therefore, CPAP should be considered in all patients with CV disease and OSA. However, at the same time, all these patients should also be given specific therapy as required for the underlying cardiac disorder. The patients should be periodically followed up to look for adherence to therapy, clinical response, side effects, and development of medical complications, if any.

Effect of Continuous Positive Airway Pressure on Cardiovascular Health in Patients with Obstructive Sleep Apnea

Numerous noncontrolled and controlled studies have shown that effective CPAP therapy has beneficial effects on HTN, HF, arrhythmias, CAD, and overall CV morbidity and mortality.

Continuous positive airway pressure reduces BP by attenuating the exaggerated SNA during sleep.[92] Several studies have shown moderate and variable effects of CPAP on BP in OSA patients.[93,94] Significant BP reductions with appropriate use of CPAP have also been observed in patients with moderate to severe OSA with difficult to control HTN.

Continuous positive airway pressure remains the treatment of choice in patients with HF and OSA. It reduces hypoxia and SNA and thus reduces nocturnal increase in BP and heart rate.[95] It also attenuates the negative intrathoracic pressure swings, which in turn, reduces the LV afterload.[96] The resultant cardiac unloading may improve LV systolic function and may improve HF, as shown in several studies.[95,97,98] In these studies, the benefit of CPAP was directly proportional to the severity of disease with greater increase in LVEF and larger BP reduction seen in patients having lower LVEF and higher AHI. The studies have also suggested that not only there is an increase in LVEF, but there is an improvement in the quality of life also (Table 2).[97,99]

Table 2: Randomized control trials evaluating the effects of CPAP on cardiac function in heart failure patients with obstructive sleep apnea						
First author (year)	Total sample size	Treatment arms	Duration (months)	Changes in		
				AHI	LVEF (%)	SBP/DBP (mmHg)
Kaneko et al., (2003)[98]	24	Control vs. CPAP	1.0	−0.5 vs. −28.8*	1.5 vs. 8.8*	6/−2 vs. −10*/−3
Mansfield et al., (2004)[97]	40	Control vs. CPAP	3.0	−8.4 vs. −21.1*	1.5 vs. 5.0†	Mean BP −6 vs. 1
Smith et al., (2007)[100]	23	Sham ACPAP vs. ACPAP	1.5	N/A vs. N/A	1.0 vs. 1.0	N/A vs. N/A
Egea et al., (2008)[99]	45	Sham CPAP vs. CPAP	3.0	−7.3 vs. −32.9	−0.5 vs. 2.2†	−1.6/1.2 vs. 0.0/0.4

*$p < 0.01$ for comparison between groups
†$p < 0.05$ for comparison between groups
ACPAP, autotitrating continuous positive airway pressure; AHI, apnea-hypopnea index; CPAP, continuous positive airway pressure; DBP, diastolic blood pressure; LVEF, left ventricular ejection fraction; N/A, data not available; SBP, systolic blood pressure.

Continuous positive airway pressure is also effective in reducing the risk of arrhythmias in patients with OSA. In patients with AF and OSA, effective CPAP therapy after cardioversion reduces the risk of recurrence of AF within 1 year as compared to untreated OSA patients.[66] Treatment of OSA also reduces the incidence and severity of ventricular arrhythmias.[60,61,101] Similarly, CPAP alone is effective in preventing bradyarrhythmias also with hardly any patient requiring permanent pacemaker implantation (in absence of underlying conduction system disease).[70]

Continuous positive airway pressure has been shown to have beneficial effects on CAD also. In some uncontrolled trials, the treatment of OSA with CPAP in patients with nocturnal angina was associated with a lower frequency of ST-segment depression and relief of nocturnal angina.[102-104] Another observational study, done in patients with CAD and OSA, showed reduction in occurrence of new adverse CV events with CPAP.[105] Finally, the beneficial effect of CPAP on subclinical atherosclerosis has already been discussed above.[89]

Specific Treatment of Cardiovascular Disorders in Patients with Obstructive Sleep Apnea

Although CPAP is the mainstay of treatment in OSA patients with CV disorders, specific CV therapy is equally important. The treatment principles are broadly same as for the patients without OSA, and the treatment guidelines and protocols for each specific disorder should be followed regardless of the presence or absence of OSA. However, there are some important aspects that merit attention.

The OSA patients who have HTN should ideally be on long-acting drugs so as to sufficiently lower BP not only during wakefulness but also during sleep. It is also important to choose a drug that does not aggravate OSA and sleepiness. Unfortunately, no antihypertensive drug is currently known to have direct effect on attenuating sleep apnea severity.[106]

In patients with HF and OSA, general measures such as fluid restriction, abstinence from sedatives, weight loss, and avoiding recumbent position during sleep are of paramount importance and should be religiously followed.[107,108] Randomized trials are needed to determine whether and by what mechanisms specific HF drugs have any direct effect on the severity of OSA.

In patients with bradyarrhythmias and OSA, it is important to decide which subset of patients may require permanent pacemaker implantation. As discussed above, most of these patients do not have heart blocks during wakefulness, do not have any brady-related symptoms and do not have any underlying conduction system disease. Moreover, there are no definite studies to suggest an increased mortality associated with bradyarrhythmias in these patients. Therefore, majority of these patients can be managed with CPAP alone.[70] However, permanent pacemaker implantation may occasionally be required in patients with persistent heart blocks despite effective CPAP therapy or in patients with poor compliance to CPAP.

CARDIOVASCULAR INVOLVEMENT IN OTHER FORMS OF SLEEP RELATED BREATHING DISORDERS

Central Sleep Apnea

Central sleep apnea (CSA) is a disorder in which the effort to breathe is absent or diminished, either intermittently or in cycles and typically for more than

10 seconds, resulting in episodic cessation of ventilation during sleep. Unlike OSA, the upper airway in CSA remains patent for most part of the respiration.

A number of clinical conditions such as HF, stroke, Parkinson's disease, brainstem injury, use of sedatives, hypothyroidism, etc. are known to result in CSA. However, in clinical practice, CSA is most frequently encountered in association with HF, LV systolic dysfunction (even in absence of overt HF), AF, and stroke.[109,110] CSA occurs in less than 1% of general population[111] but is reported in as many as 30–40% of those with HF.[112-115] In these patients, breathing during sleep has a characteristic waxing and waning pattern, with intermittent periods of central apnea or hypopnea at the nadir of ventilatory effort. This pattern is also known as Cheyne-Stokes respiration (CSR) and is typical of HF. The pathogenesis of CSA-CSR is multifactorial (Figure 2) but increased responsiveness to hyercapnia and prolonged circulation time as a result of HF appear to be the key contributors.[110,116] Even in patients with stroke, CSA appears to be a manifestation of underlying occult cardiac dysfunction, rather than the stroke itself.[117]

Cardiovascular Effects of Central Sleep Apnea

As mentioned above, CSA usually occurs as a consequence of HF and is not itself the cause of HF. However, the relationship between CSA and HF, to some extent, is bidirectional. Much like OSA, CSA also induces hypoxemia and heightened SNA that result in peripheral vasoconstriction, increased peripheral vascular resistance and activation of renin-angiotensin-aldosterone system, which lead to surges in heart rate and BP, increased myocardial oxygen demand and fluid retention. These abnormalities together result in worsening of HF and as a consequence, there is further fluid retention and pulmonary venous congestion, precipitating a vicious cycle of HF and CSA (Figure 2).[116] However, unlike OSA,

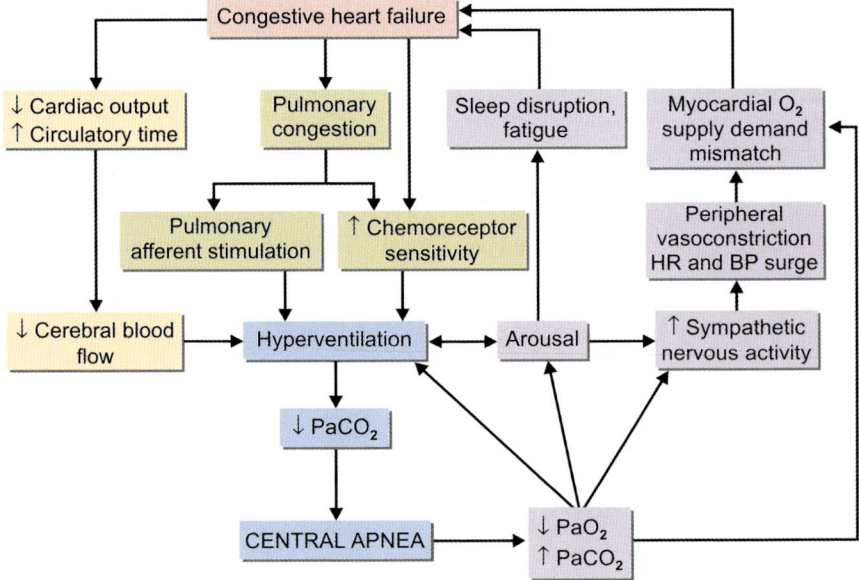

BP, blood pressure; HR, heart rate.

Figure 2: Pathophysiology of central sleep apnea in patients with heart failure.

the extremes of negative intrathoracic pressure are not a feature of CSA and, therefore, the deleterious effects on CV system are relatively less profound.

Nevertheless, regardless the role of CSA in the pathogenesis of HF, presence of CSA in HF is associated with increased CV morbidity and mortality. Compared to the patients without CSA, those with CSA have more severe HF, higher pulmonary capillary wedge pressure, greater risk of arrhythmias, and have higher mortality rate.[118-122] The risk of death in CSA is in proportion to AHI, providing further evidence of the association between CSA and adverse cardiac outcomes.[120]

Diagnosis of Central Sleep Apnea

In patients with HF, recognition of CSA is important but is challenging. Although abnormal breathing pattern may be identified on visual inspection alone, an overnight polysomnography is invariably required to confirm the diagnosis and to determine its severity. A polysomnography is also helpful in distinguishing CSA from OSA. This distinction has considerable therapeutic significance because in HF patients, OSA responds rapidly to CPAP whereas the effect of CPAP on CSA is variable and generally less satisfactory. However, it is important to remember that in many patients with HF, OSA and CSA coexist. Tkacova et al. in a small group of HF patients demonstrated that the features of OSA dominated during the early part of sleep whereas CSA-CSR became the dominant form during the latter half of night.[123] The same authors, in yet another study, demonstrated a similar progression from predominant OSA to predominant CSA occurring over a period of 1 month.[124]

Management of Central Sleep Apnea

Management of CSA in HF requires a two-pronged approach, one directed at the treatment of underlying HF and the other at the treatment of CSA itself. Standard therapeutic measures for HF such as diuretics,[118] beta-blockers,[125] and angiotensin-converting enzyme inhibitors[126] have all been demonstrated to result in improvement in CSA. However, the magnitude of such benefit and its long-term durability remain debatable. In addition, in some patients, diuretics may worsen CSA by raising $PaCO_2$ threshold for apnea, requiring necessary caution.[127] More recently, cardiac resynchronization therapy (CRT) has also been shown to have a favorable effect on AHI, oxygen saturation, and sleep quality.[128-130] These positive outcomes of CRT are believed to result from improved LV filling, better ventricular synchrony and contraction. However, over the long-term, CSA suppression may not be sustained and large-scale randomized clinical trials are needed to further evaluate the long-term effects of CRT in patients with HF and CSA.

Nocturnal O_2 supplementation for short-term period has been shown to reduce AHI in patients with HF and CSA with improved quality of life but the long-term effects on CV endpoints have not been evaluated.[131-133] Similarly, several small-scale trials have evaluated role of CPAP in these patients and have shown improvement in quality of life, LVEF, biomarkers of HF, and even cardiac mortality.[134-136] However, the results from the large, randomized trial, Canadian Continuous Positive Airway Pressure for Treatment of Central Sleep Apnea in Heart Failure (CANPAP) trial, have not shown any definite benefit.[137] This multicentric trial involved 258 patients with HF with optimized medical therapy and aimed to determine the effect of CPAP on multiple CV and CSA outcomes.

Although, the use of CPAP reduced nocturnal desaturation, improved LVEF and lowered plasma norepinephrine levels, there was no significant difference between the two groups in the primary composite end-point of mortality and cardiac transplantation at the end of 2 years of follow-up. The hospitalization rates also did not change. However, it is noteworthy that the trial was underpowered to answer many of the study questions.

Adaptive servoventilation (ASV) is a novel type of noninvasive ventilation which has been shown to be effective in patients with HF, even in cases where CPAP has failed.[138] Two trials involving HF patients with CSA have shown improvement in LVEF and suppression of CSA with ASV.[138,139] However, long-term randomized trials are needed before ASV can be routinely recommended for the treatment of CSA in HF patients.

Finally, drugs such as theophylline[140] and acetazolamide[141] have also been tried for the treatment of CSA, with variable success.

Complex Sleep Apnea

Complex sleep apnea is a form of CSA seen in patients with OSA when they are treated with CPAP.[142,143] It is specifically defined as the persistence or emergence of central apnea or hypopneas upon exposure to CPAP when obstructive events have disappeared. The clinical features of complex sleep apnea lie between those of CSA and OSA and much like other forms of sleep apnea, it can also contribute to adverse CV outcomes. However, its association with CV disease has not been adequately studied so far.

CONCLUSION

Sleep related breathing disorders are commonly occurring disorders that frequently coexist in patients with CV disease and contribute to the development and progression of cardiac disease in them. OSA is the commonest form of SRBD and is the most extensively studied with respect to CV outcomes. Evidence collected over the past few decades suggests a causal association between OSA and HTN and perhaps other CV diseases as well. This adverse outcome of OSA appears to be mediated through its typical pattern of intermittent hypoxia leading to endothelial dysfunction, oxidative stress, and inflammation. Therefore, OSA should no longer be seen only as a cause for hypersomnolence and impaired quality of life, but should also be considered to be a potential independent risk factor for CV disease.

Central sleep apnea is the second most common form of sleep apnea and the commonest type in patients with HF, in whom it appears more likely to be a manifestation of HF rather than being its cause. However, any form of sleep apnea in a patient with HF is associated with increased CV morbidity and mortality and therefore requires proper attention towards its evaluation and management.

REFERENCES

1. Leung RS, Bradley TD. Sleep apnea and cardiovascular disease. *Am J Respir Crit Care Med.* 2001;164:2147-65.
2. Hu FB, Willett WC, Manson JE, et al. Snoring and risk of cardiovascular disease in women. *J Am Coll Cardiol.* 2000;35:308-313.

3. Elmasry A, Lindberg E, Berne C, et al. Sleep-disordered breathing and glucose metabolism in hypertensive men: a population-based study. *J Intern Med.* 2001;249:153-61.
4. Coughlin SR, Mawdsley L, Mugarza JA, et al. Obstructive sleep apnoea is independently associated with an increased prevalence of metabolic syndrome. *Eur Heart J.* 2004;25:735-41.
5. Ancoli-Israel S, DuHamel ER, Stepnowsky C, et al. The relationship between congestive heart failure, sleep apnea, and mortality in older men. *Chest.* 2003;124:1400-5.
6. Quan SF, Gersh BJ. Cardiovascular consequences of sleep-disordered breathing: past, present and future: report of a workshop from the National Center on Sleep Disorders Research and the National Heart, Lung, and Blood Institute. *Circulation.* 2004;109:951-7.
7. Shahar E, Whitney CW, Redline S, et al. Sleep-disordered breathing and cardiovascular disease: cross-sectional results of the Sleep Heart Health Study. *Am J Respir Crit Care Med.* 2001;163:19-25.
8. Nieto FJ, Young TB, Lind BK, et al. Association of sleep-disordered breathing, sleep apnea, and hypertension in a large community-based study. Sleep Heart Health Study. *JAMA.* 2000;283:1829-36.
9. Hu FB, Willett WC, Colditz GA, et al. Prospective study of snoring and risk of hypertension in women. *Am J Epidemiol.* 1999;150:806-16.
10. Al-Delaimy WK, Manson JE, Willett WC, et al. Snoring as a risk factor for type II diabetes mellitus: a prospective study. *Am J Epidemiol.* 2002;155:387-93.
11. Peppard PE, Young T, Palta M, et al. Prospective study of the association between sleep-disordered breathing and hypertension. *N Engl J Med.* 2000;342:1378-84.
12. Brinker JA, Weiss JL, Lappe DL, et al. Leftward septal displacement during right ventricular loading in man. *Circulation.* 1980;61:626-33.
13. Tolle FA, Judy WV, Yu PL, et al. Reduced stroke volume related to pleural pressure in obstructive sleep apnea. *J Appl Physiol Respir Environ Exerc Physiol.* 1983;55:1718-24.
14. Parker JD, Brooks D, Kozar LF, et al. Acute and chronic effects of airway obstruction on canine left ventricular performance. *Am J Respir Crit Care Med.* 1999;160:1888-96.
15. Cargill RI, Kiely DG, Lipworth BJ. Adverse effects of hypoxaemia on diastolic filling in humans. *Clin Sci (Lond).* 1995;89:165-9.
16. Kusuoka H, Weisfeldt ML, Zweier JL, et al. Mechanism of early contractile failure during hypoxia in intact ferret heart: evidence for modulation of maximal Ca^{2+}-activated force by inorganic phosphate. *Circ Res.* 1986;59:270-82.
17. Somers VK, Mark AL, Zavala DC, et al. Contrasting effects of hypoxia and hypercapnia on ventilation and sympathetic activity in humans. *J Appl Physiol (1985).* 1989;67:2101-6.
18. Somers VK, Mark AL, Zavala DC, et al. Influence of ventilation and hypocapnia on sympathetic nerve responses to hypoxia in normal humans. *J Appl Physiol (1985).* 1989;67:2095-100.
19. Horner RL, Brooks D, Kozar LF, et al. Immediate effects of arousal from sleep on cardiac autonomic outflow in the absence of breathing in dogs. *J Appl Physiol (1985).* 1995;79:151-62.
20. Frattola A, Parati G, Cuspidi C, et al. Prognostic value of 24-hour blood pressure variability. *J Hypertens.* 1993;11:1133-7.
21. Palatini P, Penzo M, Racioppa A, et al. Clinical relevance of nighttime blood pressure and of daytime blood pressure variability. *Arch Intern Med.* 1992;152:1855-60.
22. Ponikowski P, Anker SD, Chua TP, et al. Depressed heart rate variability as an independent predictor of death in chronic congestive heart failure secondary to ischemic or idiopathic dilated cardiomyopathy. *Am J Cardiol.* 1997;79:1645-50.
23. Singh JP, Larson MG, Tsuji H, et al. Reduced heart rate variability and new-onset hypertension: insights into pathogenesis of hypertension: the Framingham Heart Study. *Hypertension.* 1998;32:293-7.
24. Dean RT, Wilcox I. Possible atherogenic effects of hypoxia during obstructive sleep apnea. *Sleep.* 1993;16:15-21.
25. Halliwell B. The role of oxygen radicals in human disease, with particular reference to the vascular system. *Haemostasis.* 1993;23 Suppl 1:118-26.
26. Venugopal SK, Devaraj S, Yuhanna I, et al. Demonstration that C-reactive protein decreases eNOS expression and bioactivity in human aortic endothelial cells. *Circulation.* 2002;106:1439-41.

27. El-Solh AA, Mador MJ, Sikka P, et al. Adhesion molecules in patients with coronary artery disease and moderate-to-severe obstructive sleep apnea. *Chest.* 2002;121:1541-7.
28. Ohga E, Nagase T, Tomita T, et al. Increased levels of circulating ICAM-1, VCAM-1, and L-selectin in obstructive sleep apnea syndrome. *J Appl Physiol (1985).* 1999;87:10-4.
29. Chin K, Ohi M, Kita H, et al. Effects of NCPAP therapy on fibrinogen levels in obstructive sleep apnea syndrome. *Am J Respir Crit Care Med.* 1996;153:1972-6.
30. Yokoe T, Minoguchi K, Matsuo H, et al. Elevated levels of C-reactive protein and interleukin-6 in patients with obstructive sleep apnea syndrome are decreased by nasal continuous positive airway pressure. *Circulation.* 2003;107:1129-34.
31. Kato M, Roberts-Thomson P, Phillips BG, et al. Impairment of endothelium-dependent vasodilation of resistance vessels in patients with obstructive sleep apnea. *Circulation.* 2000;102:2607-10.
32. Schulz R, Schmidt D, Blum A, et al. Decreased plasma levels of nitric oxide derivatives in obstructive sleep apnoea: response to CPAP therapy. *Thorax.* 2000;55:1046-51.
33. Gjorup PH, Sadauskiene L, Wessels J, et al. Abnormally increased endothelin-1 in plasma during the night in obstructive sleep apnea: relation to blood pressure and severity of disease. *Am J Hypertens.* 2007;20:44-52.
34. Sprague RS, Thiemermann C, Vane JR. Endogenous endothelium-derived relaxing factor opposes hypoxic pulmonary vasoconstriction and supports blood flow to hypoxic alveoli in anesthetized rabbits. *Proc Natl Acad Sci USA.* 1992;89:8711-5.
35. Leeman M, de Beyl VZ, Biarent D, et al. Inhibition of cyclooxygenase and nitric oxide synthase in hypoxic vasoconstriction and oleic acid-induced lung injury. *Am J Respir Crit Care Med.* 1999;159:1383-90.
36. Phillips BG, Narkiewicz K, Pesek CA, et al. Effects of obstructive sleep apnea on endothelin-1 and blood pressure. *J Hypertens.* 1999;17:61-6.
37. Eisensehr I, Ehrenberg BL, Noachtar S, et al. Platelet activation, epinephrine, and blood pressure in obstructive sleep apnea syndrome. *Neurology.* 1998;51:188-95.
38. Sanner BM, Konermann M, Tepel M, et al. Platelet function in patients with obstructive sleep apnoea syndrome. Eur Respir J. 2000;16:648-52.
39. Wessendorf TE, Thilmann AF, Wang YM, et al. Fibrinogen levels and obstructive sleep apnea in ischemic stroke. *Am J Respir Crit Care Med.* 2000;162:2039-42.
40. Hoffstein V, Herridge M, Mateika S, et al. Hematocrit levels in sleep apnea. *Chest.* 1994;106:787-91.
41. He J, Kryger MH, Zorick FJ, et al. Mortality and apnea index in obstructive sleep apnea. Experience in 385 male patients. *Chest.* 1988;94:9-14.
42. Haas DC, Foster GL, Nieto FJ, et al. Age-dependent associations between sleep-disordered breathing and hypertension: importance of discriminating between systolic/diastolic hypertension and isolated systolic hypertension in the Sleep Heart Health Study. *Circulation.* 2005;111:614-21.
43. Gami AS, Hodge DO, Herges RM, et al. Obstructive sleep apnea, obesity, and the risk of incident atrial fibrillation. *J Am Coll Cardiol.* 2007;49:565-71.
44. Lavie P, Lavie L, Herer P. All-cause mortality in males with sleep apnoea syndrome: declining mortality rates with age. *Eur Respir J.* 2005;25:514-20.
45. Silverberg DS, Oksenberg A, Iaina A. Sleep-related breathing disorders as a major cause of essential hypertension: fact or fiction? *Curr Opin Nephrol Hypertens.* 1998;7:353-7.
46. Williams AJ, Houston D, Finberg S, et al. Sleep apnea syndrome and essential hypertension. *Am J Cardiol.* 1985;55:1019-22.
47. Lavie P, Ben-Yosef R, Rubin AE. Prevalence of sleep apnea syndrome among patients with essential hypertension. *Am Heart J.* 1984;108:373-6.
48. Kales A, Bixler EO, Cadieux RJ, et al. Sleep apnoea in a hypertensive population. *Lancet.* 1984;2:1005-8.
49. Fletcher EC, DeBehnke RD, Lovoi MS, et al. Undiagnosed sleep apnea in patients with essential hypertension. *Ann Intern Med.* 1985;103:190-5.
50. Logan AG, Perlikowski SM, Mente A, et al. High prevalence of unrecognized sleep apnoea in drug-resistant hypertension. *J Hypertens.* 2001;19:2271-7.

51. Goodfriend TL, Calhoun DA. Resistant hypertension, obesity, sleep apnea, and aldosterone: theory and therapy. *Hypertension.* 2004;43:518-24.
52. Calhoun DA, Nishizaka MK, Zaman MA, et al. Aldosterone excretion among subjects with resistant hypertension and symptoms of sleep apnea. *Chest.* 2004;125:112-7.
53. Pratt-Ubunama MN, Nishizaka MK, Boedefeld RL, et al. Plasma aldosterone is related to severity of obstructive sleep apnea in subjects with resistant hypertension. *Chest.* 2007;131:453-9.
54. Mayer J, Becker H, Brandenburg U, et al. Blood pressure and sleep apnea: results of long-term nasal continuous positive airway pressure therapy. *Cardiology.* 1991;79:84-92.
55. Chobanian AV, Bakris GL, Black HR, et al. The Seventh Report of the Joint National Committee on Prevention, Detection, Evaluation, and Treatment of High Blood Pressure: the JNC 7 report. *JAMA.* 2003;289:2560-72.
56. Kario K, Shimada K, Pickering TG. Abnormal nocturnal blood pressure falls in elderly hypertension: clinical significance and determinants. *J Cardiovasc Pharmacol.* 2003;41 Suppl 1:S61-6.
57. Portaluppi F, Provini F, Cortelli P, et al. Undiagnosed sleep-disordered breathing among male nondippers with essential hypertension. *J Hypertens.* 1997;15:1227-33.
58. Verdecchia P, Schillaci G, Guerrieri M, et al. Circadian blood pressure changes and left ventricular hypertrophy in essential hypertension. *Circulation.* 1990;81:528-36.
59. Shepard JW, Garrison MW, Grither DA, et al. Relationship of ventricular ectopy to oxyhemoglobin desaturation in patients with obstructive sleep apnea. *Chest.* 1985;88:335-40.
60. Javaheri S. Effects of continuous positive airway pressure on sleep apnea and ventricular irritability in patients with heart failure. *Circulation.* 2000;101:392-7.
61. Harbison J, O'Reilly P, McNicholas WT. Cardiac rhythm disturbances in the obstructive sleep apnea syndrome: effects of nasal continuous positive airway pressure therapy. *Chest.* 2000;118:591-5.
62. Monahan K, Storfer-Isser A, Mehra R, et al. Triggering of nocturnal arrhythmias by sleep-disordered breathing events. *J Am Coll Cardiol.* 2009;54:1797-804.
63. Gami AS, Howard DE, Olson EJ, et al. Day-night pattern of sudden death in obstructive sleep apnea. *N Engl J Med.* 2005;352:1206-14.
64. Wolk R, Kara T, Somers VK. Sleep-disordered breathing and cardiovascular disease. *Circulation.* 2003;108:9-12.
65. Patel D, Mohanty P, Di Biase L, et al. Safety and efficacy of pulmonary vein antral isolation in patients with obstructive sleep apnea: the impact of continuous positive airway pressure. *Circ Arrhythm Electrophysiol.* 2010;3:445-51.
66. Kanagala R, Murali NS, Friedman PA, et al. Obstructive sleep apnea and the recurrence of atrial fibrillation. *Circulation.* 2003;107:2589-94.
67. Guilleminault C, Connolly SJ, Winkle RA. Cardiac arrhythmia and conduction disturbances during sleep in 400 patients with sleep apnea syndrome. *Am J Cardiol.* 1983;52:490-4.
68. Hoffstein V, Mateika S. Cardiac arrhythmias, snoring, and sleep apnea. *Chest.* 1994;106:466-71.
69. Koehler U, Becker HF, Grimm W, et al. Relations among hypoxemia, sleep stage, and bradyarrhythmia during obstructive sleep apnea. *Am Heart J.* 2000;139:142-8.
70. Becker H, Brandenburg U, Peter JH, et al. Reversal of sinus arrest and atrioventricular conduction block in patients with sleep apnea during nasal continuous positive airway pressure. *Am J Respir Crit Care Med.* 1995;151:215-8.
71. Grimm W, Hoffmann J, Menz V, et al. Electrophysiologic evaluation of sinus node function and atrioventricular conduction in patients with prolonged ventricular asystole during obstructive sleep apnea. *Am J Cardiol.* 1996;77:1310-4.
72. Wang H, Parker JD, Newton GE, et al. Influence of obstructive sleep apnea on mortality in patients with heart failure. *J Am Coll Cardiol.* 2007;49:1625-31.
73. Sin DD, Fitzgerald F, Parker JD, et al. Risk factors for central and obstructive sleep apnea in 450 men and women with congestive heart failure. *Am J Respir Crit Care Med.* 1999;160:1101-6.
74. Javaheri S, Parker TJ, Liming JD, et al. Sleep apnea in 81 ambulatory male patients with stable heart failure. Types and their prevalences, consequences, and presentations. *Circulation.* 1998;97:2154-9.

75. Shepard JW Jr, Pevernagie DA, Stanson AW, et al. Effects of changes in central venous pressure on upper airway size in patients with obstructive sleep apnea. *Am J Respir Crit Care Med.* 1996;153:250-4.
76. Alex CG, Onal E, Lopata M. Upper airway occlusion during sleep in patients with Cheyne-Stokes respiration. *Am Rev Respir Dis.* 1986;133:42-5.
77. Younes M. The physiologic basis of central apnea and periodic breathing. *Curr Pulmonol.* 1989;10:265-326.
78. Sanner BM, Konermann M, Doberauer C, et al. Sleep-disordered breathing in patients referred for angina evaluation—association with left ventricular dysfunction. *Clin Cardiol.* 2001;24:146-50.
79. Peker Y, Kraiczi H, Hedner J, et al. An independent association between obstructive sleep apnoea and coronary artery disease. *Eur Respir J.* 1999;14:179-84.
80. Mooe T, Rabben T, Wiklund U, et al. Sleep-disordered breathing in men with coronary artery disease. *Chest.* 1996;109:659-63.
81. Schafer H, Koehler U, Ewig S, et al. Obstructive sleep apnea as a risk marker in coronary artery disease. *Cardiology.* 1999;92:79-84.
82. Punjabi NM, Caffo BS, Goodwin JL, et al. Sleep-disordered breathing and mortality: a prospective cohort study. *PLoS medicine.* 2009;6:e1000132.
83. Mooe T, Franklin KA, Holmstrom K, et al. Sleep-disordered breathing and coronary artery disease: long-term prognosis. *Am J Respir Crit Care Med.* 2001;164:1910-3.
84. Peker Y, Hedner J, Norum J, et al. Increased incidence of cardiovascular disease in middle-aged men with obstructive sleep apnea: a 7-year follow-up. *Am J Respir Crit Care Med.* 2002;166:159-65.
85. Peker Y, Hedner J, Kraiczi H, et al. Respiratory disturbance index: an independent predictor of mortality in coronary artery disease. *Am J Respir Crit Care Med.* 2000;162:81-6.
86. Nakashima H, Katayama T, Takagi C, et al. Obstructive sleep apnoea inhibits the recovery of left ventricular function in patients with acute myocardial infarction. *Eur Heart J.* 2006;27:2317-22.
87. Minoguchi K, Yokoe T, Tazaki T, et al. Increased carotid intima-media thickness and serum inflammatory markers in obstructive sleep apnea. *Am J Respir Crit Care Med.* 2005;172:625-30.
88. Drager LF, Bortolotto LA, Lorenzi MC, et al. Early signs of atherosclerosis in obstructive sleep apnea. *Am J Respir Crit Care Med.* 2005;172:613-8.
89. Drager LF, Bortolotto LA, Figueiredo AC, et al. Effects of continuous positive airway pressure on early signs of atherosclerosis in obstructive sleep apnea. *Am J Respir Crit Care Med.* 2007;176:706-12.
90. Stein JH, Korcarz CE, Hurst RT, et al. Use of carotid ultrasound to identify subclinical vascular disease and evaluate cardiovascular disease risk: a consensus statement from the American Society of Echocardiography Carotid Intima-Media Thickness Task Force Endorsed by the Society for Vascular Medicine. *J Am Soc Echocardiogr.* 2008;21:93-111.
91. Mancia G, De Backer G, Dominiczak A, et al. 2007 Guidelines for the management of arterial hypertension: The Task Force for the Management of Arterial Hypertension of the European Society of Hypertension (ESH) and of the European Society of Cardiology (ESC). *Eur Heart J.* 2007;28:1462-536.
92. Somers VK, Dyken ME, Clary MP, et al. Sympathetic neural mechanisms in obstructive sleep apnea. *J Clin Invest.* 1995;96:1897-904.
93. Haentjens P, Van Meerhaeghe A, Moscariello A, et al. The impact of continuous positive airway pressure on blood pressure in patients with obstructive sleep apnea syndrome: evidence from a meta-analysis of placebo-controlled randomized trials. *Arch Intern Med.* 2007;167:757-64.
94. Bazzano LA, Khan Z, Reynolds K, et al. Effect of nocturnal nasal continuous positive airway pressure on blood pressure in obstructive sleep apnea. *Hypertension.* 2007;50:417-23.
95. Usui K, Bradley TD, Spaak J, et al. Inhibition of awake sympathetic nerve activity of heart failure patients with obstructive sleep apnea by nocturnal continuous positive airway pressure. *J Am Coll Cardiol.* 2005;45:2008-11.

96. Tkacova R, Rankin F, Fitzgerald FS, et al. Effects of continuous positive airway pressure on obstructive sleep apnea and left ventricular afterload in patients with heart failure. *Circulation.* 1998;98:2269-75.
97. Mansfield DR, Gollogly NC, Kaye DM, et al. Controlled trial of continuous positive airway pressure in obstructive sleep apnea and heart failure. *Am J Respir Crit Care Med.* 2004;169:361-6.
98. Kaneko Y, Floras JS, Usui K, et al. Cardiovascular effects of continuous positive airway pressure in patients with heart failure and obstructive sleep apnea. *N Engl J Med.* 2003; 348:1233-41.
99. Egea CJ, Aizpuru F, Pinto JA, et al. Cardiac function after CPAP therapy in patients with chronic heart failure and sleep apnea: a multicenter study. *Sleep Med.* 2008;9:660-6.
100. Smith LA, Vennelle M, Gardner RS, et al. Auto-titrating continuous positive airway pressure therapy in patients with chronic heart failure and obstructive sleep apnoea: a randomized placebo-controlled trial. *Eur Heart J.* 2007;28:1221-7.
101. Ryan CM, Usui K, Floras JS, et al. Effect of continuous positive airway pressure on ventricular ectopy in heart failure patients with obstructive sleep apnoea. *Thorax.* 2005; 60:781-5.
102. Franklin KA, Nilsson JB, Sahlin C, et al. Sleep apnoea and nocturnal angina. *Lancet.* 1995;345:1085-7.
103. Philip P, Guilleminault C. ST segment abnormality, angina during sleep and obstructive sleep apnea. *Sleep.* 1993;16:558-9.
104. Peled N, Abinader EG, Pillar G, et al. Nocturnal ischemic events in patients with obstructive sleep apnea syndrome and ischemic heart disease: effects of continuous positive air pressure treatment. *J Am Coll Cardiol.* 1999;34:1744-9.
105. Milleron O, Pilliere R, Foucher A, et al. Benefits of obstructive sleep apnoea treatment in coronary artery disease: a long-term follow-up study. *Eur Heart J.* 2004;25:728-34.
106. Kraiczi H, Hedner J, Peker Y, et al. Comparison of atenolol, amlodipine, enalapril, hydrochlorothiazide, and losartan for antihypertensive treatment in patients with obstructive sleep apnea. *Am J Respir Crit Care Med.* 2000;161:1423-8.
107. Issa FG, Sullivan CE. Alcohol, snoring and sleep apnea. *J Neurol Neurosurg Psychiatry.* 1982;45:353-9.
108. Smith PL, Gold AR, Meyers DA, et al. Weight loss in mildly to moderately obese patients with obstructive sleep apnea. *Ann Intern Med.* 1985;103:850-5.
109. Somers VK, White DP, Amin R, et al. Sleep apnea and cardiovascular disease: an American Heart Association/american College Of Cardiology Foundation Scientific Statement from the American Heart Association Council for High Blood Pressure Research Professional Education Committee, Council on Clinical Cardiology, Stroke Council, and Council On Cardiovascular Nursing. In collaboration with the National Heart, Lung, and Blood Institute National Center on Sleep Disorders Research (National Institutes of Health). *Circulation.* 2008;118:1080-111.
110. Kasai T, Floras JS, Bradley TD. Sleep apnea and cardiovascular disease: a bidirectional relationship. *Circulation.* 2012;126:1495-510.
111. Bixler EO, Vgontzas AN, Ten Have T, et al. Effects of age on sleep apnea in men: I. Prevalence and severity. *Am J Respir Crit Care Med.* 1998;157:144-8.
112. Yumino D, Wang H, Floras JS, et al. Prevalence and physiological predictors of sleep apnea in patients with heart failure and systolic dysfunction. *J Card Fail.* 2009;15: 279-85.
113. Lofaso F, Verschueren P, Rande JL, et al. Prevalence of sleep-disordered breathing in patients on a heart transplant waiting list. *Chest.* 1994;106:1689-94.
114. Javaheri S, Parker TJ, Wexler L, et al. Occult sleep-disordered breathing in stable congestive heart failure. *Ann Intern Med.* 1995;122:487-92.
115. Cripps T, Rocker G, Stradling J. Nocturnal hypoxia and arrhythmias in patients with impaired left ventricular function. *Br Heart J.* 1992;68:382-6.
116. Yumino D, Bradley TD. Central sleep apnea and Cheyne-Stokes respiration. *Proceedings of the American Thoracic Society.* 2008;5:226-36.

117. Nopmaneejumruslers C, Kaneko Y, Hajek V, et al. Cheyne-Stokes respiration in stroke: relationship to hypocapnia and occult cardiac dysfunction. *Am J Respir Crit Care Med.* 2005;171:1048-52.
118. Solin P, Bergin P, Richardson M, et al. Influence of pulmonary capillary wedge pressure on central apnea in heart failure. *Circulation.* 1999;99:1574-9.
119. Javaheri S, Shukla R, Zeigler H, et al. Central sleep apnea, right ventricular dysfunction, and low diastolic blood pressure are predictors of mortality in systolic heart failure. *J Am Coll Cardiol.* 2007;49:2028-34.
120. Lanfranchi PA, Braghiroli A, Bosimini E, et al. Prognostic value of nocturnal Cheyne-Stokes respiration in chronic heart failure. *Circulation.* 1999;99:1435-40.
121. Hanly PJ, Zuberi-Khokhar NS. Increased mortality associated with Cheyne-Stokes respiration in patients with congestive heart failure. *Am J Respir Crit Care Med.* 1996;153:272-6.
122. Corra U, Pistono M, Mezzani A, et al. Sleep and exertional periodic breathing in chronic heart failure: prognostic importance and interdependence. *Circulation.* 2006;113:44-50.
123. Tkacova R, Niroumand M, Lorenzi-Filho G, et al. Overnight shift from obstructive to central apneas in patients with heart failure: role of PCO_2 and circulatory delay. *Circulation.* 2001;103:238-43.
124. Tkacova R, Wang H, Bradley TD. Night-to-night alterations in sleep apnea type in patients with heart failure. *J Sleep Res.* 2006;15:321-8.
125. Tamura A, Kawano Y, Naono S, et al. Relationship between beta-blocker treatment and the severity of central sleep apnea in chronic heart failure. *Chest.* 2007;131:130-5.
126. Walsh JT, Andrews R, Starling R, et al. Effects of captopril and oxygen on sleep apnoea in patients with mild to moderate congestive cardiac failure. *Br Heart J.* 1995;73:237-41.
127. Nakayama H, Smith CA, Rodman JR, et al. Effect of ventilatory drive on carbon dioxide sensitivity below eupnea during sleep. *Am J Respir Crit Care Med.* 2002;165:1251-60.
128. Oldenburg O, Faber L, Vogt J, et al. Influence of cardiac resynchronisation therapy on different types of sleep disordered breathing. *Eur J Heart Fail.* 2007;9:820-6.
129. Stanchina ML, Ellison K, Malhotra A, et al. The impact of cardiac resynchronization therapy on obstructive sleep apnea in heart failure patients: a pilot study. *Chest.* 2007;132:433-9.
130. Sinha AM, Skobel EC, Breithardt OA, et al. Cardiac resynchronization therapy improves central sleep apnea and Cheyne-Stokes respiration in patients with chronic heart failure. *J Am Coll Cardiol.* 2004;44:68-71.
131. Staniforth AD, Kinnear WJ, Starling R, et al. Effect of oxygen on sleep quality, cognitive function and sympathetic activity in patients with chronic heart failure and Cheyne-Stokes respiration. *Eur Heart J.* 1998;19:922-8.
132. Franklin KA, Eriksson P, Sahlin C, et al. Reversal of central sleep apnea with oxygen. *Chest.* 1997;111:163-9.
133. Sasayama S, Izumi T, Matsuzaki M, et al. Improvement of quality of life with nocturnal oxygen therapy in heart failure patients with central sleep apnea. *Circ J.* 2009;73:1255-62.
134. Sin DD, Logan AG, Fitzgerald FS, et al. Effects of continuous positive airway pressure on cardiovascular outcomes in heart failure patients with and without Cheyne-Stokes respiration. *Circulation.* 2000;102:61-6.
135. Tkacova R, Liu PP, Naughton MT, et al. Effect of continuous positive airway pressure on mitral regurgitant fraction and atrial natriuretic peptide in patients with heart failure. *J Am Coll Cardiol.* 1997;30:739-45.
136. Naughton MT, Liu PP, Bernard DC, et al. Treatment of congestive heart failure and Cheyne-Stokes respiration during sleep by continuous positive airway pressure. *Am J Respir Crit Care Med.* 1995;151:92-7.
137. Bradley TD, Logan AG, Kimoff RJ, et al. Continuous positive airway pressure for central sleep apnea and heart failure. *N Engl J Med.* 2005;353:2025-33.
138. Teschler H, Dohring J, Wang YM, et al. Adaptive pressure support servo-ventilation: a novel treatment for Cheyne-Stokes respiration in heart failure. *Am J Respir Crit Care Med.* 2001;164:614-9.
139. Philippe C, Stoica-Herman M, Drouot X, et al. Compliance with and effectiveness of adaptive servoventilation versus continuous positive airway pressure in the treatment of Cheyne-Stokes respiration in heart failure over a six month period. *Heart.* 2006;92:337-42.

140. Javaheri S, Parker TJ, Wexler L, et al. Effect of theophylline on sleep-disordered breathing in heart failure. *N Engl J Med*. 1996;335:562-7.
141. Javaheri S. Acetazolamide improves central sleep apnea in heart failure: a double-blind, prospective study. *Am J Respir Crit Care Med*. 2006;173:234-7.
142. Wang J, Wang Y, Feng J, et al. Complex sleep apnea syndrome. *Patient Prefer Adherence*. 2013;7:633-41.
143. Morgenthaler TI, Kagramanov V, Hanak V, et al. Complex sleep apnea syndrome: is it a unique clinical syndrome? *Sleep*. 2006;29:1203-9.

CHAPTER 10

Systemic Effects of Sleep Related Breathing Disorders: Noncardiac

Gopi C Khilnani, Neetu Jain

INTRODUCTION

Obstructive sleep apnea (OSA) has emerged as a highly prevalent problem with pervasive, far reaching implications which are frequently encountered in clinical practice. It is estimated that the prevalence of OSA in obese adults ranges from 11% to 46% in women and 33% to 77% in men.[1] Moreover, with the ongoing epidemic of obesity, the prevalence is increasing all over the world. Over the past decade, there has been rising interest in systemic derangements associated with OSA. Though a wealth of both epidemiologic and experimental data have implicated OSA as a key culprit in increasing cardiovascular risk,[2-4] other systemic effects of OSA like those on metabolic, cerebrovascular etc. are increasingly being recognized. The biggest challenge lies in disentangling these relationships and implicating OSA as independent risk factor for these systemic effects notwithstanding the common risk factors. This can only happen when the underlying pathophysiological mechanisms are clear and treatment of OSA by continuous positive airway pressure (CPAP) shows convincing improvement. However, one thing is certain that OSA is emerging as a disorder with multisystem involvement, with several effects on many important organ-systems.

Obstructive sleep apnea is a state of intense local and systemic inflammation.[5] Its pathophysiology is strongly related with inflammatory cytokines in literature (Figure 1).[6,7] First evidence of inflammation of upper airways in patients with OSAS was obtained by Rubinstien in 1995 when he found polymorphonuclear leukocytes in their nasal mucosa.[8] Later many studies supported the presence of nasal and oropharyngeal inflammation in OSA. Intermittent hypoxia and reoxygenation may trigger a proinflammatory state by release of inflammatory markers like tumor necrosis factor-α (TNFα).[9] Obesity and mechanical stress upon upper airways due to snoring have also been proposed as cause of inflammation in OSA. However, much less data is available on effects of CPAP on airway inflammation and consistent improvement is not seen in studies.[10,11]

METABOLIC EFFECTS OF OSA

There is increase in the prevalence of obesity all over the world including developing countries. The consequences of obesity are manifold which include hypertension, type 2 diabetes, glucose intolerance, insulin resistance, and sleep

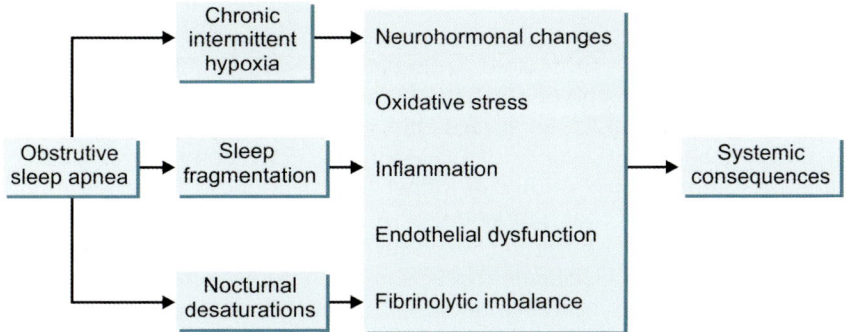

Figure 1: Mechanisms leading to systemic consequences of obstructive sleep apnea.

apnea. OSA has been found to be independently associated with individual components of metabolic dysfunction as well as increased prevalence of metabolic syndrome.[12-15] The prevalence of metabolic syndrome in patients with OSA varies between 50% to more than 80% among various studies.[13-21] Patients with severe OSA showed significantly higher metabolic index as compared to patients with mild to moderate OSA. However, this independent association was not strongly replicated in the studies which tested effect of CPAP use in such patients but emerging data points towards improvement in metabolic parameters.[22-25]

Obstructive Sleep Apnea and Type 2 diabetes Mellitus

It is becoming increasingly evident that normal sleep has an important role in glucose homeostasis.[26-29] It has been suggested that even partial loss of sleep is associated with glucose intolerance and abnormal sleep wake cycle can disrupt the corticotropic, thyrotropic, and somatotropic pathways.[30,31] Disruption of normal sleep wake cycle is an essential part of sleep apnea syndrome. A large number of studies have inferred that OSA is associated with diabetes, insulin resistance, and glucose intolerance independent of obesity.[32,33] These two conditions share similar risk factors such as male sex, advancing age, and obesity especially the abdominal adiposity. The prevalence of type 2 diabetes mellitus in OSA varies for 15–30% in various studies depending on study population, definition of OSA severity and methods to diagnose type 2 diabetes mellitus.[34-39] Few studies have reported relationship between OSA severity and the prevalence of diabetes.[36,38,40,41] This was found to be more evident in patients with excessive sleepiness which may be associated with adverse metabolic outcomes.[38] At the same time increasing severity of oxygen desaturations and intermittent nocturnal hypoxia was found to be associated with increased risk of developing type 2 diabetes.[42,43] Finally, type 2 diabetes was found to be more prevalent in patients with OSA but it is still not clear whether OSA leads to development of type 2 diabetes.

On the other hand, the prevalence of OSA in diabetes is as high as 71% combining the results of five important studies.[44-48] However, a retrospective analysis which included a large number of patients, showed that only 18% of the diabetic patients carried the diagnosis of OSA.[49] This shows that OSA is largely underestimated in patients with diabetes.

In the patients already diagnosed with diabetes, it is thought that OSA adversely affects the glycemic control which is directly related with severity of OSA.[50,51] Compared with patients without OSA the adjusted mean glycosylated hemoglobin (HbA1c) was 7.3% in mild OSA, 7.7% in moderate OSA, and 9.7% in severe OSA.[52] It was found that a most robust relationship between severity of OSA and glycemic control was observed with polysomnographic studies of longer than 4 hours.[34] There is sufficient evidence to suggest that untreated OSA may be associated with poorer glycemic control. These findings may have clinical implications in patients with type 2 diabetes especially those who are not controlled with adequate pharmacological and non-pharmacological therapy. Management of OSA with CPAP may emerge as adjuvant therapeutic strategy in such patients for better glycemic control. Many uncontrolled and randomized controlled trial have examined the role of CPAP in glycemic control. Most employed a sham CPAP in control arm and most of these studies were done in men. Only two of these reported positive findings during the study period.[53,54]

Insulin Resistance and Glucose Intolerance in Obstructive Sleep Apnea

Prevalence of impaired fasting glucose or impaired glucose tolerance is significantly higher in patients with OSA, ranging from 20–67%.[35,40,55,56] The degree of this association is similar in obese and non-obese patients.[56] Hence, the patients with OSA have lower insulin sensitivity as compared to patients without OSA after adjusting for the confounders. In a recent study, it was found that patients with mild, moderate, or severe OSA showed a 26.7%, 36.5%, and 43.7% decrease in insulin sensitivity after controlling for the common factors such as age, gender, race, and percentage body fat.[57] It was found that insulin resistance in OSA patients is independently associated with the severity of nocturnal desaturations and intermittent hypoxia.[58] Overall, studies strongly support association between OSA and insulin resistance and glucose intolerance with central adiposity being an important confounder.[34,59]

Potential Mechanisms

The two important attributes of OSA, intermittent hypoxia and sleep fragmentation, can lead to derangement in glucose metabolism by several mechanisms including activations of sympathetic nervous system and hypothalamic-pituitary axis, and changes in the inflammatory pathways.[60-63] Other possible mechanisms include hypoxic injury to pancreas and potential alteration in central pathways for glycemic control.[64]

Obstructive Sleep Apnea and Metabolic Consequence of Obesity

It is seen that OSA and obesity share some mechanisms, with a potential synergistic effects when the two conditions are seen together.[1,65] It was seen that patients with OSA have higher visceral fat accumulation, though subcutaneous fat may not be much different and similarly the amount of abdominal visceral fat showed more correlation with severity of OSA than body mass index (BMI).[66,67] Increased neck circumference which is a marker of visceral adiposity is frequently associated with OSA.[68]

Obstructive Sleep Apnea and Liver Damage

Liver steatosis is an important consequence of metabolic syndrome. A few studies have reported worsening of liver function in obese patients with OSA.[68] Those with OSA have higher shift from simple steatosis to nonalcoholic steatohepatitis (NASH) as compared with other obese patients. Chronic intermittent hypoxia is considered as most important underlying pathogenetic mechanism for liver involvement in patients with OSA.[69] Morbidly obese patients with OSA who underwent bariatric surgery were studied and on liver biopsy and polysomnography a strong association between nocturnal intermittent hypoxia and liver abnormalities was elucidated.[70,71]

There is little literature on liver function and morphology in non-morbidly obese patients with OSA. There is still no literature on the role of CPAP as a treatment strategy in such patients.

Management Considerations

Several studies have examined the role of CPAP in improving glycemic control, insulin sensitivity, and glucose intolerance. None of the studies found any benefit with the use of CPAP in patients with metabolic derangements other then the subset with hypertension.[72-74] Similar results were replicated by the studies looking at the visceral adiposity and no difference is seen with the use of CPAP. Still CPAP is the most important intervention to improve quality of life in these individuals. Second important management strategy, is lifestyle modification which mainly consists of diet and exercise and finally overall behavioral modification. There is lack of data on specific dietary intervention, exercise strategy, or intensity of weight loss recommended for these patients. Obesity is the most modifiable factor among these patients and a 10% weight loss translates in 26% reduction in the severity of OSA.[75] Emphasis of the lifestyle modification should be on reduction of central adiposity and visceral fat.[76] Several randomized control trial have compared the benefits of intensive lifestyle changes and routine care in these patients.[76-78] Definite benefit was reported with very low calorie diets, supervised exercise programs, and tailored dietary advice. However, a typical profile of an OSA patient with day time sleepiness and lack of energy may compromise ability of individuals to sustain such programs. Hence, individually tailored exercise plans are required.[79]

It is recommended that these patients should receive individually tailored integrated health services which include lifestyle modifications along with CPAP and these strategies should be supervised to ensure adherence.

NEUROCOGNITIVE EFFECTS

It is known for sometime now, that neurocognitive deficits occur with high frequency in patients with OSA.[80] The prevalence of neurocognitive dysfunction due to sleep related breathing disorders (SRBD) may be high because of the high prevalence of SRBD in the population and most of it being untreated.[81] Both males as well as females are affected. It was found to be more common with middle-aged though children are also at risk. Some cognitive dysfunction is seen in children who snore without significant OSA, hence even those with mild symptoms are at risk.[82] However, exact prevalence of these symptoms amongst patients with OSA is not known. A prospective study has shown that almost one in four patients with OSA suffers from cognitive dysfunction.[83] It has been found to be associated with specific neurocognitive problems such as verbal fluency, memory, attention, and perception.[83]

Patterns of Cognitive Impairment in Obstructive Sleep Apnea: Which Domains?

Most commonly reported cognitive deficits in sleep apnea patients are decreased attention and vigilance.[84] Thus, practically most important impairment affecting the normal life is the driving performance and is found in almost all untreated OSA patients.[85] Two areas of neurocognitive abnormalities have been studied: "cognitive function" and "psychomotor performance". The cognitive function includes attention, memory and executive functions while overall intelligence is spared.[84,86,87] The effect of OSAS on visual and verbal memory is not well established, however, is known to cause decline in reasoning, comprehension and learning.[80,88,89] It significantly impairs these higher executive functions. Involvement of prefrontal cortex, particularly the dorsolateral part and anterior cingulated has been found on functional brain imaging.[90-92] It is found that prefrontal cortex requires restoration by consolidated sleep and there are metabolic changes after sleep deprivation which was confirmed on functional neuroimaging studies.[80] While talking about the specifically affected neuropsychological domain one must take in to account underlying cognitive slowing which may be affecting all the domains.

It seems the cognitive functions that are related to attention are impaired the most which include attention span, divided attention, and sustained attention.[93] Fine motor coordination is impaired although motor speed is unaffected.[87,94] Sustained attention or vigilance is measured by Steer clear performance test and Psychomotor vigilance test (Table 1).[95]

Table 1: Tests for neurocognitive dysfunction	
Wechsler Adult Intelligence Scale-Revised	Test for intelligence
	Measures four indices: • Verbal comprehension • Working memory • Perceptual reasoning • Processing speed
Psychomotor vigilance task	Test for vigilance or sustained attention
	Patient has to press a button when a light appear randomly every few seconds for 5–10 minutes
Steer clear performance test	Test for vigilance or sustained attention
	Patient presses a button to avoid obstacles that appear randomly in two lanes
Repetitive finger tapping	Test for motor functioning
	One has to press a switch repeatedly as fast as possible with index finger
Digit span	Test for working and short-term memory
	Depends upon strings of digits of increasing length one can recall in correct serial order or reverse order after hearing or seeing them

Obstructive sleep apnea is typically associated with mild cognitive dysfunction which is measurable, may be a part of aging process in which functional abilities are spared. It is important as it may be a risk factor for Alzheimer's disease.[96] So the patients who show mild cognitive dysfunction should be evaluated for OSA considering the treatability of this condition.

The Relationship Between the Obstructive Sleep Apnea and Neurocognitive Dysfunction

While most of the studies link severity of OSA and cognitive dysfunction, a recent study found no correlation between apnea-hypopnea index and cognitive dysfunction, however, it linked cognitive abnormalities in patients with OSA with oxygen desaturation.[97] This point towards variability in literature while linking these two disorders.

Other important consideration while exploring this relationship between OSA and cognitive impairment is the overlapping risk factors (Table 2). These should be understood before establishing OSA as the cause of deficits such as attention, memory, and executive functions. It may be possible that a pre-existing cognitive impairment due to one of the risk factors may be exaggerated by OSA.[98-107] Hence, presence of sleep disordered breathing may be a double insult to brain which compromises its compensatory mechanisms to minimize challenge to cognitive function.

Pathophysiology

Repeated obstructive events lead to hypoxemia, hypercapnia, and increased sympathetic activity. These obstructions are followed by arousals. This cycle of repeated obstruction and arousal leads to disturbed sleep architecture and cognitive decline.[108] Overall, sleep fragmentation, sleep deprivation, and excessive daytime sleepiness have been proposed as possible mechanism of

Table 2: Common risk factors for cognitive impairment and OSA[98-107]	
Genetics	Down syndrome
	Craniofacial abnormalities
	ApoE4 gene abnormality
Co-morbidities	Diabetes
	Hypertension
	Obesity
	Hypothyroidism
	Stroke
	CAD
Demographic profile	Advancing Age
	Male sex
Severity of OSA	Nocturnal intermittent hypoxia
	Sleep fragmentation
	Low Mean nocturnal SpO$_2$
	Excessive day time sleepiness

CAD, coronary artery disease; OSA, obstructive sleep apnea.

neurocognitive decline mainly due to impact on attention. At the same time, cognitive decline correlated with mean nocturnal SpO$_2$.[109] Excessive daytime somnolence needs special mention as it may be responsible for some of the unique feature of neurocognitive decline in OSA.

Another proposed mechanism is endothelial dysfunction due to hypoxia and reperfusion injury which leads to increased lipid peroxidation.[110,111] Oxidative stress leads to formation of reactive oxygen species or free radicals, which can in turn cause brain injury and induce a state of chronic inflammation.[112] Underlying mechanism for endothelium dysfunction may be an imbalance between vasoconstrictor (Endothelin-I, thromboxane) and vasodilator substances (nitric oxide, prostacyclin). Nitric oxide levels are found to be decreased in patients with OSA.[113]

Management Recommendations

Whenever a clinician is evaluating a case of OSA, the neuropsychological effects must be considered. Patients may have long-term problems in scholastic performance, occupation, and relationship. Sleep specialist should in all patients enquire about vigilance, executive functioning, and motor coordination. Patients may have problems related to memory as well though actual effect is unclear. Cognitive evaluation of the patient should be performed to include direct assessment of vigilance, executive functioning, and motor functioning. Tests such as Wechsler Adult Intelligence Scale-Revised, the Psychomotor Vigilance Task, the Steer Clear Performance Test, and tests of repetitive finger tapping may be used for neurocognitive assessment (Table 1).[86,88,114-116] The reverse is also important that people who have unexplained poor vigilance and compromised executive and motor function should be screened for SRBDs and should be referred to sleep specialists. In conclusion, whenever psychiatric or cognitive disabilities are found in relation with OSA, the SRBD must be treated. Functional neuroimaging studies are experimental and mostly used for research purpose. Presently these are not recommended for diagnosis of cognitive impairment in OSA.

Management

Continuous positive airway pressure is the mainstay for treatment for these patients. Several randomized trial have shown improvement in cognitive function after CPAP therapy as compared with untreated patients.[117-119] In some studies, cognitive function has shown only partial recovery even after resolution of day time somnolence with CPAP. Though Epworth sleepiness scores and attention problems improved with CPAP therapy, executive task performance remained impaired. In patients whom there is evidence that these symptoms are unresolved even after initiation CPAP for OSA, they should assessed thoroughly even after successful treatment and referred to mental health professionals as deemed necessary. Medications such as modafinil, armodafinil, and caffeine have found to improve attention, wakefulness, and memory when used as additional treatment in patients with OSA who shows partial response to CPAP. Several randomized control trials have shown that treatment with modafinil shows improved performance on psychomotor vigilance tests, fewer attention lapses and decreased reaction time.[120,121] This on practical level translates into better driving performance. Similar improvement in attention, memory, and vigilance are shown with use armodofinil and caffeine.[122,123]

OBSTRUCTIVE SLEEP APNEA AND PSYCHIATRIC DISORDERS

Obstructive sleep apnea has been linked with depression in many studies.[124,125] Depression is also defined as fatigue or energy loss or diminished ability to think or focus which is similar to OSA. Hence it is very difficult to establish a cause-effect relationship or an independent association due to uncanny similarities in the basic clinical manifestation of these two disorders.

The prevalence of these symptoms varies in these patients for 7% to 63%.[126-128] Coleman et al. found that more than one-third patients visiting sleep clinics with insomnia had psychiatric problems and more than half of these patients have major depressive symptoms.[129] Other psychiatric disorders associated with OSA include paranoia and personality disorders.[130] These patients were found to have higher mean apnea-hypopnea index (AHI) and showed improvement with use CPAP.[131,132] They were also found to have longer mean rapid eye movement (REM) sleep episode and greater sleep fragmentation. The degree of daytime sleepiness didn't correlate well with the degree of depression. The diagnostic utility of symptoms like tiredness, weight change, and sleep disturbance if limited in this population with overlap. Other symptoms which are not shared by these two disorders like excessive crying, self-blame etc. may be more useful.

It is recommended that all patients with OSA should be assessed by a psychiatrist to assess associated mental illnesses such as depression. If a patient does not respond to therapy via CPAP, pharmacotherapy may be recommended.

Cerebrovascular Consequences of Obstructive Sleep Apnea

The prevalence of OSA in patients with stroke and transient ischemic attack is greater than that of general population. Patients with stroke are 3–4 times more likely to have OSA than matched controls.[133,134] Sixty to seventy percent of people with stroke and transient ischemic attacks have AHI more than 10.[134,135] Obstructive sleep apneas are seven times more common than central apnea in patients with stroke.[135] The stroke risk is estimated to increase 6% with every unit increase in AHI between 5 and 25.[136] Similar results were reported by various studies and it was seen that the odds of stroke increase with increasing AHI.[137] Central apneas were infrequently seen in association with stroke.[137] However, determining OSA as a cause of stroke is difficult as the risk factors are similar for both the conditions. Further, most of the studies are done in patients, who already had stroke so it is difficult to determine if OSA was precedent to stroke. Nevertheless, it was found that even after adjustment for confounder and comorbidities, OSA was independently associated with stroke with compelling evidence.[2,136,138]

Obstructive sleep apnea is not only a risk factor for stroke it also compounds the effect of stroke and increases the risk of subsequent stroke. It increases the length of hospital stay and likelihood of death at 6 months.[139,140]

Cerebrovascular blood flow is compromised by OSA in patients with stroke. During an episode of apnea, pO_2 and pH decrease while pCO_2 increase leading to dilation cerebral vasculature in the healthy area resulting in stealing blood away from already compromised regions causing greater damage.[141] This is known as "Reversed Robin Hood Syndrome."[142] There is a sharp swing in blood pressure during an apneic episode consisting of rapid rise in blood pressure followed by rapid fall.[143,144] This exposes the vasculature to damaging pressures, resulting in endothelial damage and disruption of blood-brain barrier. The sharp decline leaves brain vulnerable to ischemia, leading to lacunar infarcts, small vessel disease, and leukoaraiosis.[145-147] Several molecular and cellular mechanisms are also involved like oxidative stress, inflammation, sympathetic activation, hypercoagulation, endothelial dysfunction, platelet aggregation, and metabolic dysfunction.[146,148]

Continuous positive airway pressure therapy especially in the acute stage after stroke is the mainstay of management. Although evidence in the literature is encouraging but it is not convincing regarding the beneficial effects of CPAP in patients with stroke and OSA.[149,150] In acute phase already compromised rates of blood flow to brain can be negatively affected by OSA. CPAP prevent blood steal by healthy areas of brain. Hence, CPAP therapy is important in acute phase to limit the damage to already involved region of brain.[151]

In a study by Martinez-Gracia it was found that subsequent cerebrovascular events were 5 times less in patient with stroke and OSA who used CPAP.[152] Hence, CPAP is likely to protect against newer vascular events after stroke. It is recommended for all patients of stroke with OSA. Compliance to CPAP is found to be similar or lower is these patients as compared with those without stroke.[153,154]

OBSTRUCTIVE SLEEP APNEA AND GASTROESOPHAGEAL REFLUX DISEASE

Gastroesophageal reflux disease (GERD) is a chronic disease characterized by acidic gastric content reflux in the esophagus leading to heartburn, regurgitation, pain in abdomen etc. It is a common condition all over the world and has similar risk factors as OSA which includes obesity, male sex, and alcoholism. It has been linked to OSA in many studies.[155,156] The frequency of nocturnal GERD in OSA patients ranges from 54% to 76%.[157] OSA has been found to be increasingly associated with *Helicobacter pylori* infection which has causative association with GERD.[158] In a study with 228 subjects, no correlation was seen between severity of OSA and severity of GERD related symptoms.[159] Despite this significant association, a cause-effect relationship is still not established. Several pathophysiological mechanisms have been proposed, one includes bronchial microaspiration of gastric contents leading to exudative mucosa reaction that partially obstructs the airway leading to OSA. Another theory is that reflux into hypopharynx cause inflammation which leads to weakening and edema worsening upper airway obstruction.[160] It is hypothesized that the negative intrathoracic pressure generated during inspiration is transmitted to the intrathoracic esopahgus leading to relaxation of lower esophageal sphincter and GERD. CPAP causes passive elevation of intraesophageal pressure and probably constriction of the esophageal sphincter. Hence, CPAP used for management of OSA is likely to improve GERD symptoms and acidic pH.[155,157,161] As GERD has impact on upper airway, in theory antireflux therapy should improve OSA symptoms but the evidence in favor of it is not convincing.[161,162] Nonetheless preliminary studies show that this kind of treatment may reduce some of the symptoms of OSA, hence further long-term studies are needed to elucidate effect of antireflux therapy on OSA related morbidity and mortality.

Impact of Obstructive Sleep Apnea on Chronic Kidney Disease

Obstructive sleep apnea is known to cause hypoxemia induce endothelial dysfunction, accelerated atherosclerosis, and altered cardiovascular hemodynamics which makes it a potential risk factor for renal disorders as well. The literature now suggests that it may disproportionately common among the patients with chronic kidney diseases (CKD) affecting almost 50% of the individual suffering from end stage renal disease (ESRD).[163,164] Patients suffering from OSA were found to have higher serum creatinine level.[165] Nocturnal hypoxia, AHI and desaturation index are important predictors of renal function decline.[166,167] Obesity is a risk factor for glomerular hyper filtration and proteinuria, hence is a potential confounder. Few studies have analyzed independent effect of OSA on CKD.[168,169] These studies showed improvement in proteinuria with treatment of OSA.

Chronic kidney disease leads to fluid overload and in recumbent position this fluid may accumulate in the neck area causing increased upper airway resistance leading to OSA. Hence, CKD is a risk factor for OSA. It was found that serum urea was predictive of OSA and it was more prevalent among patients with ESRD than less severe CKD.[170] AHI improves with nocturnal renal replacement therapy.[163]

ERECTILE DYSFUNCTION

Sleep apnea seems to have independent effect on sexual function in men but is largely confounded by obesity which has major role both in OSA and erectile dysfunction. Association of OSA and erectile dysfunction is frequent with almost 70% patients with OSA having erectile dysfunction.[171] The well established male preponderance in OSA points towards the role of gonadal hormones. Testosterone is known to increase the ventilatory response to hypoxia in hypogonadal men which may exacerbate sleep apnea by driving CO_2 below the apnea threshold. Few studies have examined the role of testosterone in upper airway resistance.[172] Decreased morning testosterone level is seen in male apneics.[173] Hypoxia may be a factor in reducing the testosterone levels regardless of obesity.[171] Other factors have also been studied. Nitric oxide which is responsible for vasodilation and erection is lowered in OSA. Hypoxia may cause release of endothelin which with strong vasoconstrictor activity may affect penile vasculature. Endothelial dysfunction seems to be one of the most important factors responsible for erectile dysfunction. According to meta-analysis, use of CPAP results in significant improvement.[174]

OTHER POTENTIAL CONSEQUENCES OF OBSTRUCTIVE SLEEP APNEA

Obstructive sleep apnea has been found to be associated with high risk for osteoporosis.[175] The nature of this association needs to be clarified and potential confounders need to elucidated. The effect of CPAP on bone mineral density and bone quality need further research also the potential pathogenic mechanism behind this association need to be addressed.

Obstructive sleep apnea has been found to be associated with awakening headaches which may be mild to moderate in severity, usually occur for about 30 minutes after getting up. Eighty percent of these headaches respond to treatment of OSA with CPAP.[176] A relationship has been documented between OSA and growth retardation among children. There was improvement in height after treatment of OSA.[177]

CONCLUSION

Obstructive sleep apnea is fast emerging as a multisystem disorder with far reaching consequences on the various organ systems of the body. While the inflammatory cascade is held responsible for these effects, the exact pathogenetic mechanisms still need to be elucidated.

REFERENCES

1. Young T, Peppard PE, Taheri S. Excess weight and sleep-disordered breathing. *J Appl Physiol* (1985). 2005;99(4):1592-9.
2. Yaggi HK, Concato J, Kernan WN, et al. Obstructive sleep apnea as a risk factor for stroke and death. *N Engl J Med.* 2005;353(19):2034-41.
3. Young T, Finn L, Peppard PE, et al. Sleep disordered breathing and mortality: eighteen-year follow-up of the Wisconsin sleep cohort. *Sleep.* 2008;31(8):1071-8.
4. Redline S, Yenokyan G, Gottlieb DJ, et al. Obstructive sleep apnea-hypopnea and incident stroke: the sleep heart health study. *Am J Respir Crit Care Med.* 2010;182(2):269-77.
5. Alam I, Lewis K, Stephens JW, et al. Obesity, metabolic syndrome and sleep apnoea: all pro-inflammatory states. *Obes Rev.* 2007;8(2):119-27.
6. Krueger JM, Obal FJ, Fang J, et al. The role of cytokines in physiological sleep regulation. *Ann N Y Acad Sci.* 2001;933:211-21.
7. Entzian P, Linnemann K, Schlaak M, et al. Obstructive sleep apnea syndrome and circadian rhythms of hormones and cytokines. *Am J Respir Crit Care Med.* 1996;153(3):1080-6.
8. Rubinstein I. Nasal inflammation in patients with obstructive sleep apnea. *Laryngoscope.* 1995;105(2):175-7.
9. Minoguchi K, Tazaki T, Yokoe T, et al. Elevated production of tumor necrosis factor-alpha by monocytes in patients with obstructive sleep apnea syndrome. *Chest.* 2004;126(5):1473-9.
10. Skoczynski S, Ograbek-Krol M, Tazbirek M, et al. Short-term CPAP treatment induces a mild increase in inflammatory cells in patients with sleep apnoea syndrome. *Rhinology.* 2008;46(2):144-50.
11. Devouassoux G, Levy P, Rossini E, et al. Sleep apnea is associated with bronchial inflammation and continuous positive airway pressure-induced airway hyper-responsiveness. *J Allergy Clin Immunol.* 2007;119(3):597-603.
12. Coughlin SR, Mawdsley L, Mugarza JA, et al. Obstructive sleep apnoea is independently associated with an increased prevalence of metabolic syndrome. *Eur Heart J.* 2004;25(9):735-41.
13. Lam JC, Lam B, Lam CL, et al. Obstructive sleep apnea and the metabolic syndrome in community-based Chinese adults in Hong Kong. *Respir Med.* 2006;100(6):980-7.
14. Sasanabe R, Banno K, Otake K, et al. Metabolic syndrome in Japanese patients with obstructive sleep apnea syndrome. *Hypertens Res.* 2006;29(5):315-22.
15. Gruber A, Horwood F, Sithole J, et al. Obstructive sleep apnoea is independently associated with the metabolic syndrome but not insulin resistance state. *Cardiovasc Diabetol.* 2006;5:22.
16. Drager LF, Queiroz EL, Lopes HF, et al. Obstructive sleep apnea is highly prevalent and correlates with impaired glycemic control in consecutive patients with the metabolic syndrome. *J Cardiometab Syndr.* 2009;4(2):89-95.
17. Parish JM, Adam T, Facchiano L. Relationship of metabolic syndrome and obstructive sleep apnea. *J Clin Sleep Med.* 2007;3(5):467-72.
18. Shiina K, Tomiyama H, Takata Y, et al. Concurrent presence of metabolic syndrome in obstructive sleep apnea syndrome exacerbates the cardiovascular risk: a sleep clinic cohort study. *Hypertens Res.* 2006;29(6):433-41.

19. Peled N, Kassirer M, Shitrit D, et al. The association of OSA with insulin resistance, inflammation and metabolic syndrome. *Respir Med.* 2007;101(8):1696-701.
20. Agrawal S, Sharma SK, Sreenivas V, et al. Prevalence of metabolic syndrome in a north Indian hospital-based population with obstructive sleep apnoea. *Indian J Med Res.* 2011;134(5):639-44.
21. Akahoshi T, Uematsu A, Akashiba T, et al. Obstructive sleep apnoea is associated with risk factors comprising the metabolic syndrome. *Respirology.* 2010;15(7):1122-6.
22. Coughlin SR, Mawdsley L, Mugarza JA, et al. Cardiovascular and metabolic effects of CPAP in obese males with OSA. *Eur Respir J.* 2007;29(4):720-7.
23. Ambrosetti M, Lucioni AM, Conti S, et al. Metabolic syndrome in obstructive sleep apnea and related cardiovascular risk. *J Cardiovasc Med (Hagerstown).* 2006;7(11):826-9.
24. Oktay B, Akbal E, Firat H, et al. CPAP treatment in the coexistence of obstructive sleep apnea syndrome and metabolic syndrome, results of one year follow up. *Acta Clin Belg.* 2009;64(4):329-34.
25. Mota PC, Drummond M, Winck JC, et al. APAP impact on metabolic syndrome in obstructive sleep apnea patients. *Sleep Breath.* 2010;15(4):665-72.
26. VanHelder T, Symons JD, Radomski MW. Effects of sleep deprivation and exercise on glucose tolerance. *Aviat Space Environ Med.* 1993;64(6):487-92.
27. Spiegel K, Leproult R, L'Hermite-Baleriaux M, et al. Leptin levels are dependent on sleep duration: relationships with sympathovagal balance, carbohydrate regulation, cortisol, and thyrotropin. *J Clin Endocrinol Metab.* 2004;89(11):5762-71.
28. Kahn SE, Prigeon RL, McCulloch DK, et al. Quantification of the relationship between insulin sensitivity and beta-cell function in human subjects. Evidence for a hyperbolic function. *Diabetes.* 1993;42(11):1663-72.
29. Catalano PM, Tyzbir ED, Wolfe RR, et al. Carbohydrate metabolism during pregnancy in control subjects and women with gestational diabetes. *Am J Physiol.* 1993;264(1 Pt 1):E60-7.
30. Spiegel K, Leproult R, Colecchia EF, et al. Adaptation of the 24-h growth hormone profile to a state of sleep debt. *Am J Physiol Regul Integr Comp Physiol.* 2000;279(3):R874-83.
31. Irwin MR, Wang M, Campomayor CO, et al. Sleep deprivation and activation of morning levels of cellular and genomic markers of inflammation. *Arch Intern Med.* 2006;166(16):1756-62.
32. Punjabi NM, Ahmed MM, Polotsky VY, et al. Sleep-disordered breathing, glucose intolerance, and insulin resistance. *Respir Physiol Neurobiol.* 2003;136(2-3):167-78.
33. Ip M, Mokhlesi B. Sleep and glucose intolerance/diabetes mellitus. *Sleep Med Clin.* 2007;2(1):19-29.
34. Pamidi S, Tasali E. Obstructive sleep apnea and type 2 diabetes: is there a link? *Front Neurol.* 2012;3:126.
35. Meslier N, Gagnadoux F, Giraud P, et al. Impaired glucose-insulin metabolism in males with obstructive sleep apnoea syndrome. *Eur Respir J.* 2003;22(1):156-60.
36. Reichmuth KJ, Austin D, Skatrud JB, et al. Association of sleep apnea and type II diabetes: a population-based study. *Am J Respir Crit Care Med.* 2005;172(12):1590-5.
37. Mahmood K, Akhter N, Eldeirawi K, et al. Prevalence of type 2 diabetes in patients with obstructive sleep apnea in a multi-ethnic sample. *J Clin Sleep Med.* 2009;5(3):215-21.
38. Ronksley PE, Hemmelgarn BR, Heitman SJ, et al. Obstructive sleep apnoea is associated with diabetes in sleepy subjects. *Thorax.* 2009;64(10):834-9.
39. Fredheim JM, Rollheim J, Omland T, et al. Type 2 diabetes and pre-diabetes are associated with obstructive sleep apnea in extremely obese subjects: a cross-sectional study. *Cardiovasc Diabetol.* 2011;10:84.
40. Tamura A, Kawano Y, Watanabe T, et al. Relationship between the severity of obstructive sleep apnea and impaired glucose metabolism in patients with obstructive sleep apnea. *Respir Med.* 2008;102(10):1412-6.
41. Samson P, Casey KR, Knepler J, et al. Clinical characteristics, comorbidities, and response to treatment of veterans with obstructive sleep apnea, Cincinnati Veterans Affairs Medical Center, 2005-2007. *Prev Chronic Dis.* 2012;9:E46.
42. Lindberg E, Theorell-Haglow J, Svensson M, et al. Sleep apnea and glucose metabolism: a long-term follow-up in a community-based sample. *Chest.* 2012;142(4):935-42.

43. Muraki I, Tanigawa T, Yamagishi K, et al. Nocturnal intermittent hypoxia and the development of type 2 diabetes: the Circulatory Risk in Communities Study (CIRCS). *Diabetologia.* 2010;53(3):481-8.
44. Resnick HE, Redline S, Shahar E, et al. Diabetes and sleep disturbances: findings from the Sleep Heart Health Study. *Diabetes Care.* 2003;26(3):702-9.
45. Einhorn D, Stewart DA, Erman MK, et al. Prevalence of sleep apnea in a population of adults with type 2 diabetes mellitus. *Endocr Pract.* 2007;13(4):355-62.
46. Foster GD, Sanders MH, Millman R, et al. Obstructive sleep apnea among obese patients with type 2 diabetes. *Diabetes Care.* 2009;32(6):1017-9.
47. Laaban JP, Daenen S, Leger D, et al. Prevalence and predictive factors of sleep apnoea syndrome in type 2 diabetic patients. *Diabetes Metab.* 2009;35(5):372-7.
48. Aronsohn RS, Whitmore H, Van Cauter E, et al. Impact of untreated obstructive sleep apnea on glucose control in type 2 diabetes. *Am J Respir Crit Care Med.* 2010;181(5):507-13.
49. Heffner JE, Rozenfeld Y, Kai M, et al. Prevalence of diagnosed sleep apnea among patients with type 2 diabetes in primary care. *Chest.* 2012;141(6):1414-21.
50. Pillai A, Warren G, Gunathilake W, et al. Effects of sleep apnea severity on glycemic control in patients with type 2 diabetes prior to continuous positive airway pressure treatment. *Diabetes Technol Ther.* 2011;13(9):945-9.
51. Fendri S, Rose D, Myambu S, et al. Nocturnal hyperglycaemia in type 2 diabetes with sleep apnoea syndrome. *Diabetes Res Clin Pract.* 2011;91(1):e21-3.
52. Aronsohn RS, Whitmore H, Van Cauter E, Tasali E. Impact of untreated obstructive sleep apnea on glucose control in type 2 diabetes. *Am J Respir Crit Care Med.* 2010;181(5):507-13.
53. Lam JC, Lam B, Yao TJ, et al. A randomised controlled trial of nasal continuous positive airway pressure on insulin sensitivity in obstructive sleep apnoea. *Eur Respir J.* 2010;35(1):138-45.
54. Weinstock TG, Wang X, Rueschman M, et al. A controlled trial of CPAP therapy on metabolic control in individuals with impaired glucose tolerance and sleep apnea. *Sleep.* 2012;35(5):617-25B.
55. Fredheim JM, Rollheim J, Omland T, et al. Type 2 diabetes and pre-diabetes are associated with obstructive sleep apnea in extremely obese subjects: a cross-sectional study. *Cardiovasc Diabetol.* 2011;10:84.
56. Seicean S, Kirchner HL, Gottlieb DJ, et al. Sleep-disordered breathing and impaired glucose metabolism in normal-weight and overweight/obese individuals: the Sleep Heart Health Study. *Diabetes Care.* 2008;31(5):1001-6.
57. Punjabi NM, Beamer BA. Alterations in Glucose Disposal in Sleep-disordered Breathing. *Am J Respir Crit Care Med.* 2009;179(3):235-40.
58. Oltmanns KM, Gehring H, Rudolf S, et al. Hypoxia causes glucose intolerance in humans. *Am J Respir Crit Care Med.* 2004;169(11):1231-7.
59. Kono M, Tatsumi K, Saibara T, et al. Obstructive sleep apnea syndrome is associated with some components of metabolic syndrome. *Chest.* 2007;131(5):1387-92.
60. Dimsdale JE, Coy T, Ziegler MG, et al. The effect of sleep apnea on plasma and urinary catecholamines. *Sleep.* 1995;18(5):377-81.
61. Narkiewicz K, Somers VK. Sympathetic nerve activity in obstructive sleep apnoea. *Acta Physiol Scand.* 2003;177(3):385-90.
62. Marrone O, Riccobono L, Salvaggio A, et al. Catecholamines and blood pressure in obstructive sleep apnea syndrome. *Chest.* 1993;103(3):722-7.
63. Parlapiano C, Borgia MC, Minni A, et al. Cortisol circadian rhythm and 24-hour Holter arterial pressure in OSAS patients. *Endocr Res.* 2005;31(4):371-4.
64. Lechin F, van der Dijs B. Central nervous system circuitry involved in the hyperinsulinism syndrome. *Neuroendocrinology.* 2006;84(4):222-34.
65. Sharma SK, Kumpawat S, Banga A, et al. Prevalence and risk factors of obstructive sleep apnea syndrome in a population of Delhi, India. *Chest.* 2006;130(1):149-56.
66. Vgontzas AN, Papanicolaou DA, Bixler EO, et al. Sleep apnea and daytime sleepiness and fatigue: relation to visceral obesity, insulin resistance, and hypercytokinemia. *J Clin Endocrinol Metab.* 2000;85(3):1151-8.

67. Fantuzzi G. Adipose tissue, adipokines, and inflammation. *J Allergy Clin Immunol.* 2005;115(5):911-9; quiz 20.
68. Bonsignore MR, Borel AL, Machan E, et al. Sleep apnoea and metabolic dysfunction. *Eur Respir Rev.* 2013;22(129):353-64.
69. Mirrakhimov AE, Polotsky VY. Obstructive sleep apnea and non-alcoholic Fatty liver disease: is the liver another target? *Front Neurol.* 2012;3:149.
70. Aron-Wisnewsky J, Minville C, Tordjman J, et al. Chronic intermittent hypoxia is a major trigger for non-alcoholic fatty liver disease in morbid obese. *J Hepatol.* 2012;56(1):225-33.
71. Polotsky VY, Patil SP, Savransky V, et al. Obstructive sleep apnea, insulin resistance, and steatohepatitis in severe obesity. *Am J Respir Crit Care Med.* 2009;179(3):228-34.
72. Becker HF, Jerrentrup A, Ploch T, et al. Effect of nasal continuous positive airway pressure treatment on blood pressure in patients with obstructive sleep apnea. *Circulation.* 2003;107(1):68-73.
73. Montserrat JM, Ferrer M, Hernandez L, et al. Effectiveness of CPAP treatment in daytime function in sleep apnea syndrome: a randomized controlled study with an optimized placebo. *Am J Respir Crit Care Med.* 2001;164(4):608-13.
74. Douglas NJ, Engleman HM. Effects of CPAP on vigilance and related functions in patients with the sleep apnea/hypopnea syndrome. *Sleep.* 2000;23 Suppl 4:S147-9.
75. Peppard PE, Young T, Palta M, et al. Longitudinal study of moderate weight change and sleep-disordered breathing. *JAMA.* 2000;284(23):3015-21.
76. Despres JP, Lemieux I, Prud'homme D. Treatment of obesity: need to focus on high risk abdominally obese patients. *BMJ.* 2001;322(7288):716-20.
77. Foster GD, Borradaile KE, Sanders MH, et al. A randomized study on the effect of weight loss on obstructive sleep apnea among obese patients with type 2 diabetes: the Sleep AHEAD study. *Arch Intern Med.* 2009;169(17):1619-26.
78. Tuomilehto HP, Seppa JM, Partinen MM, et al. Lifestyle intervention with weight reduction: first-line treatment in mild obstructive sleep apnea. *Am J Respir Crit Care Med.* 2009;179(4):320-7.
79. Kline CE, Crowley EP, Ewing GB, et al. Blunted heart rate recovery is improved following exercise training in overweight adults with obstructive sleep apnea. *Int J Cardiol.* 2013;167(4):1610-5.
80. Beebe DW, Gozal D. Obstructive sleep apnea and the prefrontal cortex: towards a comprehensive model linking nocturnal upper airway obstruction to daytime cognitive and behavioral deficits. *J Sleep Res.* 2002;11(1):1-16.
81. Young T, Palta M, Dempsey J, et al. The occurrence of sleep-disordered breathing among middle-aged adults. *N Engl J Med.* 1993;328(17):1230-5.
82. Brockmann PE, Urschitz MS, Schlaud M, et al. Primary snoring in school children: prevalence and neurocognitive impairments. *Sleep Breath.* 2012;16(1):23-9.
83. Antonelli Incalzi R, Marra C, Salvigni BL, et al. Does cognitive dysfunction conform to a distinctive pattern in obstructive sleep apnea syndrome? *J Sleep Res.* 2004;13(1):79-86.
84. Mazza S, Pepin JL, Naegele B, et al. Most obstructive sleep apnoea patients exhibit vigilance and attention deficits on an extended battery of tests. *Eur Respir J.* 2005;25(1):75-80.
85. Lloberes P, Levy G, Descals C, et al. Self-reported sleepiness while driving as a risk factor for traffic accidents in patients with obstructive sleep apnoea syndrome and in non-apnoeic snorers. *Respir Med.* 2000;94(10):971-6.
86. Archbold KH, Borghesani PR, Mahurin RK, et al. Neural activation patterns during working memory tasks and OSA disease severity: preliminary findings. *J Clin Sleep Med.* 2009;5(1):21-7.
87. Bedard MA, Montplaisir J, Richer F, et al. Obstructive sleep apnea syndrome: pathogenesis of neuropsychological deficits. *J Clin Exp Neuropsychol.* 1991;13(6):950-64.
88. Naismith S, Winter V, Gotsopoulos H, et al. Neurobehavioral functioning in obstructive sleep apnea: differential effects of sleep quality, hypoxemia and subjective sleepiness. *J Clin Exp Neuropsychol.* 2004;26(1):43-54.
89. Wong KK, Grunstein RR, Bartlett DJ, et al. Brain function in obstructive sleep apnea: results from the Brain Resource International Database. *J Integr Neurosci.* 2006;5(1):111-21.

90. O'Donoghue FJ, Briellmann RS, Rochford PD, et al. Cerebral structural changes in severe obstructive sleep apnea. *Am J Respir Crit Care Med.* 2005;171(10):1185-90.
91. Macey PM, Henderson LA, Macey KE, et al. Brain morphology associated with obstructive sleep apnea. *Am J Respir Crit Care Med.* 2002;166(10):1382-7.
92. Morrell MJ, McRobbie DW, Quest RA, et al. Changes in brain morphology associated with obstructive sleep apnea. *Sleep Med.* 2003;4(5):451-4.
93. Beebe DW, Groesz L, Wells C, et al. The neuropsychological effects of obstructive sleep apnea: a meta-analysis of norm-referenced and case-controlled data. *Sleep.* 2003;26(3):298-307.
94. Greenberg GD, Watson RK, Deptula D. Neuropsychological dysfunction in sleep apnea. *Sleep.* 1987;10(3):254-62.
95. Sforza E, Haba-Rubio J, De Bilbao F, et al. Performance vigilance task and sleepiness in patients with sleep-disordered breathing. *Eur Respir J.* 2004;24(2):279-85.
96. Caselli RJ. Obstructive sleep apnea, apolipoprotein E e4, and mild cognitive impairment. *Sleep Med.* 2008;9(8):816-7.
97. Quan SF, Chan CS, Dement WC, et al. The association between obstructive sleep apnea and neurocognitive performance--the Apnea Positive Pressure Long-term Efficacy Study (APPLES). *Sleep.* 2011;34(3):303-14B.
98. Ayalon L, Ancoli-Israel S, Drummond SP. Obstructive sleep apnea and age: a double insult to brain function? *Am J Respir Crit Care Med.* 2010;182(3):413-9.
99. Petersen RC, Roberts RO, Knopman DS, et al. Prevalence of mild cognitive impairment is higher in men. The Mayo Clinic Study of Aging. *Neurology.* 2010;75(10):889-97.
100. Guindalini C, Colugnati FA, Pellegrino R, et al. Influence of genetic ancestry on the risk of obstructive sleep apnoea syndrome. *Eur Respir J.* 2010;36(4):834-41.
101. Kadotani H, Kadotani T, Young T, et al. Association between apolipoprotein E epsilon4 and sleep-disordered breathing in adults. *JAMA.* 2001;285(22):2888-90.
102. Elias MF, Elias PK, Sullivan LM, et al. Lower cognitive function in the presence of obesity and hypertension: the Framingham heart study. *Int J Obes Relat Metab Disord.* 2003;27(2):260-8.
103. Trois MS, Capone GT, Lutz JA, et al. Obstructive sleep apnea in adults with Down syndrome. *J Clin Sleep Med.* 2009;5(4):317-23.
104. Elmasry A, Lindberg E, Berne C, et al. Sleep-disordered breathing and glucose metabolism in hypertensive men: a population-based study. *J Intern Med.* 2001;249(2):153-61.
105. Parra O, Arboix A, Bechich S, et al. Time course of sleep-related breathing disorders in first-ever stroke or transient ischemic attack. *Am J Respir Crit Care Med.* 2000;161(2 Pt 1):375-80.
106. Osterweil D, Syndulko K, Cohen SN, et al. Cognitive function in non-demented older adults with hypothyroidism. *J Am Geriatr Soc.* 1992;40(4):325-35.
107. Redline S, Yenokyan G, Gottlieb DJ, et al. Obstructive sleep apnea-hypopnea and incident stroke: the sleep heart health study. *Am J Respir Crit Care Med.* 2010;182(2):269-77.
108. Ramesh V, Nair D, Zhang SX, et al. Disrupted sleep without sleep curtailment induces sleepiness and cognitive dysfunction via the tumor necrosis factor-alpha pathway. *J Neuroinflammation.* 2012;9:91.
109. Alchanatis M, Zias N, Deligiorgis N, et al. Comparison of cognitive performance among different age groups in patients with obstructive sleep apnea. *Sleep Breath.* 2008;12(1):17-24.
110. Lavie L. Obstructive sleep apnoea syndrome—an oxidative stress disorder. *Sleep Med Rev.* 2003;7(1):35-51.
111. Lavie L, Vishnevsky A, Lavie P. Evidence for lipid peroxidation in obstructive sleep apnea. *Sleep.* 2004;27(1):123-8.
112. Dyugovskaya L, Lavie P, Lavie L. Increased adhesion molecules expression and production of reactive oxygen species in leukocytes of sleep apnea patients. *Am J Respir Crit Care Med.* 2002;165(7):934-9.
113. Ip MS, Lam B, Chan LY, et al. Circulating nitric oxide is suppressed in obstructive sleep apnea and is reversed by nasal continuous positive airway pressure. *Am J Respir Crit Care Med.* 2000;162(6):2166-71.

114. Sforza E, Haba-Rubio J, De Bilbao F, et al. Performance vigilance task and sleepiness in patients with sleep-disordered breathing obstructive sleep apnea, apolipoprotein E e4, and mild cognitive impairment. *Eur Respir J.* 2004;24(2):279-85.
115. Findley L, Unverzagt M, Guchu R, et al. Vigilance and automobile accidents in patients with sleep apnea or narcolepsy. *Chest.* 1995;108(3):619-24.
116. Bedard MA, Montplaisir J, Malo J, et al. Persistent neuropsychological deficits and vigilance impairment in sleep apnea syndrome after treatment with continuous positive airways pressure (CPAP). *J Clin Exp Neuropsychol.* 1993;15(2):330-41.
117. Henke KG, Grady JJ, Kuna ST. Effect of nasal continuous positive airway pressure on neuropsychological function in sleep apnea-hypopnea syndrome. A randomized, placebo-controlled trial. *Am J Respir Crit Care Med.* 2001;163(4):911-7.
118. Lim W, Bardwell WA, Loredo JS, et al. Neuropsychological effects of 2-week continuous positive airway pressure treatment and supplemental oxygen in patients with obstructive sleep apnea: a randomized placebo-controlled study. *J Clin Sleep Med.* 2007;3(4):380-6.
119. Barnes M, Houston D, Worsnop CJ, et al. A randomized controlled trial of continuous positive airway pressure in mild obstructive sleep apnea. *Am J Respir Crit Care Med.* 2002;165(6):773-80.
120. Bittencourt LR, Lucchesi LM, Rueda AD, et al. Placebo and modafinil effect on sleepiness in obstructive sleep apnea. *Prog Neuropsychopharmacol Biol Psychiatry.* 2008;32(2):552-9.
121. Dinges DF, Weaver TE. Effects of modafinil on sustained attention performance and quality of life in OSA patients with residual sleepiness while being treated with nCPAP. *Sleep Med.* 2003;4(5):393-402.
122. Norman D, Bardwell WA, Loredo JS, et al. Caffeine intake is independently associated with neuropsychological performance in patients with obstructive sleep apnea. *Sleep Breath.* 2008;12(3):199-205.
123. Roth T, Rippon GA, Arora S. Armodafinil improves wakefulness and long-term episodic memory in nCPAP-adherent patients with excessive sleepiness associated with obstructive sleep apnea. *Sleep Breath.* 2008;12(1):53-62.
124. Ohayon MM. Epidemiology of depression and its treatment in the general population. *J Psychiatr Res.* 2007;41(3-4):207-13.
125. Harris M, Glozier N, Ratnavadivel R, et al. Obstructive sleep apnea and depression. *Sleep Med Rev.* 2009;13(6):437-44.
126. Saunamaki T, Jehkonen M. Depression and anxiety in obstructive sleep apnea syndrome: a review. *Acta Neurol Scand.* 2007;116(5):277-88.
127. Ohayon MM. The effects of breathing-related sleep disorders on mood disturbances in the general population. *J Clin Psychiatry.* 2003;64(10):1195-200; quiz, 274-6.
128. Schroder CM, O'Hara R. Depression and Obstructive Sleep Apnea (OSA). *Ann Gen Psychiatry.* 2005;4:13.
129. Coleman RM, Roffwarg HP, Kennedy SJ, et al. Sleep-wake disorders based on a polysomnographic diagnosis. A national cooperative study. *JAMA.* 1982;247(7):997-1003.
130. Derderian SS, Bridenbaugh RH, Rajagopal KR. Neuropsychologic symptoms in obstructive sleep apnea improve after treatment with nasal continuous positive airway pressure. *Chest.* 1988;94(5):1023-7.
131. Millman RP, Fogel BS, McNamara ME, et al. Depression as a manifestation of obstructive sleep apnea: reversal with nasal continuous positive airway pressure. *J Clin Psychiatry.* 1989;50(9):348-51.
132. Diamanti C, Manali E, Ginieri-Coccossis M, et al. Depression, physical activity, energy consumption, and quality of life in OSA patients before and after CPAP treatment. *Sleep Breath.* 2012;17(4):1159-68.
133. Dyken ME, Somers VK, Yamada T, et al. Investigating the relationship between stroke and obstructive sleep apnea. *Stroke.* 1996;27(3):401-7.
134. Bassetti C, Aldrich MS. Sleep apnea in acute cerebrovascular diseases: final report on 128 patients. *Sleep.* 1999;22(2):217-23.
135. Johnson KG, Johnson DC. Frequency of sleep apnea in stroke and TIA patients: a meta-analysis. *J Clin Sleep Med.* 2010;6(2):131-7.

136. Redline S, Yenokyan G, Gottlieb DJ, et al. Obstructive sleep apnea-hypopnea and incident stroke: the sleep heart health study. *Am J Respir Crit Care Med.* 2010;182(2):269-77.
137. Shahar E, Whitney CW, Redline S, et al. Sleep-disordered breathing and cardiovascular disease: cross-sectional results of the Sleep Heart Health Study. *Am J Respir Crit Care Med.* 2001;163(1):19-25.
138. Munoz R, Duran-Cantolla J, Martinez-Vila E, et al. Severe sleep apnea and risk of ischemic stroke in the elderly. *Stroke.* 2006;37(9):2317-21.
139. Turkington PM, Allgar V, Bamford J, et al. Effect of upper airway obstruction in acute stroke on functional outcome at 6 months. *Thorax.* 2004;59(5):367-71.
140. Sahlin C, Sandberg O, Gustafson Y, et al. Obstructive sleep apnea is a risk factor for death in patients with stroke: a 10-year follow-up. *Arch Intern Med.* 2008 11;168(3):297-301.
141. Faraci FM. Breathe, breathe in the air: the ins and outs of hypoxia take their toll. *Hypertension.* 2012;60(1):22-4.
142. Alexandrov AV, Nguyen HT, Rubiera M, et al. Prevalence and risk factors associated with reversed Robin Hood syndrome in acute ischemic stroke. *Stroke.* 2009;40(8):2738-42.
143. Balfors EM, Franklin KA. Impairment of cerebral perfusion during obstructive sleep apneas. *Am J Respir Crit Care Med.* 1994;150(6 Pt 1):1587-91.
144. Klingelhofer J, Hajak G, Sander D, et al. Assessment of intracranial hemodynamics in sleep apnea syndrome. *Stroke.* 1992;23(10):1427-33.
145. Bonnin-Vilaplana M, Arboix A, Parra O, et al. Sleep-related breathing disorders in acute lacunar stroke. *J Neurol.* 2009;256(12):2036-42.
146. Culebras A. Sleep and stroke. *Semin Neurol.* 2009;29(4):438-45.
147. Harbison J, Gibson GJ, Birchall D, et al. White matter disease and sleep-disordered breathing after acute stroke. *Neurology.* 2003;61(7):959-63.
148. Li Y, Veasey SC. Neurobiology and neuropathophysiology of obstructive sleep apnea. *Neuromolecular Med.* 2012;14(3):168-79.
149. Somers VK, White DP, Amin R, et al. Sleep apnea and cardiovascular disease: an American Heart Association/american College Of Cardiology Foundation Scientific Statement from the American Heart Association Council for High Blood Pressure Research Professional Education Committee, Council on Clinical Cardiology, Stroke Council, and Council On Cardiovascular Nursing. In collaboration with the National Heart, Lung, and Blood Institute National Center on Sleep Disorders Research (National Institutes of Health). *Circulation.* 2008;118(10):1080-111.
150. Parra O, Sanchez-Armengol A, Bonnin M, et al. Early treatment of obstructive apnoea and stroke outcome: a randomised controlled trial. *Eur Respir J.* 2011;37(5):1128-36.
151. Barlinn K, Alexandrov AV. Sleep-disordered breathing and arterial blood flow steal represent linked therapeutic targets in cerebral ischaemia. *Int J Stroke.* 2011;6(1):40-1.
152. Martinez-Garcia MA, Galiano-Blancart R, Roman-Sanchez P, et al. Continuous positive airway pressure treatment in sleep apnea prevents new vascular events after ischemic stroke. *Chest.* 2005;128(4):2123-9.
153. Wessendorf TE, Wang YM, Thilmann AF, et al. Treatment of obstructive sleep apnoea with nasal continuous positive airway pressure in stroke. *Eur Respir J.* 2001;18(4):623-9.
154. Minnerup J, Ritter MA, Wersching H, et al. Continuous positive airway pressure ventilation for acute ischemic stroke: a randomized feasibility study. *Stroke.* 2012;43(4):1137-9.
155. Kerr P, Shoenut JP, Millar T, et al. Nasal CPAP reduces gastroesophageal reflux in obstructive sleep apnea syndrome. *Chest.* 1992;101(6):1539-44.
156. Gonzalez ER, Castell DO. Respiratory complications of gastroesophageal reflux. *Am Fam Physician.* 1988;37(2):169-72.
157. Green BT, Broughton WA, O'Connor JB. Marked improvement in nocturnal gastro-esophageal reflux in a large cohort of patients with obstructive sleep apnea treated with continuous positive airway pressure. *Arch Intern Med.* 2003;163(1):41-5.
158. Unal M, Ozturk L, Ozturk C, et al. The seroprevalence of Helicobacter pylori infection in patients with obstructive sleep apnoea: a preliminary study. *Clin Otolaryngol Allied Sci.* 2003;28(2):100-2.
159. Valipour A, Makker HK, Hardy R, et al. Symptomatic gastroesophageal reflux in subjects with a breathing sleep disorder. *Chest.* 2002;121(6):1748-53.

160. Crausaz FM, Favez G. Aspiration of solid food particles into lungs of patients with gastroesophageal reflux and chronic bronchial disease. *Chest.* 1988;93(2):376-8.
161. Ing AJ, Ngu MC, Breslin AB. Obstructive sleep apnea and gastroesophageal reflux. *Am J Med.* 2000;108 Suppl 4a:120S-5S.
162. Steward DL. Pantoprazole for sleepiness associated with acid reflux and obstructive sleep disordered breathing. *Laryngoscope.* 2004;114(9):1525-8.
163. Unruh ML. Sleep apnea and dialysis therapies: things that go bump in the night? *Hemodial Int.* 2007;11(4):369-78.
164. Sim JJ, Rasgon SA, Kujubu DA, et al. Sleep apnea in early and advanced chronic kidney disease: Kaiser Permanente Southern California cohort. *Chest.* 2009;135(3):710-6.
165. Agrawal V, Vanhecke TE, Rai B, et al. Albuminuria and renal function in obese adults evaluated for obstructive sleep apnea. *Nephron Clin Pract.* 2009;113(3):c140-7.
166. Ahmed SB, Ronksley PE, Hemmelgarn BR, et al. Nocturnal hypoxia and loss of kidney function. *PLoS One.* 2011;6(4):e19029.
167. Chou YT, Lee PH, Yang CT, et al. Obstructive sleep apnea: a stand-alone risk factor for chronic kidney disease. *Nephrol Dial Transplant.* 2011;26(7):2244-50.
168. Chaudhary BA, Sklar AH, Chaudhary TK, Kolbeck RC, Speir WA, Jr. Sleep apnea, proteinuria, and nephrotic syndrome. *Sleep.* 1988;11(1):69-74.
169. Sklar AH, Chaudhary BA. Reversible proteinuria in obstructive sleep apnea syndrome. *Arch Intern Med.* 1988;148(1):87-9.
170. Markou N, Kanakaki M, Myrianthefs P, et al. Sleep-disordered breathing in nondialyzed patients with chronic renal failure. *Lung.* 2006;184(1):43-9.
171. Gambineri A, Pelusi C, Pasquali R. Testosterone levels in obese male patients with obstructive sleep apnea syndrome: relation to oxygen desaturation, body weight, fat distribution and the metabolic parameters. *J Endocrinol Invest.* 2003;26(6):493-8.
172. Cistulli PA, Grunstein RR, Sullivan CE. Effect of testosterone administration on upper airway collapsibility during sleep. *Am J Respir Crit Care Med.* 1994;149(2 Pt 1):530-2.
173. Grunstein RR, Handelsman DJ, Lawrence SJ, et al. Neuroendocrine dysfunction in sleep apnea: reversal by continuous positive airways pressure therapy. *J Clin Endocrinol Metab.* 1989;68(2):352-8.
174. Xu J, Huang P, Song B, et al. Effect of continuous positive airway pressure on erectile dysfunction in patients with obstructive sleep apnea syndrome: a meta-analysis. *Zhonghua Nan Ke Xue.* 2013;19(1):77-81.
175. Uzkeser H, Yildirim K, Aktan B, et al. Bone mineral density in patients with obstructive sleep apnea syndrome. *Sleep Breath.* 2013;17(1):339-42.
176. Loh NK, Dinner DS, Foldvary N, et al. Do patients with obstructive sleep apnea wake up with headaches? *Arch Intern Med.* 1999;159(15):1765-8.
177. Bar A, Tarasiuk A, Segev Y, et al. The effect of adenotonsillectomy on serum insulin-like growth factor-I and growth in children with obstructive sleep apnea syndrome. *J Pediatr.* 1999;135(1):76-80.

CHAPTER 11

Positive Airway Pressure Treatment in Obstructive Sleep Apnea

Vijay K Chennamchetty, Maramreddy Aparna, Praveen SV

INTRODUCTION

Obstructive sleep apnea (OSA)/hypopnea syndrome is a disorder that is characterized by intermittent and recurrent upper airway closure during sleep that results in sleep fragmentation, intermittent hypoxemia/hypercapnia, and increased sympathetic nervous system activation. OSA is associated with daytime sleepiness, cognitive defects, increased risk of cardiovascular disease, hypertension, stroke, and glucose intolerance.

The application of nasal continuous positive airway pressure (nCPAP) therapy for sleep apnea was first described in 1981 by Sullivan and colleagues (Figure 1).[1] In their case series report, five patients who had severe OSA were treated with CPAP applied through the nares. Their use of lower pressure levels completely prevented upper airway occlusion and allowed uninterrupted sleep. Since then, it has become the medical therapy of choice for OSA. The basic principle by which conventional positive airway pressure (PAP) systems employed to treat

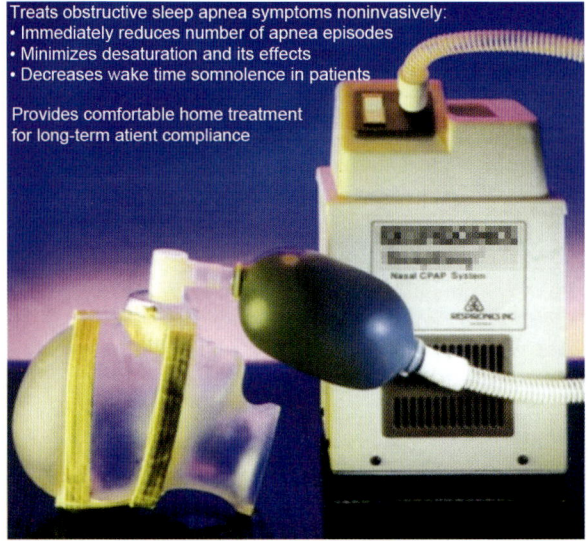

Figure 1: Sullivans 1981 nasal continuous positive airway pressure.

OSA consists of a generator that directs air under pressure to flow into the patient via a tubing and an interface (vide infra). This pressurized air pneumatically splints the upper airway, thereby maintaining patency of upper airway and facilitating the flow under decreased resistance. Thus, splinting of upper airway constitutes the primary mechanism of therapeutic action of any PAP therapy. After initial publication of CPAP effectiveness, evidence exists from multiple randomized studies showing benefit of PAP therapy regarding subjective daytime sleepiness, alertness, and improvement in overall quality of life. Treatment with PAP should ideally be approached on a case-by-case basis. A multidisciplinary approach should be used in the management of these patients. Patients should be educated about the function, care, and maintenance of their equipment, the benefits of PAP therapy, and potential problems. Long-term management of OSA and PAP therapy requires a structured, multidisciplinary approach to monitor and treat patients with OSA. The team usually contains sleep physician, sleep technician, psychiatrist, and a respiratory therapist.

POSITIVE AIRWAY PRESSURE THERAPY MODALITIES TO TREAT OBSTRUCTIVE SLEEP APNEA

Positive airway pressure therapy goes beyond CPAP alone. Bilevel PAP, end-expiratory pressure relief, and autotitrating PAP (APAP) devices may also be used in the management of OSA. Adaptive servoventilation (ASV) may also be used but is typically reserved for complicated central sleep apnea (CSA) and/or Cheyne-Stokes respiration (CSR).

- **Apnea-hypopnea index:** Total number of apneas plus hypopneas/number of hours of sleep
- **Respiratory disturbance index:** The total of apneas, hypopneas, and respiratory event-related arousals/number of hours of sleep.

The indication for treatment of OSA is dependent on a thorough clinical history and clinical signs along with objective evaluation via a polysomnogram.[2] The severity of sleep apnea is measured through apnea-hypopnea index (AHI) and respiratory disturbance index (RDI).

Sleep apnea severity is classified based on AHI/RDI into mild, moderate, and severe. Mild if AHI or RDI is from 5 to 15, moderate is 15 to 29, and severe is 30 or greater.

Continuous positive airway pressure: This modality of PAP therapy delivers the same magnitude of pressure to the patient during both inspiration and expiration. Conventional CPAP or fixed pressure CPAP is the standard PAP therapy to which all other modalities are compared.

Continuous positive airway pressure is currently the "gold standard" for treatment of moderate-to-severe OSA (AHI > 15). It also can be used as adjunctive therapy in the management of blood pressure that is difficult to control.

Current guidelines recommend that treatment of OSA should be advised and offered when the following criteria on polysomnography have been met:[3]
- Apnea-hypopnea index or a RDI greater than or equal to 15 events per hour; or
- Apnea-hypopnea index (or RDI) greater than or equal to 5, and less than 15 events per hour with documentation demonstrating any of the following symptoms.

Excessive daytime sleepiness, as documented by either a score of greater than 10 on the Epworth Sleepiness Scale (ESS) or inappropriate daytime napping (e.g., during driving, conversation, or eating) or sleepiness that interferes with daily activities; or impaired cognition or mood disorders; or hypertension; or ischemic heart disease or history of stroke; or cardiac arrhythmias, or pulmonary hypertension.

Bilevel positive pressure (bilevel PP): Bilevel PP provides the ability to independently adjust the inspiratory and expiratory pressure such that the pressure delivered during exhalation is less than that during inhalation.[4] Setting the expiratory positive airway pressure (EPAP) at a level that prevents upper airway occlusion during or at end-expiration permits the patient to generate inspiratory airflow or volume at the initiation of inspiratory effort, and this triggers delivery of inspiratory positive airway pressure (IPAP), which supports upper airway patency during inspiratory phases of breathing cycle. A setting of sufficient level of IPAP augments upper airway patency and thus eliminates partial obstructions leading to hypopneas as well. If the set EPAP is suboptimal, which can lead to occlusion of airway at end expiration, IPAP would not be triggered and eventually leads to apparent apnea.

Most bilevel PP devices can be used in three modes:
1. Spontaneous mode, where IPAP is delivered in response to a patient trigger.
2. Spontaneous-timed mode, where the patient may trigger the delivery of IPAP, but in addition, the clinician can set the device so that IPAP is delivered at prescribed intervals if patient does not trigger the device in that specified interval.
3. Timed mode, where the IPAP is delivered with a clinician set frequency and the patient cannot initiate delivery. The tendency for patient device asynchrony is greater with this mode.

Bilevel PAP devices can also be used to augment spontaneous patient respirations, as part of the treatment plan for certain pulmonary conditions, and can also be used for complicated OSA. In patients with coexisting disease comorbidities such as chronic obstructive pulmonary disease (COPD), neuromuscular disease, and thoracic restrictive diseases, bilevel ventilation may be beneficial.[5] The use of these noninvasive positive pressure ventilation (NIPPV) respiratory assist devices for the treatment of patients with severe COPD is considered medically necessary when all of the following are met:
- An arterial blood gas $PaCO_2$, done while awake and breathing the individual's usual FIO_2, is 52 mmHg
- Sleep oximetry demonstrates oxygen saturation 88% for at least 5 continuous minutes, done while breathing oxygen at 2 L/min or the individual's usual FIO_2 (whichever is higher).

In patients with OSA and neuromuscular disease, the following criteria may be used for bilevel ventilation initiation:[5,6]

- The patient has been diagnosed with a progressive neuromuscular disease (e.g., amyotrophic lateral sclerosis) or a severe thoracic cage abnormality (e.g., post-thoracoplasty for tuberculosis)
- Chronic obstructive pulmonary disease does not contribute significantly to the individual's pulmonary limitation; and one or more of the following criteria are met:

- An arterial blood gas $PaCO_2$ level is greater than or equal to 45 mmHg, done while awake and breathing the patient's usual FIO_2
- Sleep oximetry demonstrates an oxygen saturation less than or equal to 88% for at least 5 continuous minutes, done while breathing the patient's usual FIO_2
- Maximal inspiratory pressure is less than 60 cm H_2O or forced vital capacity is less than 50% of predicted for patients with a progressive neuromuscular disease.

Bilevel PAP can also play a role in the management of patients diagnosed with OSA in the perioperative setting with the aforementioned comorbidities and/or in whom CPAP is not indicated or has failed.[7]

Another large group that may benefit from NIPPV is those with obesity hypoventilation syndrome (OHS). OHS is a diagnosis of exclusion. Clinical features of OHS include symptoms of daytime hypercapnia (such as fatigue and morning headache), right-sided heart failure/cor pulmonale, $PaCO_2$ of 45 mmHg or more, hypoxia during wakefulness and sleep (arterial oxygen saturation <90%), greater than 10 mmHg increase in the $PaCO_2$ during sleep (the primary manifestation), and respiratory acidosis (pH <7.3) during sleep. There is increased risk that OSA/OHS can lead to chronic respiratory failure in these individuals. Although CPAP may be used to also treat many OHS patients, some will require bilevel PP.[8,9]

Autotitrating Positive Airway Pressure

Autotitrating devices employ algorithms to detect impending collapse or instability of the upper airway and adjust the amount of pressure that is delivered to maintain the airway patency. Once airway stability is attained, the pressure gradually decreases until an impending collapse is detected. The delivered pressure is then augmented as per algorithm. Thus, the device pressure floats over the night as per change in airway dynamics of the patient in real time. By the way the APAP devices change pressure as per patients' requirements (various body positions, different stages of sleep, alcohol intake, and nasal congestion), it appears that they reduce the overall pressure to which patients are exposed and thereby increase comfort, satisfaction, and adherence to therapy. A review of meta-analysis of APAP reveals that APAP devices may provide alleviation of OSA and perceived daytime sleepiness in comparison with standard fixed CPAP devices with a mean pressure that is about 2 cm H_2O lower.[4]

Pressure Relief Positive Airway Pressure

Pressure relief devices provide expiratory pressure relief that is proportional to expiratory flow, while pressure rises to the prescribed EPAP level at end-expiration. In expiratory pressure relief device, the pressure relief occurs at end-inspiration. The reduction of pressure at the beginning of expiration is intended to reduce the sensation of breathing against high pressure without causing the upper airways to collapse.[4] Pressure relief CPAP was effective in reducing sleep-disordered breathing (SDB) events as compared to standard CPAP.[4]

Adaptive Servoventilation

To certain extent, CPAP and bilevel PP therapy are helpful in management of Cheyne-Stokes breathing (CSB) and CSA. CSB is a subtype of CSA constituted by periodic breathing in which central apneas and hypopneas alternate with periods of hyperventilation in a crescendo/decrescendo ventilatory pattern. CSA-CSR is found most commonly in association with systolic heart failure. Majority of patients who have central apneas can also have some obstructive physiology. Sometimes, there may be no clinical benefits to CPAP or on the contrary patients may experience worsening of these conditions upon conventional CPAP or bilevel PP therapy. Adaptive servoventilation has been introduced to primarily address these variants of clinical scenarios like CSB in the context of heart failure, idiopathic CSA, and complex CSA. By definition in complex CSA, patients most often have classic OSA on diagnostic polysomnography but exhibit disruptive central apneas when CPAP is initiated.[10] Hence, complex CSA is also called as treatment-emergent CSA.

Adaptive servoventilation uses an automatic, minute ventilation targeted device that performs breath-to-breath analysis and adjusts its settings accordingly. Depending on either flow or minute ventilation, the device will automatically adjust the amount of pressure support it delivers to maintain a certain flow or minute ventilation. ASV has been shown to be more effective than CPAP in treating patients with CSB and CSA.[11] ASV has also been shown to be effective in patients with CSA.

COMPLIANCE

Compliance with PAP is a multistep process, beginning with acceptance of the therapy. On an average, acceptance of the need for CPAP use at home ranges from 70% to 80% of patients.[12,13] Adherence to PAP is the ongoing use of PAP at home and tolerance of potential side effects associated with usage.[12,14] Currently accepted measures of adequate adherence are the use of PAP for at least 4 hours a night on 70% of the nights. In general, patients overestimate their use of PAP therapy by over an hour per night.[15] Patterns of patient adherence to PAP therapy develop early in the course of treatment, typically within the first week.[16,17]

The presence of self-reported daytime sleepiness[18-20] as well as subjective improvement in sleep quality and daytime sleepiness[21-23] may correlate with increased PAP adherence. The lack of symptoms prior to evaluation of OSA may predict poor compliance to PAP therapy.[24] Other predictors like age, gender, education, marital status, physiologic parameters, severity of sleep apnea or nocturnal hypoxemia, ESS score, or CPAP pressures have assessed in various studies and shown to be not helpful to predict patients compliance prior to beginning of PAP therapy.

A linear dose response relationship was found between increased use of PAP therapy per night and achieving normal levels of objective and subjective daytime sleepiness. The maximum effect observed at 7 hours of use per night and thereafter the outcome plateaued for measures of functional status.[25] Symptoms can recur with a single missed night.[26] When followed up for an year, 25% of patients may discontinue PAP therapy.[19] Problems with compliance of PAP therapy are similar to compliance to any other medical therapy. Studies comparing compliance of multiple medications ranging from antihypertensives, inhalers, home oxygen, antiepileptics, and others have shown compliance rates of 50–80%.[27] Few studies have shown that the patients having more compliance with medications are equally compliant with CPAP. In a study, patients with low medication adherence demonstrated a 40.1% probability of using CPAP for 4 hours a day or longer compared with 55.2% for subjects with adequate medication adherence. Married patients were more adherent to medications and CPAP.[28]

A task force of the American Academy of Sleep Medicine (AASM) recently published guidelines for the evaluation, management, and long-term care of OSA in adults.[3] The guidelines recommended a multidisciplinary approach to patient care involving a sleep specialist, nursing, respiratory therapy, sleep technicians, and the patient's primary care physician.

Patterns of adherence develop within the first week of starting PAP usage[16,17] and discontinuing CPAP is associated with lower hours of use early in the course of treatment.[19,29,30] This finding suggests that to promote good compliance, patients should receive some contact within the first week of receiving CPAP to evaluate hours of use, improvement or lack of improvement in symptoms, potential side effects of treatment, and any necessary interventions. Sleep physicians should help their patients obtain good patient compliance early in the treatment course, so that this will possibly be maintained in the long-term. A study of a population based CPAP program achieved compliance rates of 84% at 6 months. These patients underwent an educational session before starting CPAP, telephone contact daily during the first week, and clinic visits at weeks 2 and 4, and months 3 and 6.[31] Current recommendations are for follow-up visits annually, based on the patient's early adherence, tolerance, and improvement in symptoms.[32] In every follow-up visit, compliance report should be reviewed and a thorough discussion about possible side effects that affect tolerance and adherence should be made. Side effects include mask discomfort, claustrophobia, pressure discomfort, nasal obstruction, and dryness.

MASK INTERFACES

Successful use of PAP therapy requires an adequate and comfortable mask interface. It has been noted that the type of mask interface prescribed may have a significant impact on influencing acceptance and adherence to CPAP therapy. The pros and cons of different mask interfaces are discussed below.

Nasal Mask

The nasal interface was first described in 1981.[1] The nasal mask seals around the bridge of the nose superiorly, above the superior lips inferiorly, and just lateral to the medial cheeks bilaterally (Figure 2). Typically, the smallest mask size that encompasses the nose without pinching the nares is used. The nasal mask is frequently the first choice offered to patients.[33] Patients can expectorate and can speak, and it allows more physiologic breathing.

In a small study, 16 patients who were on nasal mask were randomized to nasal mask or full face mask for two separate nights. Both interfaces were found to be equally effective in maintaining nocturnal gas exchange and preventing SDB.

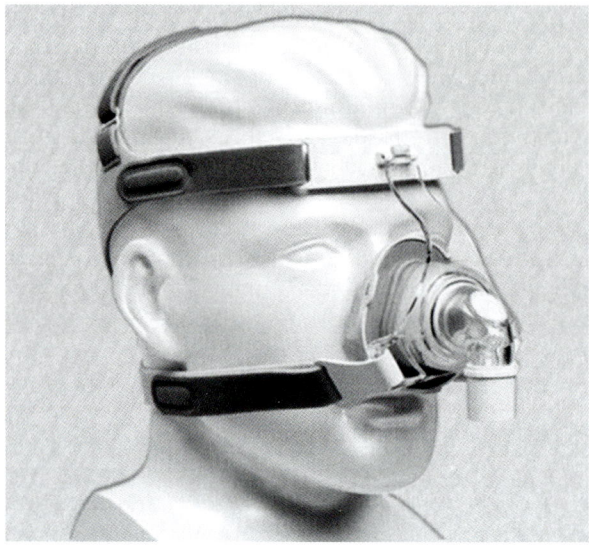

Figure 2: Nasal continuous positive air pressure mask.

However, the nasal mask provided fewer air leaks. Also, there was a subjective increase in comfort on the nasal mask as found by the visual analog score.[34]

Full Face Mask/Oronasal Mask

A full face mask seals across the forehead, around the temples and the chin, encompassing the eyes, nose, and mouth (Figure 3). Oronasal masks, which are more commonly used, seal around the bridge of the nose to the chin, encompassing the nose and mouth (Figure 4). A full face or oronasal mask may be indicated when mouth leaks are significant and prevents adequate ventilator support. Adequate ventilator support is particularly relevant for predominant nocturnal mouth breathers. In the first randomized controlled trial, Teo and colleagues[35] studied 24 patients who underwent 2 consecutive CPAP titration

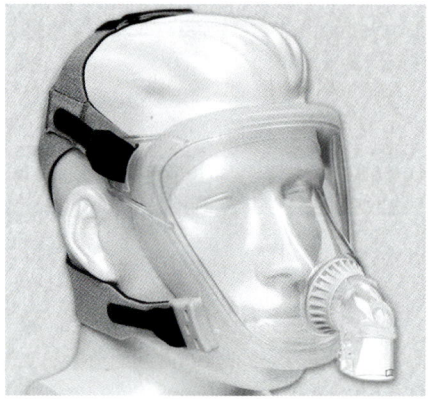

Figure 3: Full face mask.

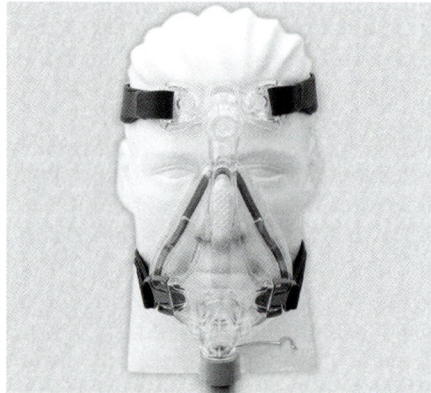

Figure 4: Oronasal mask.

studies and were randomized to a nasal mask with chin strap or oronasal mask. The patients completed a visual analog scale after each study. There was no difference in sleep quality; however, there was a higher leak noted in the oronasal mask. Patients also rated the nasal masks higher in satisfaction because they were better fitting and more comfortable. The AHI was higher while using an oronasal mask even though the CPAP pressures were similar. Simultaneous application of pressure via an oronasal mask in the nose and mouth may lead to posterior displacement of upper airway structures, resulting in reduced airway opening. The tongue may fall back due to airway pressure while using an oronasal mask in some patients, potentially leading to failure of CPAP therapy.[36] A large study compared nasal mask, nasal pillows, and an oronasal mask in a randomized trial during CPAP titration. The final AHI did not differ between the three groups. Oronasal mask use led to higher mask leakage compared with nasal pillows but not nasal mask. Importantly, considerably higher pressures were needed when oronasal mask was used.[37] In these patients, CPAP pressure requirements were higher on an average by 2.8 cm H_2O in the moderate OSA patients and by 6 cm H_2O in the severe OSA patients. There was no difference in pressures needed when either a nasal mask or nasal pillows were used, similar to the results of the Ryan study.[38] These findings may imply inadequacy of pressures while switching over from a nasal mask or pillows to an oronasal mask without a change in CPAP pressure.

Oral Mask

Oral masks are butterfly-shaped interfaces that rest in the oral vestibule between the lips and the teeth (Figure 5).

This device ensures that the desired airway pressure is delivered with minimal leakage.[39] In a small study of seven patients, the oral mask was found to have pressure-flow relationships with PAP comparable to the nasal interface.[40]

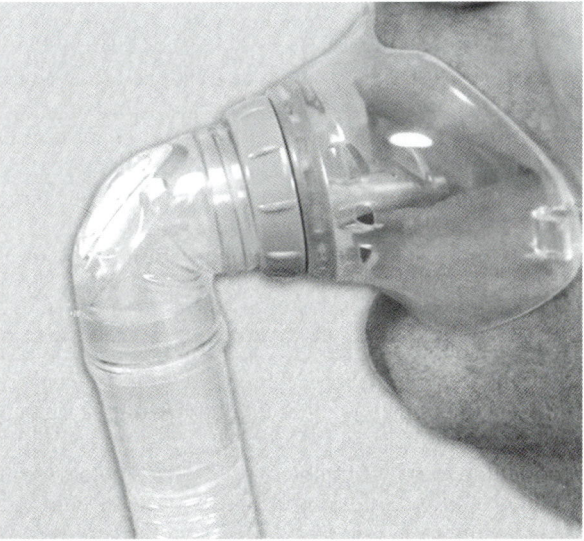

Figure 5: Oral mask.

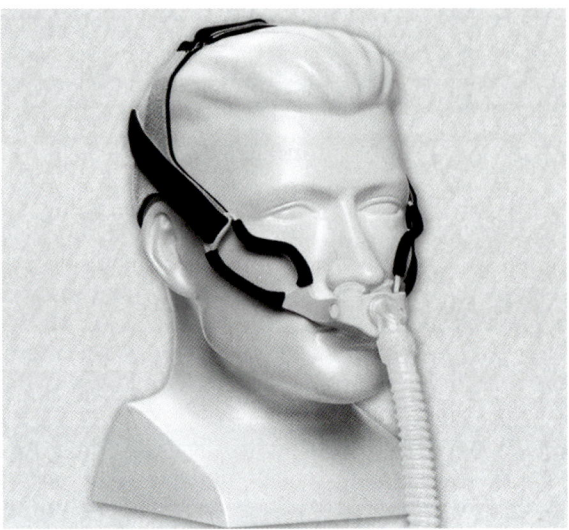

Figure 6: Nasal pillows.

Beecroft and colleagues[39] compared the oral mask to nasal and oronasal interface devices. The available data from small studies[39] in patients with a new diagnosis of OSA with a 6-month follow-up revealed no significant difference in the proportion of nonadherence between the groups. Patients did appreciate the lack of headgear and reported higher satisfaction with the oral Mask. The common adverse effect noted includes a choking sensation. Oral mask appears to be better interface than oronasal mask for nasal CPAP intolerable patients.

Nasal Pillows

Nasal pillows (Figure 6) can be used when there is pressure sore on the nasal bridge or patients who do not tolerate nasal masks. Massie et al. compared nasal pillows to nasal masks in 39 patients in a 6-week randomized, crossover study. This study showed a significant increase in percentage of days used in the nasal pillows group compared with the nasal mask group. There was no difference in the ESS and the Functional Outcomes of Sleep Questionnaire (FOSQ) between the 2 groups. They noted that the nasal pillows may not be appropriate for patients with higher CPAP pressures as there were concerns of the mask seal and the possibility of inadequate pressure delivery.

They concluded that nasal pillows are well tolerated as patients have reported less discomfort with their use, and is an effective interface for patients with OSA at a CPAP pressure of less than or equal to 14 cm H_2O.

More recently in 2011, Ryan and colleagues studied 21 patients in an 8-week crossover design with randomization to nasal pillows or nasal mask. The nasal pillows had less reported pressure on the face and a significant improvement in the Social Functioning and Change of Health Score, but there was not a significant improvement in compliance. The nasal mask had less reported complaints of cold face/nose, and at the end of the trial, 12 patients stated they preferred the nasal mask over the nasal pillows. With these results, they concluded that patients should be evaluated on an individual basis for usage of nasal pillows.[36]

Combination Devices

In patients requiring high pressures, inadequate fitting of the interface may lead to CPAP intolerance and usage of alone mandibular advancement device (MAD) may be inadequate to control the SDB. There comes the role of using an MAD along with CPAP or bilevel PP via masks may be helpful.

General Considerations Including Adverse Effects of Interfaces

When prescribing any of the available interfaces for OSA, it is always preferable to follow the manufacturer's suggestion for proper sizing, avoid overtightening, and check skin regularly for signs of pressure ulcers, which may occur if the mask is too tight.[33]

Nasal Mask

The most common adverse effect is nasal congestion from the vasodilation and mucus production, which can be mitigated by using heated humidification, and treatment of allergic rhinitis. Mouth leaks occur in subjects with a tendency to sleep with open mouths but this could be alleviated by using a chin strap.[33]

Orofacial Mask

Adverse effects of full face/oronasal masks include increased dead space in which noninvasive ventilator settings may need to be adjusted.[33] Patients may have swallowing difficulties and a potential aspiration risk, especially with underlying esophageal reflux or vomiting.[33]

Oral Mask

Adverse effects of the oral mask include dental pain, orthodontic problems, nasal leaks, initial hypersalivation, and aerophagia apart from a choking sensation.

If an ulcer does develop, it is recommended to use mask or skin barriers or switch to an alternate type of interface.[33]

Edentulous patients require dentures to be worn at night for snuggly fit interface.[33]

Claustrophobia is a common complaint and a common fear to start CPAP therapy and therapy with nasal mask/nasal pillows has decreased its incidence. Patients may benefit from counseling before and during treatment of CPAP. A trial therapy of using CPAP while patient is awake may be beneficial. Desensitization has shown some ray of hope for claustrophobic patients. Means et al.[41,42] reported a case series of patients who were not adherent to CPAP because of claustrophobia. The patients were put through a graded desensitization process with the aid of a clinical psychologist. This process was successful in increasing the nights of CPAP use and hours used per night.

Silicone rubber in interfaces may lead to contact allergic dermatitis. Mask straps may contain neoprene made of dialkylthioureas and can cause a scalp allergic dermatitis.[43]

Ocular complications occur in up to 30% of patients using CPAP. These include bacterial conjunctivitis, corneal abrasions and ulcers, dry eyes, and increased ocular pressure. Nocturnal lubricants or artificial tears may provide relief from dry eyes in the morning. Nasal pillows or lowering of pressure may be necessary in other cases.

To summarize about interfaces, addressing issues concerning the interface is important for patient comfort. Though nasal mask is the commonest prescribed interface, any intolerance to given interface has to be addressed on a case-to-case basis. However, compliance and effectiveness has not been shown to be superior for any one type of interface.

VARIED DEVICES TO IMPROVE COMPLIANCE

As alternatives to conventional CPAP, devices such as bilevel PP, APAP, expiratory pressure relief PAP and ASV are used to improve patient comfort in the expectation that adherence may improve. None have been shown to improve compliance conclusively compared with traditional CPAP, but still may be used as an option in those who complain of pressure intolerance. Randomized clinical studies have demonstrated similar improvement in AHI, ESS, and FOSQ; however, no difference in compliance was found at 30 days or at 1 year.[44,45] These trials were done in patients new to PAP therapy.

Bilevel PAP may be a viable option in patients who have failed CPAP due to pressure intolerance (vide supra for mechanism).

Autotitrating PAP machines (vide supra for mechanism) designed to effectively treat OSA with a lower mean pressure, which may improve pressure tolerance and increase compliance. With APAP, mean airway pressures have been reported to be less than those with fixed CPAP. There are also improvements in AHI, ESS scores, sleep architecture, quality of life, oxygen saturation, and cognitive impairment. There is mixed data showing compliance superiority of APAP devices over conventional CPAP. A meta-analysis also showed similar adherence between APAP and fixed CPAP.[46] Some studies support a patient preference of APAP over fixed CPAP, but this did not translate to better compliance. While APAP devices have not been shown to convincingly increase compliance or acceptance of CPAP therapy, APAP may have a role in those who complain of pressure intolerance, particularly in those with high pressures. APAP has a potential to use as an attended or unattended titration study to determine fixed CPAP pressure or as a way to quickly start treatment.[47,48] However, APAP is not recommended for split-night titration, or as an unattended study in those with congestive heart failure, COPD, CSA, or hypoventilation.[49]

Expiratory pressure relief (vide supra for mechanism) hopes to improve patient comfort and, in effect, adherence. One nonrandomized study showed improved compliance of 1.7 hours a night on expiratory pressure relief versus conventional CPAP at 3 months.[50] However, randomized studies have not shown a significant difference in compliance in comparison with standard CPAP for up to 6 months.[51]

Role of Cognitive Behavioral Therapy

Cognitive behavioral therapy (CBT) is based on psychosocial theories, which describe how patients who perceive more benefit have higher outcome expectation, and with more knowledge will likely be more compliant.[52] In a study published by Richards et al., the CBT intervention group used CPAP for

2.9 hours longer per night at 28 days compared with the standard group. In the intervention group 77% was using CPAP for 4 hours or longer per night compared with 31% in the standard group. CPAP refusal was 8% in the intervention group compared with 30% in the standard group. Enhancing patient perception via education and cognitive therapy, therefore, seems to be a promising way to improve adherence.

What parameters need to be assessed for patients on PAP therapy: On every follow-up visit, patients should be assessed for several OSA outcomes including adherence and tolerance of PAP therapy. These outcomes include resolution of sleepiness and snoring, OSA-specific quality of life measures, patient and spouse satisfaction with the therapy and response to therapy, avoidance of factors known to worsen OSA like alcohol intake, obtaining adequate sleep and proper sleep hygiene, as well as management in overweight patients. Some patients may have symptoms of ongoing sleepiness despite adequate PAP adherence or residual sleepiness. These patients should be evaluated for other causes of daytime sleepiness including insufficient sleep or poor sleep hygiene, mood disorders, comorbid illness and associated medication effects, as well as the possible presence of other sleep disorders. Residual sleepiness despite adequate PAP therapy, may be addressed with pharmacologic therapy.[53]

CONCLUSION

Positive airway pressure therapy is the gold standard therapy for OSA. There have been substantial developments and modifications over the past 3 decades in an effort to provide greater comfort to the patient with regard to both interface and devices. There has been an increased understanding of pathophysiology of various forms of OSA and different modalities of PAP have been developed to better address these subsets of SDB. Importantly, evidence is available through randomized controlled trials demonstrating the efficacy of PAP therapy in OSA. Sleep apnea represents a chronic disease and requires a multidisciplinary approach to proper care. This proper care in OSA patients is achieved through practicing evidence-based practice guidelines through a multidisciplinary team including sleep physician, primary care physician, and support-service providers such as nurses, sleep technicians, and respiratory therapists. The goal of the team is to educate patients on their underlying disease and provide them with the information to be involved in self-management of their disease and, using these outcome measures, develop better treatment strategies over time.

REFERENCES

1. Sullivan CE, Issa FG, Berthon-Jones M, et al. Reversal of obstructive sleep apnoea by continuous positive airway pressure applied through the nares. *Lancet*. 1981;1:862.
2. Epstein LJ, Kristo D, Strollo PJ Jr, et al. Clinical guideline for the evaluation, management and long-term care of obstructive sleep apnea in adults. *J Clin Sleep Med*. 2009;5:263.
3. Sleep-related breathing disorders in adults: recommendations for syndrome definition and measurement techniques in clinical research. The report of an American Academy of Sleep Medicine Task Force. *Sleep*. 1999;22:667.
4. Sander MH, Strollo PJ Jr, Atwood CW Jr, et al. Positive airway pressure in the treatment of sleep apnea-hypopnea In: Chokroverty S, editor. Sleep disorder medicine. 3rd ed. Saunders, Elsevier: Philadelphia; 2009; p. 2390-2.

5. Bonekat HW. Noninvasive ventilation in neuromuscular disease. *Crit Care Clin.* 1998;14:775.
6. Bradley WG, Anderson F, Bromberg M, et al. Current management of ALS: comparison of the ALS CARE Database and the AAN Practice Parameter. The American Academy of Neurology. *Neurology.* 2001;57:500.
7. Gross JB, Bachenberg KL, Benumof JL, et al. Practice guidelines for the perioperative management of patients with obstructive sleep apnea: a report by the American Society of Anesthesiologists Task Force on perioperative management of patients with obstructive sleep apnea. *Anesthesiology.* 2006;104:1081.
8. Piper AJ, Wang D, Yee BJ, et al. Randomised trial of CPAP vs bilevel support in the treatment of obesity hypoventilation syndrome without severe nocturnal desaturation. *Thorax.* 2008;63:395.
9. Mokhlesi B, Kryger MH, Grunstein RR. Assessment and management of patients with obesity hypoventilation syndrome. *Proc Am Thorac Soc.* 2008;5:218.
10. Morgenthaler TI, Kagramanov V, Hanak V, et al. Complex sleep apnea syndrome: is it a unique clinical syndrome? *Sleep.* 2006;29:1203.
11. Teschler H, Dohring J, Wang YM, et al. Adaptive pressure support servo-ventilation: a novel treatment for Cheyne-Stokes respiration in heart failure. *Am J Respir Crit Care Med.* 2001;164:614.
12. Collard P, Pieters T, Aubert G, et al. Compliance with nasal CPAP in obstructive sleep apnea patients. *Sleep Med Rev.* 1997;1:33.
13. Villar I, Izuel M, Carrizo S, et al. Medication adherence and persistence in severe obstructive sleep apnea. *Sleep.* 2009;32:623.
14. Grunstein RR. Sleep-related breathing disorders. Nasal continuous positive airway pressure treatment for obstructive sleep apnoea. *Thorax.* 1995;50:1106.
15. Kribbs NB, Pack AI, Kline LR, et al. Objective measurement of patterns of nasal CPAP use by patients with obstructive sleep apnea. *Am Rev Respir Dis.* 1993;147:887.
16. Weaver TE, Kribbs NB, Pack AI, et al. Night-tonight variability in CPAP use over the first three months of treatment. *Sleep.* 1997;20:278.
17. Budhiraja R, Parthasarathy S, Drake CL, et al. Early CPAP use identifies subsequent adherence to CPAP therapy. *Sleep.* 2007;30:320.
18. Edinger JD, Carwile S, Miller P, et al. Psychological status, syndromatic measures, and compliance with nasal CPAP therapy for sleep apnea. *Percept Mot Skills.* 1994;78:1116.
19. McArdle N, Devereux G, Heidarnejad H, et al. Long-term use of CPAP therapy for sleep apnea/hypopnea syndrome. *Am J Respir Crit Care Med.* 1999;159:1108.
20. Engleman HM, Wild MR. Improving CPAP use by patients with the sleep apnoea/hypopnoea syndrome (SAHS). *Sleep Med Rev.* 2003;7:81.
21. Drake CL, Day R, Hudgel D, et al. Sleep during titration predicts continuous positive airway pressure compliance. *Sleep.* 2003;26:308.
22. Wells RD, Freedland KE, Carney RM, et al. Adherence, reports of benefits, and depression among patients treated with continuous positive airway pressure. *Psychosom Med.* 2007;69:449.
23. Wolkove N, Baltzan M, Kamel H, et al. Long-term compliance with continuous positive airway pressure in patients with obstructive sleep apnea. *Can Respir J.* 2008;15:365.
24. Barbe F, Mayoralas LR, Duran J, et al. Treatment with continuous positive airway pressure is no effective in patients with sleep apnea but no daytime sleepiness. A randomized, controlled trial. *Ann Intern Med.* 2001;134:1015.
25. Weaver TE, Maislin G, Dinges DF, et al. Relationship between hours of CPAP use and achieving normal levels of sleepiness and daily functioning. *Sleep.* 2007;30:711.
26. Kribbs NB, Pack AI, Kline LR, et al. Effects of one night without nasal CPAP treatment on sleep and sleepiness in patients with obstructive sleep apnea. *Am Rev Respir Dis.* 1993;147:1162.
27. Osterberg L, Blaschke T. Adherence to medication. *N Engl J Med.* 2005;353:487.
28. Platt AB, Kuna ST, Field SH, et al. Adherence to sleep apnea therapy and use of lipid-lowering drugs: a study of the healthy-user effect. *Chest.* 2010;137:102.
29. Grote L, Hedner J, Grunstein R, et al. Therapy with nCPAP: incomplete elimination of sleep related breathing disorder. *Eur Respir J.* 2000;16:921.

30. Johnson MK, Carter R, Nicol A, et al. Long-term continuous positive airway pressure (CPAP) outcomes from a sleep service using limited sleep studies and daycase CPAP titration in the management of obstructive sleep apnoea/hypopnoea syndrome. *Chron Respir Dis.* 2004;1:83.
31. Sin DD, Mayers I, Man GC, et al. Long-term compliance rates to continuous positive airway pressure in obstructive sleep apnea: a population-based study. *Chest.* 2002;121:430.
32. Kushida CA, Littner MR, Morgenthaler T, et al. Practice parameters for the indications for polysomnography and related procedures: an update for 2005. *Sleep.* 2005;28:499.
33. Kryger MH, Buchanan P, Grunstein R. Principles and Practice of Sleep Medicine, 5th edition. St Louis (MO): WB Saunders; 2010. pp. 1233-49, 1318-30.
34. Willson GN, Piper AJ, Norman M, et al. Nasal versus full face mask for noninvasive ventilation in chronic respiratory failure. *Eur Respir J.* 2004;23:605-9.
35. Teo M, Amis T, Lee S, et al. Equivalence of nasal and oronasal masks during initial CPAP titration for obstructive sleep apnea syndrome. *Sleep.* 2011;34:951-5.
36. Schorr F, Genta PR, Grego´rio MG, et al. Continuous positive airway pressure delivered by oronasal mask may not be effective for obstructive sleep apnoea. *Eur Respir J.* 2012; 40(2):503-5.
37. Ebben MR, Oyegbile T, Pollak CP. The efficacy of three different mask styles on a PAP titration night. *Sleep Med.* 2012;13(6):645-9.
38. Ryan S, Garvey JF, Swan V, et al. Nasal pillows as an alternative interface in patients with obstructive sleep apnoea syndrome initiating continuous positive airway pressure therapy. *J Sleep Res.* 2011;20:367-73.
39. Beecroft J, Zanon S, Lukic D, et al. Oral continuous positive airway pressure for sleep apnea. *Chest.* 2003;124:2200-8.
40. Smith PL, O'Donnell CP, Allan L, et al. A physiologic comparison of nasal and oral positive airway pressure. *Chest.* 2003;123:689-94.
41. Edinger JD, Means MK, Stechuchak KM, et al. A pilot study of inexpensive sleep-assessment devices. *Behav Sleep Med.* 2004;2:41.
42. Means MK, Edinger JD. Graded exposure therapy for addressing claustrophobic reactions to continuous positive airway pressure: a case series report. *Behav Sleep Med.* 2007;5:105.
43. Parthasarathy S. Mask interface and CPAP adherence. *J Clin Sleep Med.* 2008;4:511-2.
44. Reeves-Hoche MK, Hudgel DW, Meck R, et al. Continuous versus bilevel positive airway pressure for obstructive sleep apnea. *Am J Respir Crit Care Med.* 1995;151:443.
45. Gay PC, Herold DL, Olson EJ. A randomized, double-blind clinical trial comparing continuous positive airway pressure with a novel bilevel pressure system for treatment of obstructive sleep apnea syndrome. *Sleep.* 2003;26:864.
46. Ayas NT, Patel SR, Malhotra A, et al. Auto-titrating versus standard continuous positive airway pressure for the treatment of obstructive sleep apnea: results of a meta-analysis. *Sleep.* 2004;27:249.
47. Berry RB, Parish JM, Hartse KM. The use of autotitrating continuous positive airway pressure for treatment of adult obstructive sleep apnea. An American Academy of Sleep Medicine review. *Sleep.* 2002;25:148.
48. d'Ortho MP. Auto-titrating continuous positive airway pressure for treating adult patients with sleep apnea syndrome. *Curr Opin Pulm Med.* 2004;10:495.
49. Morgenthaler TI, Aurora RN, Brown T, et al. Practice parameters for the use of autotitrating continuous positive airway pressure devices for titrating pressures and treating adult patients with obstructive sleep apnea syndrome: an update for 2007. An American Academy of Sleep Medicine report. *Sleep.* 2008;31:141.
50. Aloia MS, Stanchina M, Arnedt JT, et al. Treatment adherence and outcomes in flexible vs standard continuous positive airway pressure therapy. *Chest.* 2005;127:2085.
51. Dolan DC, Okonkwo R, Gfullner F, et al. Longitudinal comparison study of pressure relief (C-Flex) vs CPAP in OSA patients. *Sleep Breath.* 2009;13:73.
52. Stepnowsky CJ Jr, Marler MR, Ancoli-Israel S. Determinants of nasal CPAP compliance. *Sleep Med.* 2002;3:239.
53. Pack AI, Black JE, Schwartz JR, et al. Modafinil as adjunct therapy for daytime sleepiness in obstructive sleep apnea. *Am J Respir Crit Care Med.* 2001;164:1675.

CHAPTER 12

Pharmacotherapy

Shivani Swami, Vivek Nangia

INTRODUCTION

The mainstay of therapy for all sleep related breathing disorders is the use of positive airway pressure (PAP) devices. However, quite a large number of patients decline to use a contraption during sleep; while with others, compliance to therapy is an issue. Not all patients are candidates for a surgical intervention or an oral appliance. The success rates of sleep apnea surgery are also very variable.

Medical therapy for sleep apnea includes lifestyle modifications like weight reduction, avoidance of tobacco and alcohol, positional therapy, supplemental oxygen therapy, and pharmacotherapy. The potential mechanisms by which the pharmacological agents could benefit the patients are: maintaining patency of the upper airway during sleep, increasing respiratory drive, reducing the proportion of rapid eye movement (REM) sleep, facilitating cholinergic tone during sleep, or reducing upper airway resistance/surface tension. Unfortunately, no agent studied so far has been able to adequately prevent upper airway collapse or improve apnea-hypopnea index (AHI) sufficiently to justify its use as a primary therapy. Hence, pharmacotherapy plays a secondary or adjunctive role only.[1-3]

Pharmacological agents can broadly be classified into five categories: (1) agents that impact sleep pattern, (2) agents that promote wakefulness, (3) agents that reduce nasal air resistance and congestion, (4) agents that promote ventilation, and (5) agents that should be avoided.

AGENTS THAT IMPACT SLEEP PATTERN

Protryptyline

It is a tricyclic antidepressant known to suppress REM sleep.[4] Obstructive sleep apnea (OSA) is often the most severe during this phase and thus, reduction in REM sleep may decrease the frequency or severity of obstructive events. It also increases the tone of the upper airway dilator muscle by increasing the hypoglossal and recurrent laryngeal nerve activity.[5] However, while it may lead to reduction in the number of obstructive apneas but there may just be an increase in the number of hypopneas,[6] and hence may still result in microarousals, autonomic nervous system activation and hence deleterious cardiovascular effects. Some users have reported an improvement in daytime sleepiness.[4]

A double-blind crossover trial comparing the effect of protriptyline to placebo in 5 patients with OSA showed that protriptyline reduced REM sleep time and subjective daytime sleepiness. It also reduced REM-related apneas (16 per hour to 3 per hour), but the overall AHI changed minimally (64 per hour to 60 per hour). Three patients had a statistically significant, but probably not a clinically significant, reduction in their apnea index (AI) after 6 months of protriptyline therapy (56 versus 71 events per hour).[4]

A controlled trial randomly assigned 10 patients with OSA to receive protriptyline, acetazolamide, or placebo for two weeks. Protriptyline did not have a significant effect on symptoms or the frequency of apneas, hypopneas, arousals, or desaturations, compared to placebo.[7]

Side effects may include dry mouth, urinary hesitancy, constipation, confusion, and ataxia. It is not considered a standard form of treatment due to its lack of significant impact on obstructive sleep apnea hypopnea syndrome (OSAHS).

Serotonergic Agents

Serotonin plays a role in hypoglossal nerve function, and patients with OSA may have a central deficiency of serotonin activity, which may be partially explained by obesity and insulin resistance. Theoretically, increasing serotonin may increase genioglossal tone and thus improve OSA.[8]

Buspirone, which partly acts through the serotonin receptors in the central nervous system, augments ventilation and increases ventilator responsiveness both during sleep and wakefulness.[9,10] It is also believed to reduce the apneic threshold for carbon dioxide.

Fluoxetine was found to increase sleep latency independent of its effect on sleep-disordered breathing (SDB) but reduce the REM percentage.[11] There have been many inconclusive trials on a combination of fluoxetine and ondansetron. The best results were achieved using a combination of the selective serotonin receptor antagonist, ondansetron, and the serotonin reuptake inhibitor, fluoxetine. The trial randomly assigned 35 patients with OSA (defined as an AHI of >10 events per hour) to receive placebo, ondansetron (24 mg) alone, ondansetron (24 mg) plus fluoxetine (5 mg), or ondansetron (24 mg) plus fluoxetine (10 mg) for 28 days.[12] Only the combinations of ondansetron and fluoxetine reduced the AHI, with the combination of ondansetron (24 mg) plus fluoxetine (10 mg) having a larger magnitude of effect than the combination of ondansetron (24 mg) plus fluoxetine (5 mg). The combination of ondansetron (24 mg) plus fluoxetine (10 mg) also induced a trend towards better oxyhemoglobin saturation.[13]

Paroxitine has also been shown to increase the genioglossus inspiratory activity, but not alter the duration or number of obstructive events. In a study of 20 patients, it mildly reduced the AHI (30 vs. 36 events per hour) during non-REM sleep but had no effect on sleepiness, memory, mood, or indices of respiratory events.[14]

Mirtazapine, a newer antidepressant agent, is a 5-hydroxytryptamine-1 (5-HT$_1$) agonist and 5-HT$_2$ and 5-HT$_3$ antagonist. It also affects noradrenegic and histaminergic receptors that could enhance central respiratory drive. In low doses, it enhances the genioglossal nerve activity while in higher doses, it inhibits the same. Trials have not exhibited any benefit in treatment of OSAHS. In fact, its use was associated with weight gain and sedation, and hence worsening of sleep apnea.[15,16]

Clonidine, an alpha-2 adrenergic agonist, is also known to suppress REM sleep but has shown no benefit in AHI, mean apnea duration, and the mean lowest oxygen saturation reached. It should, in fact, be used carefully as an antihypertensive drug in patients with OSA as it can often result in severe respiratory depression and hypotension.[17] Clonidine when used as a premedication drug in patients undergoing sleep apnea surgery resulted in lesser dosages of propofol and piritamide needed for induction and anesthesia.[18]

Trazodone, which has the potential to improve OSA by increasing the arousal threshold, is yet to show any significant clinical benefit.[19]

AGENTS THAT PROMOTE WAKEFULNESS

Few patients may continue to experience excessive daytime sleepiness in spite of being on optimized PAP therapy, maintaining saturations during sleep, and an improvement in the AHI.[20] However, in such patients, other causes of sleepiness noncompliance with PAP, ill-fitting PAP masks, insufficient sleep, poor sleep hygiene, other sleep disorders such as narcolepsy or restless legs syndrome/periodic leg movements of sleep, and depression need to be ruled out before considering adjunctive therapy.[21] The purpose of medication in such patients is to target the residual daytime sleepiness. Modafinil and armodafinil are the two main stimulants used for this purpose.

Modafinil

It is believed to be a central $\alpha 1$ adrenergic agonist which induces wakefulness by inhibiting dopamine and noradrenaline reuptake transporters.[22] The effectiveness of modafinil has been demonstrated in multiple randomized trials.[23-27] One of the largest studies is a randomized double-blind crossover trial of 157 patients with OSA with persistent daytime sleepiness despite adequate conventional therapy. It lasted 12 weeks and compared modafinil (titrated upward from 200 mg to 400 mg) with placebo once daily for 12 weeks.[24] A greater proportion of patients in the modafinil group experienced resolution in the excessive daytime sleepiness than in the placebo group (51 vs. 27%), as measured by the Epworth Sleepiness Scale. Some patients reported an elevation in blood pressure attributed to modafinil use;[28] therefore, monitoring is recommended.

The peak plasma absorption for modafinil occurs at 2–4 hours and its elimination half-life is 13 hours. Hence, when administered in the morning, it typically promotes wakefulness into the early evening without disrupting nighttime sleep. Usual approach is to start at a dose of 100 mg and then titrate up to a maximum of 400 mg as needed. A divided dosing schedule with 200 mg in the morning and 200 mg in the early to mid-afternoon may benefit patients with persistent afternoon sleepiness. Patients generally report improvement within 7 days of starting therapy or increasing a dose.

Modafinil has also been used to mitigate daytime sleepiness in patients with short-term withdrawal of PAP therapy. It improves vigilance, quality of life, productivity, activity, and intimacy.[29]

Armodafinil

Armodafinil is the R- and the longer-lasting enantiomer of racemic modafinil. It appears to be similarly effective, according to randomized trials.[30,12] However, armodafinil and modafinil have never been directly compared. Armodafinil is started at 150 mg in the morning and is increased after 1 week to 250 mg, if needed.

Both modafinil and armodafinil have been known to cause severe skin hypersensitivity reactions (Stevens-Johnson syndrome and toxic epidermonecrolysis), hence patients have to be advised to discontinue the drug immediately, if they notice any rash. Rashes usually appear within the first 5 weeks of therapy. The other side effects include headache, nausea, anorexia, dry mouth, and diarrhea. Both are metabolized through the liver and thus interact with other drugs due to their effect on cytochrome P450 enzymes. It should be used cautiously in patients with heart diseases like left ventricular dysfunction and mitral valve prolapse, and those with arrhythmias as palpitations and ischemic changes have been reported.[1]

Other Stimulants

Methylphenidate stimulates the central nervous system through two possible mechanisms: a sympathomimetic effect and stimulation of the brainstem reticular activating system and cortex. Attention deficit hyperactivity disorder, narcolepsy, or mild brain injury are the common clinical conditions where it is used often. *Amphetamines* are also potent central nervous system stimulants and sympathoactive agents. Some clinicians use them as a substitute to modafinil; however, there are no clinical trials to support their use. Side effects of methylphenidate include headache, nausea, dry mouth, anorexia, and diarrhea. It should be used cautiously in patients with a history of arrhythmias or heart disease. The major toxicities of amphetamines are psychiatric (e.g., irritability and psychosis) and cardiovascular (e.g., hypertension and heart failure). Both these agents are of greater potential risk for dependency and abuse. *Caffeine* is another central nervous system stimulant; however, there is no scientific data to support its use in adults with OSA.[1]

AGENTS THAT REDUCE NASAL AIR RESISTANCE

Nasal passage offers significant amount of resistance to the airflow especially if further narrowed by the presence of rhinopathy, hypertrophied turbinates, and adenotonsillar hypertrophy. Short-acting *topical nasal decongestants* have not shown any additional benefit over positional therapy and hence are not recommended. On the contrary, they are associated with mucosal vasoconstriction followed by rebound vasodilatation thus adversely affecting the nasal patency. *Topical nasal steroid sprays*, fluticasone and budesonide, on the other hand, have been shown to favorably influence the AHI and nasal airway resistance resulting in improved daytime alertness and nasal decongestion.[31,32] In OSA, a well-known anti-inflammatory marker to get elevated is leukotrienes. Montelukast, a *leukotriene receptor antagonist*, when administered to children, with mild SDB, resulted in significantly lower AHI without changing the sleep parameters.[33] A study combining montelukast and topical steroid spray in children with residual SDB following tonsillectomy and adenoidectomy also resulted in a significantly lower AHI (0.3 vs. 4.7).[34] A Cochrane review, on intranasal corticosteroids, published in 2008, showed their significant efficacy in improving nasal obstruction symptoms and in reducing adenoid size. Consequently, this may influence the anatomic component by decreasing upper airway resistance at the nasal, adenoidal, and/or tonsillar levels. Therefore, topical nasal steroids may influence sleep apnea severity both in children and adults.[35]

AGENTS THAT PROMOTE VENTILATION

Agents that promote ventilation have not been shown to be beneficial in patients with OSA, and have a limited role in patients with central sleep apnea (CSA).

Theophylline and aminophylline act by blocking the adenosine receptors, thereby stimulating ventilatory drive. Theophylline has been used to treat patients with periodic breathing or CSA, especially Cheyne-Stokes breathing, due to left ventricular systolic dysfunction.[36] However, most of the good quality studies have reported similar negative findings.[37-39] Aminophylline also has been found to increase sleep fragmentation and hence reduce sleep efficiency.[40]

Acetazolamide is a carbonic anhydrase inhibitor and a weak diuretic. It causes mild metabolic acidosis, which stimulates respiration and decreases the frequency of central apneas.[41,42] In a crossover trial of 12 patients with CSA associated with Cheyne-Stokes breathing due to heart failure (mean AHI 55 events per hour), acetazolamide decreased the AHI (34 vs. 57 events per hour for placebo), while improving subjective sleep quality, restfulness, and fatigue as compared to placebo.[42] Another two nonrandomized trials have shown acetazolamide to be associated with reduction of the AHI and less daytime sleepiness.[41]

Donepezil is a centrally acting cholinesterase inhibitor. Cholinergic activity is known to affect upper airway opening via peripheral and central mechanisms.[43-46] A study done in 23 patients of Alzheimer's disease demonstrated significant improvement in oxygen saturation and AHI.[47] These data require confirmation with larger controlled clinical trials that measure patient-important outcomes before donepezil can be recommended for patients with OSA.

Physostigmine, a cholinergic agonist, has been investigated as possible treatments for OSA. In a single night study, 10 subjects had an AHI of 41 on physostigmine compared with 54 on placebo.[1] The greatest impact was on apneas during REM sleep, and there was an inverse relationship with body mass index, such that slimmer subjects had a greater fall in AHI. The drug was given intravenously, making it impractical for home use. There have been no studies with oral cholinergic agents.

Progestational agents are respiratory stimulants whose effect on patients with OSA is uncertain. Some studies have reported a net beneficial effect,[48,49] while others have not.[50,51] Based on these results, neither primary estrogen replacement therapy nor supplementary therapy with estrogens, whether with estrogen alone or coupled with progesterone, is recommended for the purpose of treating OSA.[21] There are also potential adverse side effects associated with the administration of estrogen replacement therapy.[52]

Doxapram is a respiratory stimulant that acts through peripheral carotid chemoreceptors. Intravenous doxapram has been shown to decrease the average length of apnea in patients with OSA.[53] Using doxapram in the perioperative period led to fewer postoperative respiratory complications (2% vs. 29%), shorter postoperative stay in the recovery room and the hospital overall.[54]

Opioid antagonists are short-acting agents that improve oxygenation, presumably, by stimulating the central nervous system by competitive inhibition of endorphins at receptor sites or by stimulating the cortex, to increase ventilation. However, they also cause significant sleep disruption. Administration of *naloxone* as intravenous infusion results in lesser oxyhemoglobin desaturation index and the severity of oxyhemoglobin desaturation episodes, along with reduction, by about 80%, in the amount of REM sleep.[55]

Nicotine also has similar effects: increase in ventilation, improved oxygenation along with significant sleep disruption.[56] Besides that, it is addictive and has numerous other side effects because of which it is not recommended for the treatment of OSA.

Greater than 25% patients of hypothyroidism suffer from OSA. Use of thyroxine in such patients, possibly by resolving macroglossia, has successfully eliminated OSA in some studies, even in the absence of weight loss. Thus, patients with coexisting OSA and hypothyroidism must be treated with thyroxine.[57]

Sabeluzole, a glutamate antagonist, and *baclofen*, a gamma-aminobutyric agent, are two other drugs which have been studied but not found to have any significant clinical benefit.

Oxygen

Hypoxemia and sleep fragmentation are considered to lead to the consequences of sleep apnea, therefore, treatment of hypoxemia through supplemental oxygen was thought of.

Earlier studies done on the effect of oxygen administration demonstrated that oxygen administration could increase apnea duration, associated hypercapnea, and respiratory acidosis.[58-60] Supplemental oxygen administration is also associated with a clinically insignificant reduction in apnea frequency though, is not effective in increasing daytime alertness.[61] However, patients with cerebrovascular disease or coronary artery disease, with oxyhemoglobin desaturation during sleep, might benefit from supplemental oxygen, provided they have only marginally elevated apneic events.[62,63] It may also be used as an adjunct to PAP therapy, in a selected few patients.[64]

There are two level II and two level III studies that show oxygen administration improves oxygenation parameters in patients with OSA.[65-68] Three of these studies involved special populations of OSA patients; one evaluated 3 patients on long-term opioid therapy,[66] one studied 43 patients who had already undergone not fully successful surgical management of OSA,[67] and one involved 8 continuous positive airway pressure (CPAP) intolerant males.[68] The remaining study primarily reported on the effect of transtracheal oxygen therapy in 4 patients, three of whom had significant obstructive lung disease.[65] Although all studies showed favorable effects on oxygenation, the effect of oxygen therapy on apneas, hypopneas, and subjective sleepiness was inconsistent.

Qnexa

It is the combination of the drugs, phentermine and topiramate, being marketed as a treatment to obesity and related conditions. Phentermine is an appetite suppressant and topiramate is an anticonvulsant, which has a weight loss side effect. It got approval from US Food and Drug Administration (FDA) on July 2012, with recommendations for post-market monitoring for cardiovascular risk and an indication against use by pregnant women.

Alternative therapies like *homeopathy and acupuncture* have also been studied to assess their role as supportive therapy. The various homeopathic drugs used are as follows:

- Arsenicum album: for respiratory disorders that worsen at night and are accompanied by fear, agitation, restlessness, weakness, and exhaustion
- Lachesis: for conditions that get worse while trying to sleep. This remedy is most appropriate for those who are intense, talkative, jealous, and may feel depressed (particularly in the morning). It may also help people who are frightened of going to sleep
- Opium: this remedy may be prescribed for individuals with sleep apnea and narcolepsy (inability to control falling asleep during the daytime). This remedy is appropriate for individuals who may be somewhat confused due to the sleep disorder
- Sambucus: for difficulty breathing at night. This remedy is most appropriate for individuals who may have nasal obstruction or asthma and actually jump up out of bed with a feeling of suffocation
- Spongia: for respiratory symptoms that are worsened by cold air and lying down. This remedy is appropriate for individuals who often feel tightness in the chest area
- Sulphur: for chronic conditions accompanied by sleep disturbances and nightmares, especially if the individual also has skin rashes that become worse with heat. This remedy is most appropriate for individuals who prefer cold temperatures and strongly dislike any kind of restriction.

Some evidence suggests that a type of acupuncture called auriculotherapy acupoint pressure may help treat sleep apnea.

AGENTS TO BE AVOIDED

Benzodiazepines, barbiturates, narcotics, and anesthetics should only be used with great caution as they destabilize the upper airway by suppressing the central nervous system.

CONCLUSION

Owing to the multiple complex pathogenetic mechanisms involved in the development of OSA, no pharmacologic agents investigated so far has been fully able to prevent or overcome upper airway obstruction, sufficient enough to justify itself as a primary therapy in the management of OSA. Pharmacotherapy is purely adjunctive. The only situation where medication is shown to be significantly beneficial is residual sleepiness despite adequate PAP therapy. Modafinil and armodofinil have shown good results in this situation. Topical nasal steroid sprays have been found to improve AHI in children or adults with perennial allergic rhinitis.

REFERENCES

1. Abad VC. Pharmacologic therapy for obstructive sleep apnea. *Sleep Med Clin.* 2013;8: 527-42.
2. Randerath WJ, Verbraecken J, Andreas S, et al. Non-CPAP therapies in obstructive sleep apnoea. *Eur Respir J.* 2011;37:1000.
3. Mason M, Welsh EJ, Smith I. Drug therapy for obstructive sleep apnoea in adults. *Cochrane Database Syst Rev.* 2013;5:CD003002.
4. Brownell LG, West P, Sweatman P, et al. Protriptyline in obstructive sleep apnea: a double blind trial. *N Engl J Med.* 1982;307:1037-42.
5. Bonora M, St John WM. Differential elevation by protriptyline and depression by diazepam of upper airway respiratory muscle activity. *Am Rev Respir Dis.* 1985;131:41-5.
6. Smith PL, Haponik EF, Allen RP, et al. The effects of protriptyline in sleep disordered breathing. *Am Rev Respir Dis.* 1983;127:8-13.
7. Whyte KF, Gould GA, Airlie MA, et al. Role of protriptyline and acetazolamide in the sleep apnea/hypopnea syndrome. *Sleep.* 1988;11:463.
8. Hudgel DW, Gordon EA, Meltzer HY. Abnormal serotonergic stimulation of cortisol production in obstructive sleep apnea. *Am J Respir Crit Care Med.* 1995;152:186.
9. Mendelson WB, Martin JV, Rapoport DM. Effects of buspirone on sleep and respiration. *Am Rev Respir Dis.* 1990;141:1527-30.
10. Garner SJ, Eldridge FL, Wagner PG, et al. Buspirone, an anxiolytic drug that stimulates respiration. *Am Rev Respir Dis.* 1989;139:946-50.
11. Hanzel DA, Proia NG, Hudgel DW. Response of OSA to fluoxetine and protriptyline. *Chest.* 1991;100:416-21.
12. Hirshkowitz M, Black JE, Wesnes K, et al. Adjunct armodafinil improves wakefulness and memory in obstructive sleep apnea/hypopnea syndrome. *Respir Med.* 2007;101:616.
13. Prasad B, Radulovacki M, Olopade C, et al. Prospective trial of efficacy and safety of ondansetron and fluoxetine in patients with obstructive sleep apnea syndrome. *Sleep.* 2010;33:982.
14. Kraiczi H, Hedner J, Dahlöf P, et al. Effect of serotonin uptake inhibition on breathing during sleep and daytime symptoms in obstructive sleep apnea. *Sleep.* 1999;22:61.
15. Marshall NS, Yee BJ, Desai AV, et al. Two randomized placebo-controlled trials to evaluate the efficacy and tolerability of mirtazapine for the treatment of obstructive sleep apnea. *Sleep.* 2008;31(6):824-31.
16. David WC, Christopher O. Efficacy of mirtazapine in obstructive sleep apnoea syndrome. *Sleep.* 2007;30:35-41.
17. Roberge RJ, Kimball ET, Rossi J, et al. Clonidine and sleep apnea syndrome interaction: antagonism with yohimbine. *J Emerg Med.* 1998;16:727.
18. Issa FG. Effect of clonidine in obstructive sleep apnea. *Am Rev Respir Dis.* 1992;145:435-9.
19. Heinzer RC, White DP, Jordan AS, et al. Trazodone increases arousal threshold in obstructive sleep apnoea. *Eur Respir J.* 2008;31(6):1308-12.
20. Pépin JL, Viot-Blanc V, Escourrou P, et al. Prevalence of residual excessive sleepiness in CPAP-treated sleep apnoea patients: the French multicentre study. *Eur Respir J.* 2009;33:1062.
21. Morgenthaler TI, Kapen S, Lee-Chiong T, et al. Practice parameters for the medical therapy of obstructive sleep apnoea. *Sleep.* 2006;29:1031-5.
22. Lyons TJ, French J. Modafinil: the unique properties of a new stimulant. *Aviat Space Environ Med.* 1991;62:432-5.
23. Kingshott RN, Vennelle M, Coleman EL, et al. Randomized, double-blind, placebo-controlled crossover trial of modafinil in the treatment of residual excessive daytime sleepiness in the sleep apnea/hypopnea syndrome. *Am J Respir Crit Care Med.* 2001;163:918.
24. Pack AI, Black JE, Schwartz JR, et al. Modafinil as adjunct therapy for daytime sleepiness in obstructive sleep apnea. *Am J Respir Crit Care Med.* 2001;164:1675.
25. Schwartz JR, Hirshkowitz M, Erman MK, et al. Modafinil as adjunct therapy for daytime sleepiness in obstructive sleep apnea: a 12-week, open-label study. *Chest.* 2003;124:2192.

26. Black JE, Hirshkowitz M. Modafinil for treatment of residual excessive sleepiness in nasal continuous positive airway pressure-treated obstructive sleep apnea/hypopnea syndrome. *Sleep.* 2005;28:464.
27. Inoue Y, Takasaki Y, Yamashiro Y. Efficacy and Safety of Adjunctive Modafinil Treatment on Residual Excessive Daytime Sleepiness among Nasal Continuous Positive Airway Pressure-Treated Japanese Patients with Obstructive Sleep Apnea Syndrome: A Double-Blind Placebo-Controlled Study. *J Clin Sleep Med.* 2013;9:751.
28. Heitmann J, Cassel W, Grote L, et al. Does short-term treatment with modafinil affect blood pressure in patients with obstructive sleep apnea? *Clin Pharmacol Ther.* 1999;65:328-35.
29. Weaver TE, Chasens ER, Arora S. Modafinil improves functional outcomes in patients with residual excessive sleepiness associated with CPAP treatment. *J Clin Sleep Med.* 2009;5:499.
30. Roth T, White D, Schmidt-Nowara W, et al. Effects of armodafinil in the treatment of residual excessive sleepiness associated with obstructive sleep apnea/hypopnea syndrome: a 12 week, multicenter, double-blind, randomized, placebo-controlled study in nCPAP-adherent adults. *Clin Ther.* 2006;28:689.
31. Canova CR, Downs SH, Knoblauch A, et al. Increased prevalence of perennial allergic rhinitis in patients with obstructive sleep apnea. *Respiration.* 2004;71:138-43.
32. Alexopoulos EI, Kaditis AG, Kalampouka E, et al. Nasal corticosteroids for children with snoring. *Pediatr Pulmonol.* 2004;38:161-7.
33. Goldbart AD, Greenberg-Dotan S, Tal A. Montelukast for children with obstructive sleep apnea: a double-blind, placebo-controlled study. *Pediatrics.* 2012;130(3):e575-80.
34. Kheirandish L, Goldbart AD, Gozal D. Intranasal steroids and oral leukotriene modifier therapy in residual sleep-disordered breathing after tonsillectomy and adenoidectomy in children. *Pediatrics.* 2006;117:e61-6.
35. Zhang L, Mendoza-Sassi RA, Ce´sar JA, et al. Intranasal corticosteroids for nasal airway obstruction in children with moderate to severe adenoidal hypertrophy. *Cochrane Database Syst Rev.* 2008;(3):CD006286.
36. Javaheri S, Parker TJ, Wexler L, et al. Effect of theophylline on sleep-disordered breathing in heart failure. *N Engl J Med.* 1996;335:562.
37. Espinoza H, Antic R, Thornton A, et al. The effects of aminophylline on sleep and sleep-disordered breathing in patients with obstructive sleep apnea syndrome. *Am Rev Respir Dis.* 1987;136:80-4.
38. Saletu B, Oberndorfer S, Anderer P, et al. Efficiency of continuous positive airway pressure versus theophylline therapy in sleep apnea: comparative sleep laboratory studies on objective and subjective sleep and awakening quality. *Neuropsychobiology.* 1999;39:151-9.
39. Hein H, Behnke G, Jorres RA, et al. The therapeutic effect of theophylline in mild obstructive sleep Apnea/Hypopnea syndrome: results of repeated measurements with portable recording devices at home. *Eur J Med Res.* 2000;5:391-9.
40. Espinoza H, Antic R, Thornton AT, et al. The effects of aminophylline on sleep and sleep disordered breathing in patients with obstructive sleep apnea syndrome. *Am Rev Respir Dis.* 1987;136(1):80-4.
41. De Backer WA, Verbraecken J, Willemen M, et al. Central apnea index decreases after prolonged treatment with acetazolamide. *Am J Respir Cri Care Med.* 1995;151(1):87.
42. Javaheri S. Acetazolamide improves central sleep apnea in heart failure: a double-blind, prospective study. *Am J Respir Crit Care Med.* 2006;173(2):234.
43. Hedner J, Kraiczi H, Peker Y, et al. Reduction of sleep disordered breathing after physostigmine. *Am J Respir Crit Care Med.* 2003;168:1246-51.
44. O'Donnell CP, Schwartz AR, Smith PL. Upper airway collapsibility: the importance of gender and adiposity. *Am J Respir Crit Care Med.* 2000;162:1606-7.
45. Bellingham MC, Ireland MF. Contribution of cholinergic systems to state dependent modulation of respiratory control. *Respir Physiol Neurobiol.* 2002;131:135-44.
46. Gilman S, Chervin RD, Koeppe RA, et al. Obstructive sleep apnea is related to a thalamic cholinergic deficit in MSA. *Neurology.* 2003;61:35-9.

47. Moraes W, Poyares D, Sukys-Claudino L, et al. Donepezil improves obstructive sleep apnea in Alzheimer disease. *Chest.* 2008;133:677-83.
48. Keefe DL, Watson R, Naftolin F. Hormone replacement therapy may alleviate sleep apnea in menopausal women: a pilot study. *Menopause.* 1999;6:196.
49. Strohl KP, Hensley MJ, Saunders NA, et al. Progesterone administration and progressive sleep apneas. *JAMA.* 1981;245:1230.
50. Cistulli PA, Barnes DJ, Grunstein RR, et al. Effect of short-term hormone replacement in the treatment of obstructive sleep apnoea in postmenopausal women. *Thorax.* 1994;49:699.
51. Rajagopal KR, Abbrecht PH, Jabbari B. Effects of medroxyprogesterone acetate in obstructive sleep apnea. *Chest.* 1986;90:815.
52. Manson JE, Martin KA. Postmenopausal hormone-replacement therapy. *N Engl J Med.* 2001;345:34-40.
53. Suratt PM, Wilhoit SC, Brown ED, et al. Effect of doxapram on obstructive sleep apnea. *Bull Eur Physiopathol Respir.* 1986;22:127-31.
54. Bamgbade OA. Advantages of doxapram for postanesthesia recovery and outcomes in bariatric surgery patients with obstructive sleep apnea. *Eur J Anaesthesiol.* 2011;28:387-91.
55. Atkinson RL, Suratt PM, Wilhoit SC, et al. Naloxone improves sleep apnea in obese humans. *Int J Obes.* 1985;9:233.
56. Hein H, Kirsten D, Jugert C, et al. Nicotine as therapy of obstructive sleep apnea? *Pneumologie.* 1995;49 Suppl 1:185.
57. Skjodt NM, Atkar R, Easton PA. Screening for hypothyroidism in sleep apnea. *Am J Respir Crit Care Med.* 1999;160:732.
58. Motta J, Guilleminault C. Effects of oxygen administration in sleep induced apneas. Guilleminault C, Dement WC (Eds). Sleep Apnea Syndromes. NY: Alan R Liss; 1978. pp. 137-44.
59. Kimoff RJ, Cheong TH, Olha AE, et al. Mechanisms of apnea termination in obstructive sleep apnea: role of chemoreceptor & mechanoreceptor stimuli. *Am J Respir Crit Care Med.* 1994;149:707-14.
60. Martin RJ, Sanders MH, Gray BA, et al. Acute and long term ventilatory effects of hyperoxia in adult sleep apnea syndrome. *Am Rev Respir Dis.* 1982;125:175-80.
61. Gold AR, Schwartz AR. The effect of chronic nocturnal oxygen administration upon sleep apnoea syndrome. *Am Rev Respir Dis.* 1986;134:925-9.
62. Hanly P, Sasson Z, Zuberi N, et al. ST segment depression during sleep in obstructive sleep apnoea. *Am J Cardiol.* 1993;71:1341-5.
63. Franklin KA, Nilsson JB, Sahlin C, et al. Sleep apnoea and nocturnal angina. *Lancet.* 1995;345:1085-7.
64. Sanders MH, Kern N. Obstructive sleep apnea treated by independently adjusted inspiratory and expiratory positive airway pressures via nasal mask: physiologic and clinical implications. *Chest.* 1990;98:317-24.
65. Chauncey J, Aldrich M. Preliminary findings in the treatment of obstructive sleep apnea with transtracheal oxygen. *Sleep.* 1990;13:167-74.
66. Farney RJ, Walker JM, Cloward TV, et al. Sleep-disordered breathing associated with long-term opioid therapy. *Chest.* 2003;123:632-9.
67. Landsberg R, Friedman M, Ascher-Landsberg J. Treatment of hypoxemia in obstructive sleep apnea. *Am J Rhinol.* 2001;15:311-3.
68. Phillips BA, Schmitt FA, Berry DT, et al. Treatment of obstructive sleep apnea: a preliminary report comparing nasal CPAP to nasal oxygen in patients with mild OSA. *Chest.* 1990;98:325-30.

CHAPTER 13

Surgical Management of Obstructive Sleep Apnea

Rajeev Kumar, Alok Thakar

INTRODUCTION

Surgical intervention is aimed at increasing the upper airway lumen either by removing the space occupying lesions, excessive lax soft tissues in upper airway, or correcting the craniofacial morphology. Although continuous positive airway pressure (CPAP) is currently considered as the standard modality of treatment for obstructive sleep apnea (OSA),[1] however, a significant percentage of patients were reported to be noncompliant to CPAP.[2] This group of patients and some other distinct subgroup of patients may benefit from surgical intervention. Obstruction is usually dynamic and may be at multiple levels. Correct identification of the multiple levels of obstruction is of utmost importance prior to any surgical intervention. Surgical expansion of the multilevel obstructions may be addressed either as a single-stage operation or in multiple-staged operations.

LEVELS OF OBSTRUCTION

Obstruction in upper airway can be anywhere between nose to larynx and can be multisegmental. However, the correct assessment of level of obstruction is reported to be difficult because of the following reasons:
- The natural sleep cannot be recreated during assessment
- The dynamic nature of upper airway is difficult to assess by any single tool.

This has led to an increased number of investigative tools used for correctly assessing the level of upper airway obstruction.

Broadly, the level of obstruction in the upper airway from nose to larynx is categorized into following subsites with the anatomical structures responsible for or contributing to OSA (Table 1). These anatomical structures are the key points where the disease process and/or anatomical variation lead to development of OSA.

EVALUATION OF LEVEL OF OBSTRUCTION

General ENT Examination

In outpatient department (OPD), a thorough ear-nose-throat (ENT) examination will give a lot of clues regarding the underlying problem. Apart from general

Surgical Management of Obstructive Sleep Apnea

Table 1: Upper airway sub-sites and corresponding anatomical structures contributing to obstructive sleep apnea

Level of obstruction	Anatomical structures involved
Nose	Nasal valve, nasal septum, turbinate, maxilla
Nasopharynx	Adenoids
Oropharynx	Soft palate, tonsils, base of tongue, lingual tonsils
Larynx	Supraglottis, glottis, subglottis
Oral cavity	Mandible

physical examination which includes height, weight, body mass index (BMI), and local examination specific to ENT needs to be done thoroughly. A look at the face will give clue regarding abnormal facial morphology including mandible, external nasal framework, and nasal valve functioning and neck circumference. The examination of the airway starts with the nose examination. During nasal examination, one needs to look at nasal valve function, deviation of nasal septum and turbinate hypertrophy. Rest of the nasal examination requires endoscopic assessment. Endoscopic examination can reveal any obstructive pathology inside the nasal cavity and nasopharynx which is the contributing factor to the development of OSA. The presence of nasal and nasopharyngeal pathologies like polyps, benign slow-growing tumors (angiofibroma, schwannoma, and fibrous dysplasia), and adenoidal hypertrophy can readily be detected with endoscopic evaluation in the OPD setting. Oral cavity examination gives a fair amount of idea regarding tongue abnormality, soft palate position in relation to tongue, tonsillar enlargement and narrow velopharynx. Apart from this, indirect laryngoscopic examination reveals lingual tonsillar hypertrophy, supraglottic, glottic and subglottic pathology (recurrent respiratory papillomatosis, bilateral cord palsy, subglottic stenosis).

Although general ENT examination helps to rule out various pathologies, the most important area of concern is oropharynx. Oropharynx is primarily an anatomical division of pharynx which consists of soft palate, base of tongue, and tonsils. This is the most difficult area to assess and treat owing to its dynamic nature during sleep, circumferential soft tissues, and physiological importance in swallowing and speech. The obstruction level in oropharynx has been further subdivided into retropalatal and retroglossal/hypopharyngeal. Most of the modern investigative tools help to find and define precise level of obstruction in this area only. The most modern and precise investigations which help the surgeon to select the area of surgical intervention are discussed in the following section.

Muller Maneuver

This procedure requires the patient to perform a "reverse valsalva". A fiberoptic nasopharyngoscope/laryngoscope (FOL) is introduced through one nostril of the patient after spraying the nostril with 10% xylocaine spray. The FOL is positioned at velopharynx and patient is instructed to breathe in with closed mouth and pinched nostrils. This maneuver will simulate the collapse of complaint tissues at the level of palate and base of tongue as occurring during sleep. The degree

Table 2: Muller maneuver		
Degree of pharyngeal collapse recorded at each level as: • 1+ minimal collapse • 2+ collapse decreasing cross-sectional area by 50% • 3+ collapse decreasing cross-sectional area by 75% • 4+ obliteration of the airway.		
Soft palate level	*Retroglossal level*	*Recommendation*
3+/4+	No collapse	Ideal case for UPPP
3+/4+	1+/2+	Suboptimal, acceptable for UPPP
<3+	>2+	Not suitable for UPPP

UPPP, uvulopalatopharyngoplasty.

of collapse will be observed at soft palate level (retropalatal collapse) and scored as per Sher's criteria (Table 2). Thereafter, the FOL is advanced further to view base of tongue collapse. The same procedure is repeated and scoring will be done for retroglossal collapse. Muller maneuver is a quick OPD procedure and is reproducible, but has the inherent disadvantage of being undertaken with the patient in an awake state rather than asleep. This procedure has been recommended before selecting the patients for uvulopalatopharyngoplasty (UPPP).[3]

Sleep Nasoendoscopy

The concept of sleep nasal endoscopy was introduced by Croft and Pringle (1991) to assess the airway collapse during sleep.[4] In this procedure, patient is either sedated or asleep. FOL is then introduced through nose and collapse of upper airway lumen is observed at retropalatal and retroglossal level. Also termed as drug-induced sleep nasoendoscopy, this investigation is becoming investigation of choice for surgeons. The advantages include: procedure simulates near natural sleep, dynamic in nature, assesses all levels of obstruction simultaneously, no radiation involved, cost-effective, and can be performed before the surgery on operation theatre table to confirm the previous assessment done for level of obstruction. A comparative study of sleep nasoendoscopy and Muller maneuver found out that Muller maneuver is less accurate in assessing sites of pharyngeal obstruction.[5] Sleep nasoendoscopy has been quoted to be quality assessment in a case of sleep-disordered breathing and fundamental before surgical intervention.[6]

Computed Tomography

The role of computed tomography (CT) in the assessment of upper airway is debatable. CT provides three-dimensional (3D) upper airway assessments along with cross-sectional narrowing at the level of palate and base of tongue/hypopharynx. The measurements are objective and can be used for comparison after surgery. Being a noninvasive method, it provides good anatomical details of craniofacial morphology as well. However, being done in an awake patient along with radiation exposure limits its routine utility for OSA. 3D CT has shown retropalatal and lateral diameter to be significantly correlated with respiratory distress index. Retropalatal space is the most relevant obstruction identified on CT.[7] The cine CT is done during sleep and is an optional tool for assessment but availability, cost, and radiation exposure again limits its routine use. The use of CT should be individualized on case basis, and generalized use in all cases is not to be encouraged.

Magnetic Resonance Imaging

Sleep magnetic resonance imaging (MRI) is a valuable tool for assessing the dynamics of upper airway during natural sleep. MRI during sleep delineates soft tissues collapse accurately along with level of obstruction. Respiratory events can be correlated with airway collapse in real time during MRI.[8] MRI is reported to be helpful in both primary and surgically failed cases. However, MRI has certain limitations including cost, availability, prolonged procedure time, and interference with implanted pacemakers and electroencephalogram. The MRI machine produces an inherited noisy environment which can disturb sleep and subsequent accurate assessment of airway. The patients suffering from claustrophobia may be unable to undergo such an evaluation.

Somnofluoroscopy

Somnofluoroscopy is a technique in which patients with OSA are observed during polysomnography (PSG) study and during an obstructive episode, the upper airway is seen using image intensifier. The findings are recorded and analyzed. Based on this technique, level of obstruction has been classified into three categories:[9]

Type 1: Obstruction occurs at the level of soft palate only.
Type 2: Obstruction occurs at the level of soft palate initially followed by closure of more distal airway.
Type 3: Obstruction initially occurs distal to soft palate. Airway at the level of soft palate may close or remain open.

Somnofluoroscopy records only two-dimensional anatomy and visualization is limited in patients with short and thick neck. The radiation exposure adds to above limitations. Therefore, its routine use for upper airway assessment in patients of OSA is not recommended.

Lateral Cephalometry

Lateral cephalometry involves radiological assessment of upper airway in which lateral X-ray of head and neck is taken in expiration phase. Relationship between various soft tissues and bony points is measured to evaluate level of airway obstruction. The measurements including length of soft palate (distance between posterior nasal spine and tip of soft palate), posterior airway space (narrowest dimension in hypopharynx) and position of hyoid relative to mandibular plane is calculated.[9] Length of mandible has been shown to correlate significantly with OSA.[10] These parameters have been used to evaluate the success of maxillomandibular surgeries undertaken to correct airway narrowing. Cephalometry allows assessment of maxillomandibular hypoplasia and used routinely before corrective surgeries. Routine use of cephalometry is not required for all cases of OSA.

Pharyngeal Manometry

Pharyngeal manometry involves continuous pressure recording during sleep at various level in upper airway. Usually, three catheters are employed to measure the upper airway pressure. The level of obstruction determined usually falls into two groups: one group has level of obstruction at velopharyngeal level while other group has level of obstruction at base of tongue level or multisegmental. The former group is considered ideal candidate for UPPP.[9] Pharyngeal manometry has shown diagnostic accuracy for hypopharyngeal obstruction in UPPP failure patients.[11] It has the advantages of being cost-effective, well tolerated during sleep and correlates well with PSG. Pharyngeal manometry is a good investigative tool but is not routinely used for assessment for OSA patients.

TREATMENT

The treatment for OSA is essentially nasal continuous positive airway pressure (nCPAP). The surgical intervention is limited to two subgroups of patient:
1. With definitive obstructive upper airway pathology
2. Those that are noncompliant to CPAP.

Corrective Nasal Surgical Procedures

The role of nasal surgery in the management of OSA is limited but potentially helpful (Table 3). Corrective surgical procedures on deviated nasal septum (DNS) and hypertrophied turbinates can alleviate symptoms of snoring and mild sleep apnea but cannot cure moderate to severe OSA.[12] However, it has been reported in literature that treating the obstructive nasal pathology (DNS, hypertrophied turbinates, nasal polyposis) helps to improve the compliance to nCPAP by reducing nasal airway resistance.[13,14]

The nasal surgeries like septoplasty for DNS, inferior turbinate reduction for hypertrophied turbinates and functional endoscopic sinus surgery for nasal polyposis can be done on day care basis either under local anesthesia or general anesthesia. The benefit of such surgeries can be estimated by comparing preoperative and postoperative pressure requirements for nCPAP.

Table 3: Common nasal surgical procedures for obstructive sleep apnea patients

Pathology	Surgical procedure	Surgical modalities/approaches	Complications
Deviated nasal septum	Septoplasty	Conventional/open Endoscopic	Synechiae formation Septal perforation
Turbinate hypertrophy	Turbinate reduction	Submucosal diathermy Cryosurgery Laser surgery	Rehypertrophy Nasal crusting
	Turbinate resection	Partial excision Submucosal turbinectomy Radical turbinectomy	Atrophic rhinitis
Nasal polyposis Allergic fungal rhinosinusitis	Sinus surgery	Functional endoscopic sinus surgery External/open approach	Hemorrhage Orbital hematoma Intracranial infection

The obstructive pathology commonly seen at the level of nasopharynx is adenoidal tissue hypertrophy. This is commonly seen in pediatric age group along with tonsillar hypertrophy. However, endoscopic evaluation of nasopharynx must be done to rule out adenoidal tissue hypertrophy and must be surgically addressed if present.

Tonsillectomy

The role of tonsillectomy in the management of OSA in adult population is limited. Tonsillar hypertrophy is commonly seen in pediatric population and rarely in adult population. However, whenever it is present as an obstructive pathology, surgical resection of the tonsils can alleviate or improve the symptoms of OSA.[15] Tonsillectomy has reported to improve compliance for nCPAP in previously noncompliant patients.[16] The common indications for tonsillectomy in OSA patients are: (1) substantial tonsillar hypertrophy and (2) as a component of UPPP procedure. There are numerous surgical procedures described in literature for performing tonsillar resection with certain advantages over other procedure. The common among those are mentioned below:
- "Cold Steel" tonsillectomy
- Coblation tonsillectomy
- Radiofrequency-assisted tonsillotomy
- Diathermy tonsillectomy
- Laser tonsillectomy
- Ultrasonic/harmonic scalpel tonsillectomy.

The most common complications include hemorrhage (primary and secondary) and postoperative pain. The role of tonsillectomy is well established in pediatric population. In selected adult population with OSA having enlarged tonsils (grade III or IV) tonsillectomy is recommended.

Uvulopalatopharyngoplasty

Uvulopalatopharyngoplasty is a surgical procedure aimed at correcting retropalatal obstruction. The procedure involves surgical removal of tonsils, part of anterior and posterior tonsillar pillars, part of soft palate and uvula.[9] The anterior and posterior tonsillar pillars are sutured together and posterior soft palate mucosa is sutured with anterior soft palate mucosa. The procedure is aimed at removing the excessive lax tissues at the level of velopharynx. By performing the UPPP, the cross-sectional area of velopharynx is increased. UPPP is helpful in those OSA patients who primarily have retropalatal obstruction only. The preoperative selection of patients for this procedure is of utmost importance. Patients who have undergone UPPP and failed to improve were retrospectively evaluated and found to have multisegmental levels of obstruction. The success rate of UPPP has been reported to be variable.[17] Favorable factors associated with UPPP success have been a BMI between 28 and 30, apnea-hypopnea index (AHI) less than 25, large tonsils, a favorable Mueller's maneuver (as per Sher's criteria), and isolated retropalatal obstruction on sleep endoscopy.[17] Reported complications have included nasal regurgitation of fluids, dryness of the throat, rhinolalia aperta, taste disturbance, and velopharyngeal stenosis. It has also been noted to sometimes affect nCPAP compliance owing to persistent dry throat and leak of air.[18]

The key for success of UPPP is correct patient selection and requires meticulous preoperative diagnostic workup.

Tongue Base Reduction with or without Hyoid Suspension

Tongue base reduction with temperature-controlled radiofrequency is performed by introduction of the probe into tongue base and raising the probe temperature up to 40–70°C. This results in formation of plasma field at probe tip consisting of highly ionized particles which breaks down the molecular bonds between cells. This procedure results in reduction of tongue base. The role of tongue base reduction in OSA patients is validated by few studies.[19,20] However, studies have shown low success rate and relapse on long-term follow-up for tongue base reduction in isolation.[21] Tongue base reduction with radiofrequency can be done in selected subgroup of patients with isolated retroglossal obstruction and mild-to-moderate OSA. Postoperative complications including pain are limited (<5%). One major complication includes tongue base abscess formation which requires incision and drainage. Speech and swallowing is generally unaffected.[18] On other hand, hyoid bone suspension aims to prevent collapse of tongue base during sleep. In this procedure, hyoid bone is suspended to thyroid cartilage surgically to improve retroglossal/hypopharyngeal space. The procedure may be undertaken in isolation for tongue base obstruction,[22-24] or as a component of multilevel surgery (MLS).[25,26] Temporary dysphagia up to 4 weeks, aspiration, hematomas, seromas, and articulation problems has been reported as complications associated with hyoid bone suspension.[18]

Tongue Base Resection and Other Procedures for Retroglossal Obstruction

Retroglossal/hypopharyngeal obstruction is considered the most difficult to treat level of obstruction surgically. Literature is filled with numerous surgical procedures aiming to correct retroglossal collapse during sleep. These procedures include laser midline glossectomy, tongue base reduction with hyoepiglottoplasty, lingualplasty, lingual tonsillectomy, palatopharyngoglossoplasty, uvulopalatopharyngoglossoplasty, glossopexia, and tongue base suspension.[18] All these procedures were reported to help improve symptoms of OSA, but the long-term results were reported to be low. These procedures on soft tissue of tongue base have not been recommended as an isolated treatment option for patients with moderate-to-severe OSA. However, these procedures can be combined with other procedures like UPPP and nasal surgery in case of multilevel obstruction.

Genioglossus Advancement

The genioglossus advancement aims to improve the retroglossal/hypopharyngeal space by surgically advancing the genioglossus muscle and its attachment on genial tubercle. The genial tubercle is a bony projection on the inner cortex of mandible on which the genioglossus muscle is attached. A window is created by bicortical osteotomy centered over genial tubercle and genial tubercle with genioglossus muscle attached to it is pulled forward through the bony window and rotated and fixed over mandible. This surgical procedure has shown efficacy in improvement of OSA symptoms when combined with other surgeries for multisegmental obstruction.[27,28] However, literature found inadequate data to support the use of genioglossus advancement as an isolated procedure in moderate-to-severe OSA patients.

Maxillomandibular Advancement

Maxillomandibular advancement (MMA) aims to achieve enlargement of the upper airway at retropalatal and retroglossal level through expansion of the skeletal framework. The ideal candidate for this surgical procedure is patients who have documented mandibular and maxillary retrusion. Apart from this, some selected patients who are noncompliant to nCPAP can be considered. The procedure requires bilateral sagittal split osteotomies on mandibular ramus with rigid internal fixation along with Le-Fort I osteotomy with rigid internal fixation. An advancement of 10–15 mm of maxilla and mandible is considered sufficient to improve the airway.[18,29,30] The efficacy of MMA has been reported to be similar to CPAP in relieving OSA symptoms.[31] Young patients with low BMI (BMI < 30) and no other comorbidities like diabetes are ideal candidates for this surgical procedure. The long-term results in MMA are reported to be stable and encouraging. The common complications include palatal perforation, maxillary pseudoarthrosis, malocclusion, transient cheek and chin hypoesthesia, and local site infection.[29,30]

Distraction Osteogenesis

Distraction osteogenesis (DOG) is a surgical procedure in which progressive lengthening of bone is achieved along with stretching of surrounding soft-tissue envelope. The concept of new bone formation and bone healing go simultaneously after activating the distraction device by 1 mm/day rate. The procedure is especially useful in patients who have severe maxillomandibular anomalies.[32,33] This procedure is generally done in syndromic pediatric population.

In selected adolescent and adult patients with OSA secondary to severe maxillomandibular hypoplasia, DOG is ideal procedure to achieve sufficient widening of the airway where MMA is not suitable option. The risk of malocclusion, length of procedure, and discomfort of the device is some of the limiting factors.[18]

Laryngeal Surgery

The laryngeal pathology resulting in OSA is generally obstructive in nature. The common pathologies seen in adult population are papilloma, bilateral abductor cord palsy, and laryngeal tumors.[34] The collapse of laryngeal apparatus during sleep is commonly seen in pediatric population and is known as laryngomalacia. This pathology is not seen in adult population per se. The diagnosis of the pathology is done with sleep endoscopy which helps evaluate the level of obstruction within the larynx. The larynx has three anatomical divisions and pathology can involve either one or more divisions. Laryngeal papillomas can involve supraglottis, glottis, and subglottis larynx and requires surgical excision for improving compromised airway. Similarly, bilateral cord palsy resulting in progressive effortful breathing can lead to OSA symptoms. Surgical laser cordectomy can be done to improve the airway. Laryngeal tumors, generally benign tumors can lead to obstruction of airway and lead to development of OSA over a period of time. These tumors need to be addressed surgically to clear the obstruction.

Multilevel Surgery

Multilevel surgery implies correction of obstructive pathology at two or more sites. The rationale for MLS is that in most of the patients with OSA, there is multisegmental disease. The common sites addressed are nasal, retropalatal, and retroglossal/hypopharyngeal. The surgical procedures can be either staged or can be done in single stage. The surgical list includes septoplasty, turbinate reduction/resection, tonsillectomy, UPPP, tongue base reduction, genioglossus advancement, and hyoid myotomy with suspension and many more. The efficacy of MLS as a viable alternative to nCPAP has been reported in prospective studies. The MLS is an option for subsets of nCPAP failure patients who are young having moderate-to-severe OSA, with BMI less than 30 kg/m² and retroglossal obstruction.[35,36] One-stage multisegmental surgery is shown to be efficacious and viable option for CPAP failure/noncompliant patients. The morbidity and complication rate is acceptable and limited.[18] The success of MLS depends on correct selection of patient, correct identification of sites of obstruction and correct surgeries chosen by the experienced surgeon.

Tracheostomy

Tracheostomy is a surgical procedure in which a stoma is created in cervical trachea usually at the level of second and third tracheal ring. It is generally done to bypass obstruction usually at the level of oropharynx and larynx. The role of tracheotomy in modern scenario is limited and generally not acceptable. Historically, tracheostomy was considered as gold standard for obstructive sleep apnea syndrome (OSAS), but CPAP has been now accepted as gold standard for management of OSAS. The morbidity associated with tracheostomy limits its utility in modern era. However, there are still few indications where tracheostomy is considered last and life-saving procedure. Patients with life-threatening cardiopulmonary complications owing to severe OSAS and not responding to CPAP or surgical options will ultimately require tracheostomy as a last resort. Tracheostomy has been reported to reduce both morbidity and mortality in OSA patients. All the parameters of OSAS improve after tracheostomy including daytime sleepiness, snoring, and AHI.[37-39] Temporary tracheostomy (for short period of time) can be required during certain surgeries done for improving retroglossal/hypopharyngeal airway.[18] Tracheostomy is a viable option for those patients where all conservative medical and surgical procedures have failed.

CONCLUSION

Surgical management for each site of obstruction needs to be standardized based on evidence. Proper selection of the patient for a given surgical intervention needs to be substantiated by various investigative tools. Surgical intervention should be tailor-made for each patient of OSA and not generalized. Surgical intervention should not be considered only as option for CPAP failures but also as a first-line therapy for selected subgroups of patients based on their preliminary evaluation. A thorough ENT evaluation is a must before putting the patient on CPAP therapy.

REFERENCES

1. Sullivan CE, Issa FG, Berthon-Jones M, et al. Reversal of obstructive sleep apnoea by continuous positive airway pressure applied through the nares. *Lancet.* 1981;1:862-5.
2. Somiah M, Taxin Z, Keating J, et al. Sleep quality, short-term and long-term CPAP adherence. *J Clin Sleep Med.* 2012;8(5):489-500.
3. Sher AE, Thorpy MJ, Shprintzen RJ, et al. Predictive value of Muller maneuver in selection of patients for uvulopalatopharyngoplasty. *Laryngoscope.* 1985;95:1483-7.
4. Croft CB, Pringle M. Sleep nasoendoscopy a technique of assessment in snoring and obstructive sleep apnoea. *Clin Otolaryngol Allied Sci.* 1991;16(5):504-9.
5. Pringle MB, Croft CB. A comparison of sleep nasendoscopy and the Muller manoeuvre. *Clin Otolaryngol Allied Sci.* 1991;16(6):559-62.
6. Kotecha BT, Hannan SA, Khalil HM, et al. Sleep nasendoscopy: a 10-year retrospective audit study. *Eur Arch Otorhinolaryngol.* 2007;264:1361-7.
7. Li HY, Chen NH, Wang CR, et al. Use of 3-dimensional computed tomography scan to evaluate upper airway patency for patients undergoing sleep disordered breathing surgery. *Otolaryngol Head Neck Surg.* 2003;129:336-42.
8. Barrera JE. Sleep magnetic resonance imaging: dynamic characteristics of the airway during sleep in obstructive sleep apnea syndrome. *Laryngoscope.* 2011;121(6):1327-35.
9. Charles CB, Pringle MB. Snoring and sleep apnoea. In: Mackay IS, Bull TR, editor. Scott-Brown's Otorhinolaryngology, Head and Neck Surgery. 6th ed. Great Britain: Butterworth-Heinemann; 1997. pp. 1-22.
10. Miles PG, Vig PS, Weyant RJ, et al. Craniofacial structure and obstructive sleep apnea syndrome: a qualitative analysis and meta-analysis of the literature. *Am J Orthod Dentofacial Orthop.* 1996;109(2):163-72.
11. Farmer WC, Giudici SC. Site of airway collapse in obstructive sleep apnea after uvulopalatopharyngoplasty. *Ann Otol Rhinol Laryngol.* 2000;109:581-4.
12. Li HY, Wang PC, Chen YP, et al. Critical appraisal and meta-analysis of nasal surgery for obstructive sleep apnea. *Am J Rhinol Allergy.* 2011;25(1):45-9.
13. Nakata S, Noda A, Yagi H, et al. Nasal resistance for determinant factor of nasal surgery in CPAP failure patients with obstructive sleep apnea syndrome. *Rhinology.* 2005;43(4):296-9.
14. Powell NB, Zonato AI, Weaver EM, et al. Radiofrequency treatment of turbinate hypertrophy in subjects using continuous positive airway pressure: a randomized, double-blind, placebo-controlled clinical pilot trial. *Laryngoscope.* 2001;111(10):1783-90.
15. Verse T, Kroker BA, Pirsiq W, et al. Tonsillectomy for treatment of obstructive sleep apnea in adults with tonsillar hypertrophy. *Laryngoscope.* 2000;110:1556-9.
16. Nakata S, Miyazaki S, Ohki M, et al. Reduced nasal resistance after simple tonsillectomy in patients with obstructive sleep apnea. *Am J Rhinol.* 2007;21:192-5.
17. Boot H, van Wegen R, Poublon RM, et al. Long term results of uvulopalatopharyngoplasty for obstructive sleep apnea syndrome. *Laryngoscope.* 2000;110:469-75.
18. Randerath WJ, Verbraecken J, Andreas S, et al. Non-CPAP therapies in obstructive sleep apnoea. *Eur Respir J.* 2011;37:1000-28.
19. Powell NB, Riley RW, Guilleminault C. Radiofrequency tongue base reduction in sleep-disordered breathing: a pilot study. *Otolaryngol Head Neck Surg.* 1999;120:656-64.
20. Stuck BA, Maurer JT, Verse T, et al. Tongue base reduction with temperature-controlled radiofrequency volumetric tissue reduction for treatment of obstructive sleep apnea syndrome. *Acta Otolaryngol.* 2002;122:531-6.
21. Li KK, Powell NB, Riley RW, et al. Temperature-controlled radiofrequency tongue base reduction for sleep-disordered breathing: long-term outcomes. *Otolaryngol Head Neck Surg.* 2002;127:230-4.
22. den Herder C, van Tinteren H, de Vries N. Hyoidthyroidpexia: a surgical treatment for sleep apnea syndrome. *Laryngoscope.* 2005;115:740-5.

23. Riley RW, Powell NB, Guilleminault C. Obstructive sleep apnea and the hyoid: a revised surgical procedure. *Otolaryngol Head Neck Surg.* 1994;111:717-21.
24. Stuck BA, Neff W, Hormann K, et al. Anatomic changes afterhyoid suspension for obstructive sleep apnea: an MRI study. *Otolaryngol Head Neck Surg.* 2005;133:397-402.
25. Baisch A, Maurer JT, Hormann K. The effect of hyoid suspension in a multilevel surgery concept for obstructive sleep apnea. *Otolaryngol Head Neck Surg.* 2006;134:856-61.
26. Yin SK, Yi HL, Lu WY, et al. Genioglossus advancement and hyoid suspension plus uvulopalatopharyngoplasty for severe OSAHS. *Otolaryngol Head Neck Surg.* 2007;136:626-31.
27. Santos Junior JF, Abrahao M, Gregorio LC, et al. Genioplasty for genioglossus muscle advancement in patients with obstructive sleep apnea-hypopnea syndrome and mandibular retrognathia. *Braz J Otorhinolaryngol.* 2007;73:480-6.
28. Kezirian EJ, Goldberg AN. Hypopharyngeal surgery in obstructive sleep apnea: an evidence-based medicine review. *Arch Otolaryngol Head Neck Surg.* 2006;132:206-13.
29. Riley RW, Powell NB, Guilleminault C. Maxillofacial surgery and obstructive sleep apnea: a review of 80 patients. *Otolaryngol Head Neck Surg.* 1989;101:353-61.
30. Li KK, Powell NB, Riley RW, et al. Long-term results of maxillomandibular advancement surgery. *Sleep Breath.* 2000;4:137-40.
31. Randerath WJ, Bauer M, Blau A, et al. Stellenwert der Nicht-nCPAP-Verfahren in der Therapie des obstruktiven Schlafapnoe-Syndroms. [Relevance of non-CPAP treatment options in the therapy of obstructive sleep apnea syndrome.] *Somnologie.* 2006;10:67-98.
32. Li KK, Riley R, Powell N. Skeletal expansion by gradual intraoral distraction osteogenesis for the treatment of obstructive sleep apnea. *Head Neck Surg.* 2002;13:119-22.
33. Ow AT, Cheung LK. Meta-analysis of mandibular distraction osteogenesis: clinical applications and functional outcomes. *Plast Reconstr Surg.* 2008;121:54e-69e.
34. Olsen KD, Suh KW, Staats BA. Surgically correctable causes of sleep apnea syndrome. *Otolaryngol Head Neck Surg.* 1981;89:726-31.
35. Lin HC, Friedman M, Chang HW, et al. The efficacy of multilevel surgery of the upper airway in adults with obstructive sleep apnea/hypopnea syndrome. *Laryngoscope.* 2008;118(5):902-8.
36. Richard W, Kox D, den Herder C, et al. One stage multilevel surgery (uvulopalatopharyngoplasty, hyoid suspension, radiofrequent ablation of the tongue base with/without genioglossus advancement), in obstructive sleep apnea syndrome. *Eur Arch Otorhinolaryngol.* 2007;264(4):439-44.
37. Guilleminault C, Cummiskey J. Progressive improvement of apnea index and ventilatory response to CO2 after tracheostomy in obstructive sleep apnea syndrome. *Am Rev Respir Dis.* 1982;126:14-20.
38. Kim SH, Eisele DW, Smith PL, et al. Evaluation of patients with sleep apnea after tracheotomy. *Arch Otolaryngol Head Neck Surg.* 1998;124(9):996-1000.
39. Thatcher GW, Maisel RH. The long-term evaluation of tracheostomy in the management of severe obstructive sleep apnea. *Laryngoscope.* 2003;113(2):201-4.

CHAPTER 14

Dental Sleep Medicine: An Overview

Anmol S Kalha, Jayan Balakrishnan

INTRODUCTION

Over the recent decades, the boundaries between dentistry and medicine have started to continuously blur. Sleep medicine reflects a larger process of integration of dentistry and orthodontics into an integrated interdisciplinary field. The oral cavity and its supporting craniofacial structures have an intricate relationship with the airway dynamics. The ability to modify form and thereby affect function has been central to dental and orthodontic management of sagittal and transverse issues in the maxillomandibular region. Strong evidence comes to light that shows an increasing efficacy of oral appliances (OAs) in mild to moderate cases of obstructive sleep apnea (OSA). To relate dental sleep medicine to a mechanical appliance-based discipline would be a fallacy. What is crucial is a mindset change and a complete understanding of the processes involved in OSA management

Dentistry's entry into management of upper airway sleep disorders has led to the development of a new speciality, i.e., *Dental Sleep Medicine*. This subspeciality involves OA therapy for OSA and snoring, maxillomandibular advancement surgeries to increase upper airway volume, cephalometric studies for airway evaluation, and most important of all, prevention of sleep disordered breathing (SDB) in children by maxillary expansion, functional appliances, adenotonsillectomy, and oral habit breaking therapy.

Dentists trained in dental sleep medicine, orthodontists, and maxillofacial surgeons are recognized members of interdisciplinary team to manage upper airway sleep disorders. OAs particularly mandibular advancement devices (MAD) have been found to be effective in mild to moderate OSA and those patients not amenable to CPAP therapy. Current literature cites the therapeutic efficacy of OA to be comparable to CPAP therapy. In certain situations, maxillomandibular advancement surgeries offer a near 100% cure like tracheotomy. It is the first line of treatment for SDB in craniofacial syndromes with severe maxillomandibular deficiencies.

UNIQUENESS OF HUMAN PHARYNX

The human pharynx is unique in animal kingdom in terms of its size, shape, and predisposition to collapsibility. In other mammals, the epiglottis is in continuation with soft palate making the nasopharynx and laryngopharynx continuous which facilitates simultaneous breathing, swallowing and good olfactory sensation acting as a preventive mechanism against predators (Figures 1 and 2).[1,2] In human neonates, the epiglottis is approximating the soft palate like other mammals in order to facilitate simultaneous suckling and breathing (Figure 3). By the end of first year the larynx in humans descend downward creating an oropharynx which helps in the development of speech and language, breathing, deglutition, and mastication.[1,2,3] The tongue in humans occupies a significant part of oropharynx

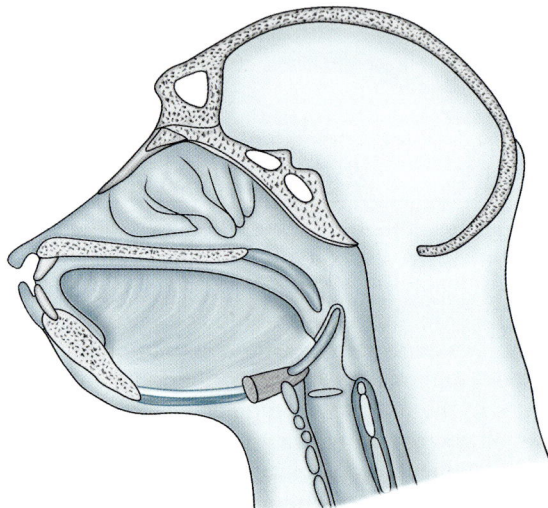

Figure 1: Diagrammatic representation of pharynx of a primate. The epiglottis is in close continuation with soft palate.

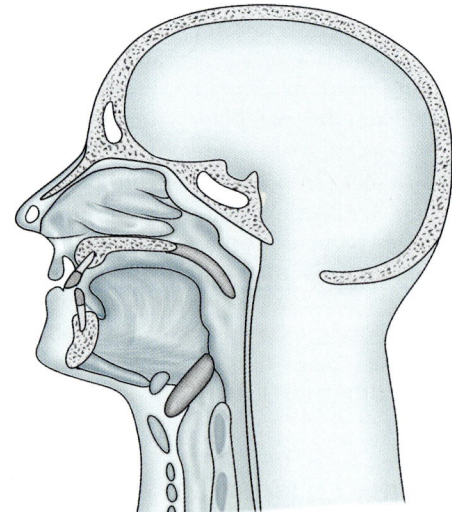

Figure 2: Diagrammatic representation of human adult pharynx. The larynx is descended creating a space between epiglottis and soft palate for creation of oropharynx.

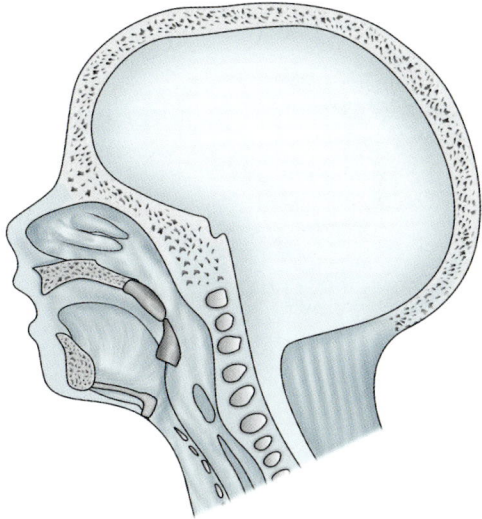

Figure 3: Diagrammatic representation of neonate pharynx. The epiglottis is in close continuation with soft palate like in primates.

unlike other mammals where tongue is restricted to oral cavity. This can be further appreciated by virtue of the facial skeleton in humans directly below the frontal bone while in other mammals it lies protruded away from the frontal bone. Due to bipedalism and erect posture of humans, the spatial position and orientation of jaws become important for head posture, breathing, phonation deglutition, and mastication.[4]

Human airway is like a collapsible tube susceptible to collapse in any region mainly in the oropharynx and hypopharynx (Figure 4). The tonicity of the various muscle groups; namely, suprahyoid, infrahyoid, tongue, soft palate, pharyngeal walls, and morphology of skeletal base impacts the patency of airway.

HISTORICAL PERSPECTIVE OF DENTAL SLEEP APPLIANCES

The dental practitioners and specialists have documented the importance of the spatial positions of the jaws with respect to collapsibility of the airway nearly a century back. In early twentieth century, the surgeons saved the life of micrognathic infants by suturing the tongue to lower lips to open and maintain the airway during sleep.[5] In 1934 Pierre Robin, a French pediatrician used mandibular anterior repositioning device for the first time in children with Pierre Robin syndrome to prevent asphyxia.[6] However, the utility of OAs was recognized by Charles Samuelson, a psychiatrist who designed a tongue retaining device for himself and documented it in 1982.[7] Since then substantial progress has been made, particularly pertaining to the utility of MADs. In 1995, a milestone review by American Association of Sleep Medicine summarized the efficacy of OAs and suggested practice parameters.[8] A decade later in 2006, the document was further revised and republished reflecting newer data in this burgeoning field.[9] Currently, there is mounting evidence with respect to efficacy

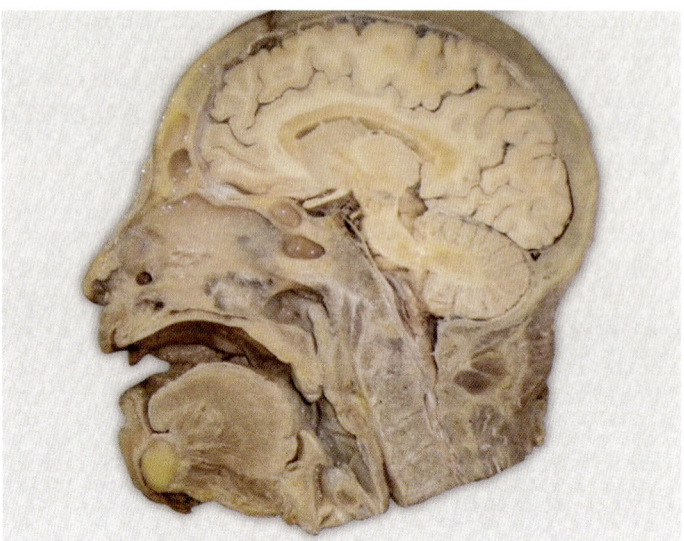

Figure 4: Longitudinal cadaveric section of human pharynx. The upper airway is like a collapsible tube, it is kept patent by various muscle groups namely tongue, suprahyoid, infrahyoid, soft palate, and pharyngeal muscles.

of OA therapy.[10-16] The basis for use of MADs for airway takes its roots from the use of functional appliances used by orthodontist for growth modification of jaws and modulating their spatial position in relation to each other and the cranium.

SLEEP MEDICINE AND DENTISTRY

Dental practitioners are stakeholders in the practice of sleep medicine by virtue of their competence and skills in changing the spatial positions of the jaws. So a new subspecialty of sleep medicine, namely, dental sleep medicine has emerged. According to American Association of Dental Sleep Medicine, "Dental Sleep Medicine is an area of practice that focuses on management of sleep related breathing disorders including snoring and OSA through the use of OA therapy and upper airway surgeries".[17]

The role of dentists in management of SDB encompasses screening for risk factors, making appropriate referrals to other medical specialties, prevention of SDB by growth modification of jaws, maxillary expansion, appropriate orthodontic intervention, comanagement with OA therapy and performing maxillomandibular surgeries to obviate craniofacial risk factors. Although international classification of sleep disorders cites nearly 100 movements and breathing disorders in sleep, dental professionals have a role to play only in the management of snoring, OSA, sleep bruxism (SB), and upper airway resistance syndrome.[18]

Craniofacial Risk Factors

Keeping in view the peculiarity of human pharynx, many craniofacial risk factors have been identified which predisposes humans to SDB. Some of the craniofacial

risk factors are mandibular retrognathism/hypoplastic mandible, inferiorly and posteriorly placed hyoid bone (Figures 5A to C), high arched palate, maxillary deficiency, long face problems/syndrome, large, mandibular tori, edentulism, and neck circumference of over 16 inches.[19,20-23] Some of the clinical signs which should be taken as clue for investigation of SDB are:
- Lip incompetency with oral breathing
- Puckering of chin
- Adenotonsillitis
- Airway grading of Mallampati more than grade III
- Allergic shiners
- Enlarged uvula
- Severe clockwise rotation of mandible
- Small nares and high and narrow nose
- Enlarged and crenated tongue.

Some studies have demonstrated an association between temporomandibular joint disorders (TMD) and SDB and hence cases with TMDs should be investigated for SDB.[24]

CLINICAL EVALUATION AND DIAGNOSIS

Besides a routine clinical examination, patient should be specifically examined for neck size, TMD, and periodontal status.[25] Gold standard for diagnosing SDB is

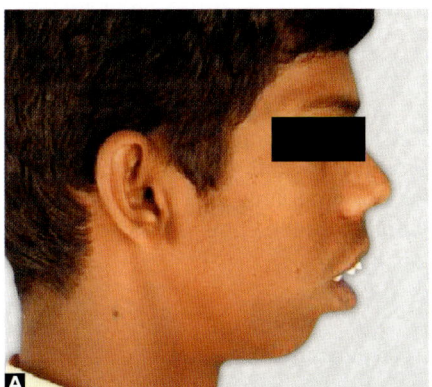

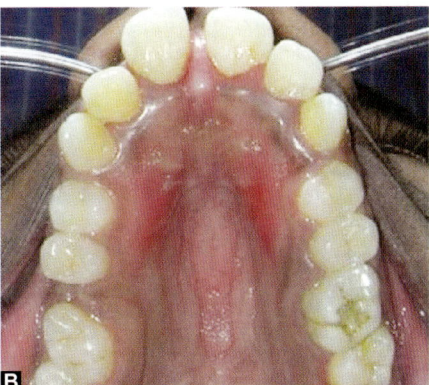

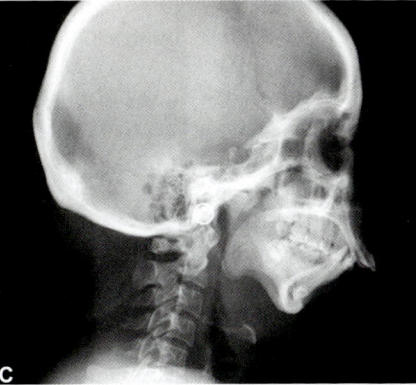

Figure 5: **A,** Profile view of a case of long face syndrome with upper airway sleep disorder. The facial feature is characterized by incompetent lips, excessive proclination of upper teeth, hypoplastic and clockwise rotation of mandible. The above are some of risk factors for upper airway collapse. **B,** Narrow and deep palatal vault are risk factors for sleep disordered breathing. **C,** Lateral cephalogram of a case of severe obstructive sleep apnea. Hypoplastic mandible, decreased oropharyngeal airway, and posteriorly and inferiorly placed hyoid bone are the classical findings.

polysomnography and prognosis and therapeutic efficacy with dental intervention can be objectively assessed by comparison of baseline and post-treatment apnea hypopnea index (AHI) scores. In addition, imaging studies, which include cephalometric radiography, computed tomography scans, magnetic ressonance imaging, and acoustic imaging techniques also play a crucial role.

Cephalograms are true lateral radiographs of skull recorded using cephalostats at end expiration. There are various cephalometric analysis for evaluation of airway. A comprehensive cephalometric analysis can provide a fairly good idea of risk factors and collapsibility of airway.[22,26-28] The cephalometric landmarks and analysis are presented in table 1. Though cephalograms are cost-effective, easily available, routinely done in dental practice but have the disadvantage of being two dimensional and recorded in erect position. Baseline cephalograms can be compared with cephalograms recorded with appliance *in situ* to assess improvement in airway dimensions and hyoid position changes (Figure 6).

Magnetic resonance imaging is useful in volumetric analysis of airway and helps in assessing the dimensions of airway in various planes (Figure 7).

Acoustic reflection technique is a newly introduced chair side evaluation method where in minimum cross-sectional area of airway can be measured using reflection of sound waves.[29] Acoustic pharyngometry is a noninvasive procedure based on acoustic reflection technology which is akin to sonar technology used in ships. Sound waves are projected down the airway and reflected back out in such a way that the pharyngometer software can analyze and quantify changes in the airway cross-sectional area. It allows users to quickly and easily measure a patient's pharyngeal airway size and stability from the oral pharyngeal junction to glottis.

Oral Appliance Therapy

American Association of Sleep Medicine has recommended prescription of mandibular repositioning appliances for mild to moderate snoring, mild to moderate OSA, and those severe cases not amenable to CPAP therapy or surgery.[8,9] There are mainly two types of appliances for upper airway disorders, the tongue retaining devices and MADs.

Tongue Retaining Devices

Tongue retaining device developed by Cartwright in 1982 consist of a hollow bulb attached to a tray that fits on mandibular and maxillary teeth and edentulous ridges (Figure 8). The patient projects tip of the tongue in hollow bulb and is retained in the bulb by suction. The research on the design of the appliance has led to development of tongue stabilizing device (AVEOTSD). This is a vestibular appliance not attached to teeth and tongue is held forward by suction. Currently, tongue retaining devices represent a tiny percentage of sleep appliances and are studied far less.

Mandibular Advancement Devices

These are removable appliances which help in placing the mandible in predetermined forward position during sleep. All MADs function to reposition and stabilize the mandible in protruded position during sleep. All MADs prevent the tongue from approaching the posterior wall of pharynx and causing obstruction. They maintain the patency of the upper airway by elevating base

Table 1: Cephalometric analysis for upper airway

S. No	Parameter	Description	Value mean
1	NAS (nasopharyngal airway space)	Measured from posterior nasal spine (PNS) to upper pharyngeal wall along palatal plane	25.9 + 2.6 mm (M) 24.1 + 2.3 mm (F)
2	SAS (superior pharyngeal airway space)/VAS (velopharyngeal airway space)	A horizontal distance from the tip of the soft palate to pharyngeal wall	9.9 + 2.8 mm (M) 9.9 + 2.4 mm (F)
3	PAS (posterior airway space)/ orophangeal airway space	Horizontal distance from the posterior margin of the tongue to pharyngeal wall measured on the Go- B line.	10.1 + 3.1 mm (M) 10.0 + 2.8 mm (F)
4	HAS (hypopharyngealairway space/MAS)	Minimum horizontal distance in the hypopharyngeal area measure from point V (intersection of tongue and epiglottis)	18.7 + 2.6 mm (M) 16.5 + 3.1 mm (F)
5	Hyoid distance (MP-H)	The perpendicular distance from mandibular plane (Go-Gn) to the anterior superior aspect of hyoid	15 mm
6	Hyoid angle	The angle from the mandibular plane (Go-Gn) to the superior aspect of the hyoid	25.42 + 7.48
7	Hyoid, C3 vertebrae and menton relationship	The perpendicular distance from H to line joining inferior-anterior tip of cervical third vertebrae (C3) to menton	H point should be on or above the line

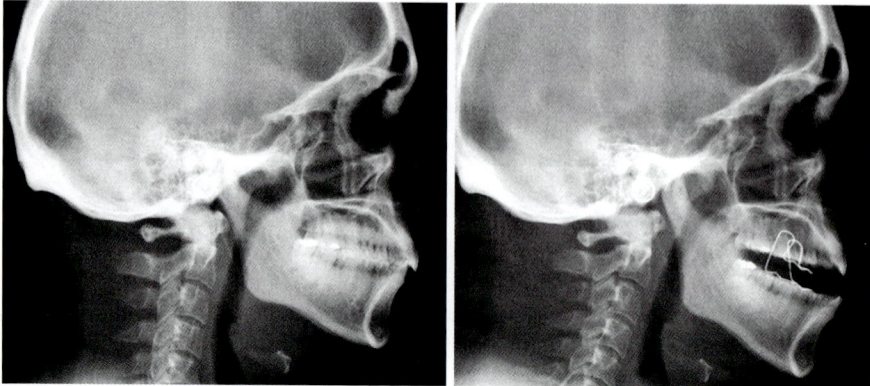

Figure 6: Photo sequence of lateral cephalograms of a patient of moderate obstructive sleep apnea with and without mandibular advancement appliance. Note the gross improvement in oropharyngeal space and hyoid positioning with mandibular advancement appliance.

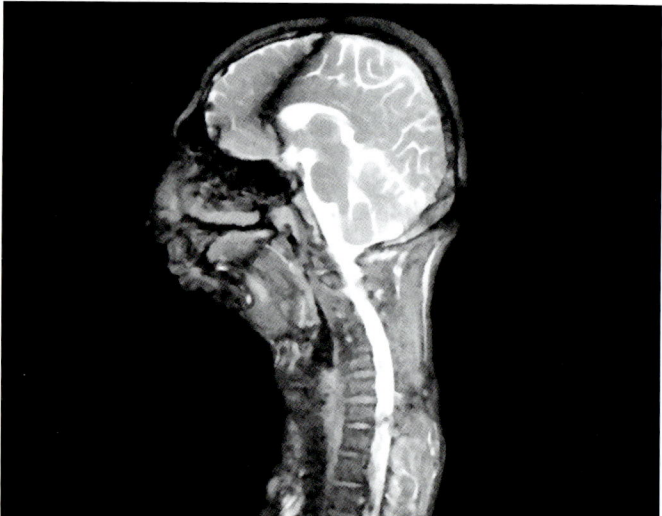

Figure 7: Magnetic resonance imaging (axial view) of a case of severe obstructive sleep apnea due to severe mandibular hypoplasia secondary to temporomandibular joint ankylosis. The upper airway dimensions are grossly reduced

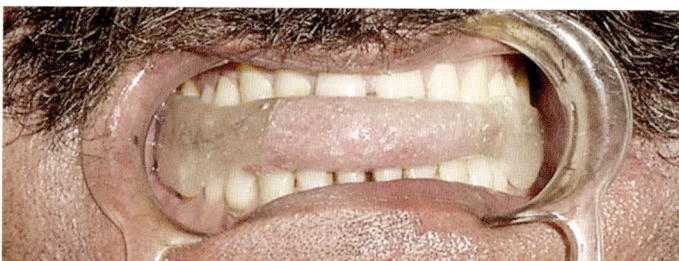

Figure 8: Tongue retaining device.

of the tongue, by tensing the palatoglossus muscle and pulling the soft palate forward, decompressing tissues around pharynx, stabilizing lateral pharyngeal walls by applying tension to pterygomandibular raphe, and splaying the tonsillar arches.[30] MADs not only enhance the oropharyngeal dimensions but also the velopharyngeal dimensions by pulling the soft palate forward due to the stretch on palatoglossus muscle.[31] They can be fixed or adjusted (Figures 9 and 10). In fixed type, the bite is recorded at the predetermined position and they are

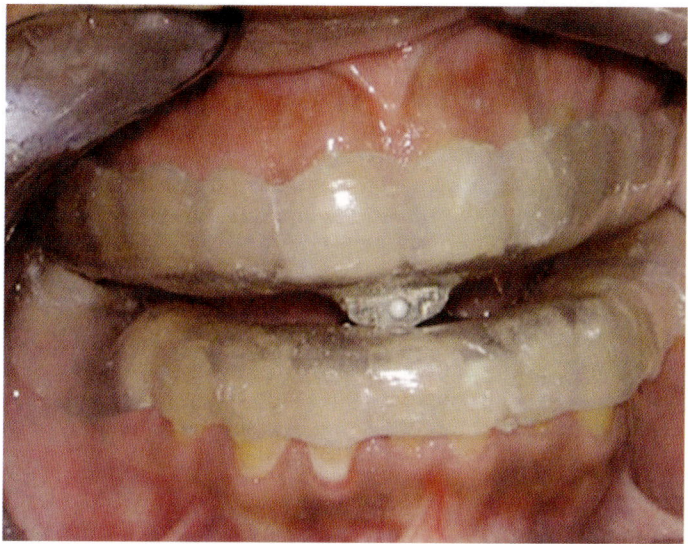

Figure 9: Intraoral view of Thornton adjustable positioner, an adjustable mandibular advancement device.

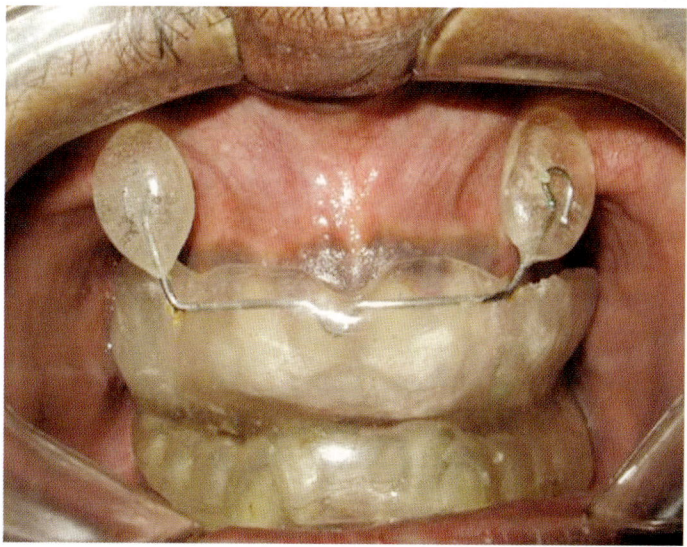

Figure 10: Mandibular advancement splint with nasal dilators.

fabricated as a single block. While the adjustable appliances are dual blocks consisting of mandibular and maxillary appliances joined by one of the several modes, including elastic or plastic connectors, metal rods and tube connectors, hook and screw connectors and acrylic resin extensions. Numerous appliance design variations exist, giving rise to plethora of MADs. To date no significant research has clearly demonstrated advantage of one appliance device over the others; however, studies suggest they may impact efficacy and tolerance.[32]

The adjustable MADs are most advantageous because they facilitate incremental advancement of mandibular position over time. In the adjustable design once satisfactory subjective improvement is achieved, objective assessment can be done by polysomnography with appliance *in situ*. If there is 50% improvement in AHI, scores the titration can be stopped; however, the mandibular protrusion should not exceed beyond 70% of maximum protrusion.

The current evidence suggests that MAD have better patient acceptance and are more successful in improving signs and symptoms of OSA.[33,34] MAD has shown to significantly improve objective sleep measurements such as AHI, arousal index, snoring, and arterial oxygenation. They significantly improve subjective and objective measurements of sleepiness, quality of life, and blood pressure. Studies also have shown that CPAP and MAD have similar improvements in cardiovascular outcomes and inflammatory markers.[35,36]

The MADs can predispose to transient TMJ discomfort, increased salivation, loosening of teeth, and change in bite, but the advantages outweigh the disadvantages on account of larger health benefits.

Maxillomandibular Surgical Advancement

Maxillomandibular advancement surgeries are basically meant to advance the skeletal bases and result in increasing the airway dimensions in all three planes;

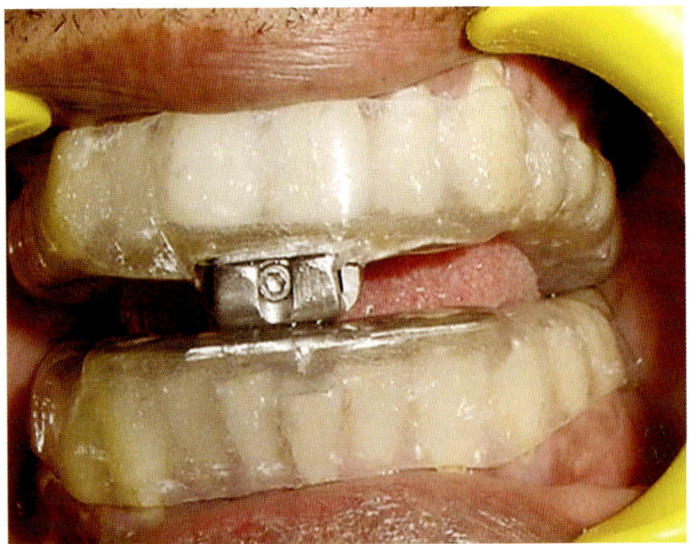

Figure 11: Intraoral view of medical dental snoring device, an adjustable mandibular advancement device.

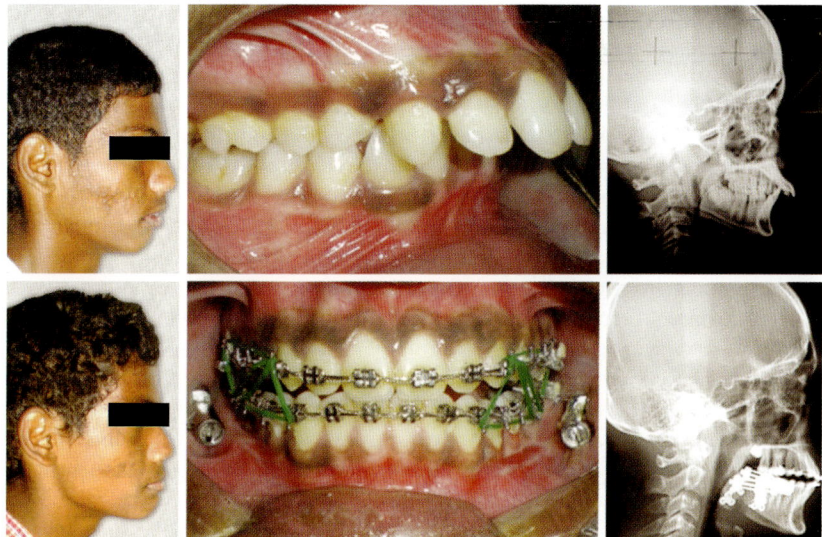

Figure 12: Photo sequence of a case of skeletal class 2 division 1 malocclusion and moderate obstructive sleep apnea due to mandibular deficiency treated by combined orthodontics and bilateral corpus distraction osteogenesis

namely, anterior, posterior, and laterally. Many of the syndromic cases like Pierre Robbins, Nager's, Pfeiffer's, Crouzon's and Apert's, and post TMJ ankylosis characterized by severe mandibular deficiency resulting in reduced airway dimensions make them susceptible to OSA. Surgical mandibular advancements by orthognathic surgeries or by distraction osteogenesis are the only viable and predictable options. Mandibular skeletal advancement is generally done by bilateral sagittal split ramus osteotomy (BSSRO). BSSRO is done with sagittal osteotomy through the ramus of the mandible and the advanced segments are fixed using titanium plates and screws (Figure 12). Effective advancement of 7–10 mm is possible with BSSRO but for larger discrepancies which are common in syndromic cases bilateral corpus distraction is the option. An Indian cephalometric-based study on 20 patients has reported an increase in posterior airway space, superior airway space, minimum airway space dimensions following mandibular advancement by BSSRO in the ratio of 1: 0.35, 1: 0.34, and 1: 024, respectively.[37] Hyoid moved superiorly and anteriorly by 2.1 mm and 2.8 mm, respectively. The authors concluded that surgical advancement of mandible in class 2 malocclusions even without symptoms of SDB can be considered as first line of prevention with respect to OSA.[37]

Distraction osteogenesis is a biological process of new bone formation between vascularized margins of osteotomized bone segments gradually separated by incremental traction.

In the current practice scenario, the corticotomy is done distal to the last molar and distracters are fixed across the corticotomy with the help of titanium screws. The distracters are placed parallel to each other and predetermined vector determined by aesthetic requirement of patients. Following the latency period of 5–7 days, the regenerate is incrementally stretched at the rate of 1 mm per day. The regenerate is moulded during distraction using intraoral elastics in various patterns in order to achieve occlusion and to optimize maxillomandibular relationship.[38,39] Distraction osteogenesis of maxillomandibular skeleton has the advantage of tissue histogenesis which minimizes post-treatment relapse. Successful correction ranging from 10 mm to 45 mm has been reported in literature.[39-41] Though tracheostomy is cited as permanent cure for severe OSA with severe mandibular retrognathism, the mandibular advancement by distraction osteogenesis provides 80–90% improvement.[40,41] Mandibular advancement also improves the position of hyoid bone. Genial advancement is often integrated with mandibular advancement or is done as isolated procedure which not only achieves chin prominence but stretches the suprahyoid muscles to correct hyoid position resulting in optimizing tongue position.

Maxillary advancement is done by LeFort I osteotomy or by midface distraction using intraoral or extraoral distraction. Maxillary deficiency is a common feature of cleft maxillary hypoplasia associated with OSA and maxillary advancement not only helps in improving esthetics but also improves airway in the velopharyngeal region.[42]

Literature sites maxillomandibular advancement as treatment option in severe OSA even if the jaws are optimally placed.[43] The genioglossus advancement procedure by rectangular osteotomy of symphyseal region is also reported to provide beneficial results in selected cases.

High arched palate with narrow maxilla in adults often lead to SDB due to lowered tongue posture and mandibular rotation. Surgically-assisted rapid palatal expansion is currently proposed as treatment option in these cases. In a landmark pilot study by Cistulli et al. on 10 adult patients who underwent surgically-assisted rapid palatal expansion concluded major reduction in snoring, OSA, and hyper somnolence.[44] Maxillary expansion increases oral space, optimizes tongue posture, increases nasal width reducing nasal resistance, and in turn improves the airway and nasal breathing (Figure 13).

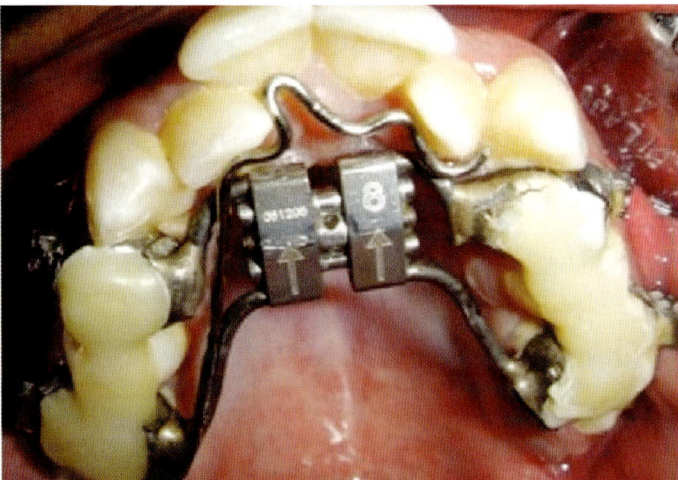

Figure 13: Intraoral view of HYRAX appliance used for rapid maxillary expansion. Rapid maxillary expansion with adenotonsillectomy is considered as first line of treatment for sleep disordered breathing in children.

PREVENTION OF SLEEP DISORDERED BREATHING IN CHILDREN

Significant component of craniofacial development occurs in first 4 years of life. Ninety percent of craniofacial development is complete by the age of 12 years, therefore, it can be concluded that morphometric features that put adults at risk of OSA or SDB are probably present as early as 12 years of age.[45,46] Hence addressing these features at an early age may significantly reduce SDB or prevent the same in the future.

An important factor in optimum development of maxilla at a very early age is breastfeeding. Breastfeeding is an important orofacial exercise required for stimulating maxillary expansion which aids in achieving normal tongue posture and propels mandibular growth.[47] Use of bottle nipple or pacifier can interfere in proper contact of tongue and its distribution of force on palate. The vacuum created by strong sucking action can increase depth of palate. Proper swallowing pattern is seen in breastfed children and is crucial for optimum craniofacial development. Tongue thrust is likely to develop in bottle fed children. Importance of breastfeeding should also be seen in light of its effects on craniofacial development and prevention of SDB.

In a classical work, Harvold and coworkers demonstrated that the obstruction of nasal airway significantly alters craniofacial growth.[48,49] Compromised/obstructed airway in children often results in craniocervical extension and forward head posture which is an adaptation for maintenance of patency of airway.[50] However, this adaptation does not happen in sleep, thus risking the child to SDB.

Adenotonsillar enlargement is one of the most common causes of airway obstruction in children leading to compromised breathing and altered craniofacial growth. Obstruction in the nasopharyngeal airway promotes oral breathing which is a sign of impending OSA. Adenotonsillectomy often improves nasal breathing, quality of sleep, and enhancement in delta sleep which increases growth hormone secretion influencing craniofacial growth.[51]

The role of combined adenotonsillectomy and RME and best sequence of the treatment have been evaluated in prepubertal children who had OSA and adenotonsillar hypertrophy. In majority of such patients, both therapeutic approaches were required to resolve OSA and the order of treatment does not appear to be important.[52] In another landmark study by Pirelli et al. in 31 children with narrow maxillae and absence of adenotonsillar hypertrophy, those undergoing RME showed a complete resolution of SDB in 6–12 months.[53] These studies suggest an important role of RME in treatment of OSA in children.

Mandibular deficiencies in growing children are best addressed by functional orthopedic appliances like activator, bionator, twin blocks, etc. The functional appliances correct mandibular deficiency by growth modification, improves tongue posture, and optimizes spatial maxillomandibular relationship (Figure 14). The effect of functional appliances on oropharyngeal airway dimensions has been assessed by Ozbek and coworkers more than a decade back. They found that these appliances significantly increase the airway space at oropharyngeal and nasopharyngeal levels.[54] A randomized controlled trial reported in 2002 involving 7-year-old children with OSA treated by functional appliances observed a significant reduction in AHI from 7.1 + 4.6 to 2.6 +2.2.[55] In a recent study, normalization of AHI was demonstrated in retrognathic adolescents with SDB in absence of tonsillar hypertrophy treated with functional orthopedic appliances.[56]

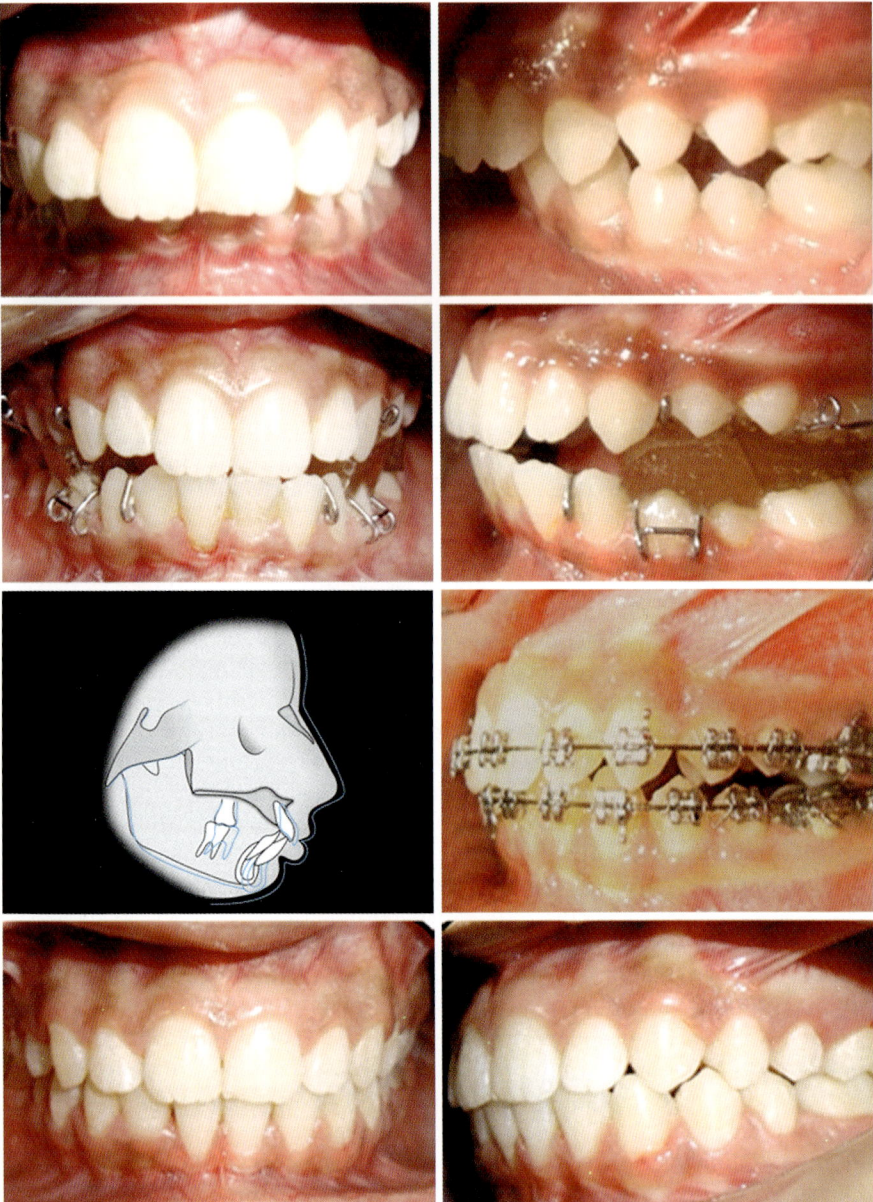

Figure 14: Intraoral photo sequence of a case of deep bite, increased overjet, and deficient mandible treated by twin block functional appliance and fixed orthodontic therapy. Optimizing mandibular growth not only improves facial aesthetics but also airway and breathing.

Therapeutic extraction of premolar teeth is one of the common procedures in orthodontics for retraction of teeth and resolving crowding. However, there are few studies and case reports which are suggestive of reduction of airway space and pharyngeal airway dimensions following extraction treatment.[57,58]

Careful consideration must be given and sleep physician must elicit history of orthodontic treatment with extraction while examining patients with OSA.

SLEEP BRUXISM

Sleep bruxism is an oral parafunctional activity that occurs when the individual is asleep. According to the American Academy of Sleep, SB is a parasomnia which is an undesirable physical phenomenon which occurs during sleep; however, the condition does not affect sleep and wakefulness.[59] The pathophysiology of this condition is not clear. It has been classified as primary (idiopathic) and secondary (iatrogenic forms). The secondary forms are associated with neurological, psychiatric, OSA, or with administration and withdrawal of drugs. Management includes behavioral and stress management, lifestyle changes, and oral hard acrylic splints to protect the teeth from grinding. The patient goes back to sleep after arousal and the cycle is repeated. Patients with SB need to be screened for other comorbid medical conditions like OSA, insomnia, attention deficit hyperactivity disorder, depression, mood disorders, and gastroesophageal reflux before undertaking any treatment approach especially pharmacotherapy.[60] MAD is one of the management options particularly when SB is associated with OSA.

CONCLUSION

Management of upper airway sleep disorders is an interdisciplinary approach. Dentists trained in sleep medicine, orthodontists, oral, and maxillofacial surgeons and prosthodontists have a crucial role in prevention, interception, and comprehensive management of snoring, OSA, and SB. Enlow and Hans in their classical book "Essentials of Facial growth" have stated that *"From the first day, all through life, the jaws help maintain the vital human airway"*.[61] So it is very important for all the stakeholders in the management of upper airway sleep disorders to acknowledge the above cited profound statement and factor in the craniofacial inputs in the diagnosis, treatment planning, and management of SDB.

REFERENCES

1. Lieberman P. Biology and evolution of language. Cambridge: Harvard University press; 1984.
2. Laitman JT1, Reidenberg JS, Marquez S, et al. What the nose knows: new understanding of Neaenderthal upper respiratory tract. *Proc Natl Acad Sci USA*. 1996;93(20):10543-5.
3. Crelin ES. The human vocal tract: anatomy function development and evolution. New York: Vantage Press; 1987.
4. Walker A, Shipman P. The wisdom of bones: in search of human origins. Vintage books, Inc New York; 1996.
5. Rogers RR. Past, present and future use of oral appliance therapies in sleep related breathing disorders. *CDA Journal*. 2012;40(2):151-7.
6. Robin P. Glossoptosis due to atresia and hypertrophy of the mandible. *Am J Dis Child*. 1934;48:541-4.
7. Cartwright RD, Samelson CF. The effects of a nonsurgical treatment for obstructive sleep apnea. The tongue retaining device. *J Am Med Assoc*. 1982;248(6):705-9.
8. American Sleep Disorder Association report: Practice parameters for the treatments of snoring and obstructive sleep apnea with oral devices. *Sleep*. 1995;18(6):511-3.

9. Ferguson KA, Cartwright R, Rogers R, et al. Oral appliances for snoring and obstructive sleep apnea: a review. *Sleep.* 2006;29(2):244-62.
10. Ferguson KA, Ono T, Lowe AA, et al. A randomized cross over study of an oral appliance vs nasal continuous positive airway pressure in treatment of mild moderate sleep apnea. *Chest.* 1996;109(5):269-75.
11. Clark GT, Blumenfeld I, Yoffe N, et al. A crossover study comparing the efficacy of continuous positive airway pressure with anterior mandibular positioning devices in patients with obstructive sleep apnea. *Chest.* 1996;109(6):1477-83.
12. Lowe AA. Dental appliances for the treatments of snoring and obstructive sleep apnea. In: Kryger M, Roth T, Dement W, editors: Principles and Practice of Sleep Medicine, 3rd edition. Philadelphia: Saunders; 2000. pp. 929-39.
13. Jayan B, Prasad BNBM, Kamat VR, et al. Therapeutic efficacy of Thornton adjustable positioner in the management of patients with severe obstructive sleep apnea–A pilot study. *India J sleep Med.* 2008;3(3):97-101.
14. Lim J, Lasserson TJ, Fleetnam J, et al. Oral appliances for obstructive sleep apnoea. *Cochrane database Syst Rev.* 2006;(1):CD004435.
15. Schwarting S, Huebers V, Helse M, et al. Position paper on the use of mandibular advancement devices in adults with sleep related breathing disorders. *Sleep breath.* 2007;11(2):125-6.
16. D Attanasio R, Dennis RB. Oral appliance therapy for sleep related breathing disorders. In: Attansio R, Dennis RB (Eds). Dental management of sleep disorders, 1st edition. Blackwell Publishing; 2010. pp. 221-63.
17. American Academy of Dental Sleep Medicine. AADSM Protocol: Oral appliance therapy for sleep disordered breathing. Available from: www.aadsm.org.
18. American Academy of Sleep Medicine. International classification of Sleep disorders, 2nd edition. Westchester, IL: American Academy of Sleep Medicine; 2005.
19. Bailey DR. Oral evaluation and upper airway anatomy associated with snoring and obstructive sleep apnea. *Dental Clin North Am.* 2001;45(4):715-32.
20. Bacon WH, Turlot JC, Krieger J, et al. Cephalometric evaluation of pharyngeal obstructive factors in patients with sleep apnea syndrome. *Angle Orthod.* 1990;60(2): 115-22.
21. deBerry-Borowiecki B, Kukwa A, Blanks RH. Cephalometric analysis for diagnosis and treatment of obstructive sleep apnea. *Laryngoscope.* 1988;98(2): 226-34.
22. Jayan B, Prasad BNBM, Atul K, et al. The role of cephalometric analysis in obese and non obese urban Indian adults with obstructive sleep apnea syndrome: A pilot study. *Indian J sleep Med.* 2007;2:59-63
23. Lowe AA, Fleetham JA, Adachi S, et al. Cephalometric and computed tomographic predictors of obstructive sleep apnea severity. *Am J Orthod Dentofacial Orthop.* 1995;107(6):589-95.
24. Merill RL. Temporomandibular disorder pain and dental treatment of obstructive sleep apnea. In Sleep Medicine and Dentistry, Dental Clinics of North America. 2012;56(2):415-33.
25. Bailey DR, Attanasio R. Screening and comprehensive evaluation for sleep related breathing disorders. In Sleep Medicine and Dentistry, Dental Clinics of North America. 2012;56(2):331-42.
26. Bacon WH, Turlot JC, Krieger J, et al. Cephalometric evaluation of pharyngeal obstructive factors in patients with sleep apnea syndrome. *Angle Orthod.* 1990;60(2):115-22.
27. Nelson S, Hans M. Contribution of craniofacial risk factors in increasing apneic activity among obese and non obese habitual snorers. *Chest.* 1997;111(1):154-62.
28. Jayan B, Kharbanda OP. Orthodontists role in upper airway sleep disorders. In: Orthodontics Diagnosis and management of malocclusion and dentofacial deformities, 2nd edition. In: OP Kharbanda (Ed). Elsevier; 2013. pp. 709-28.
29. Attanasio R, Bailey DR. Imaging for sleep related breathing disorders. In dental management of sleep disorders. In: Attanasio R, Bailey DR (Eds). Wiley-Blackwell; 2010. pp. 151-63
30. Mohsenin N, Mostofi MT, Mohsenin V. The role of oral appliances in treating obstructive sleep apnea. *J Am Dent Assoc.* 2003;134(4):442-9.

31. Johal A, Battagel JM. Current principles in the management of obstructive sleep apnea with mandibular advancement appliances. *British Dental Journal*. 2001;190(10):532-6.
32. Ahrens A, McGrath C, Hagg U. Subjective efficacy of Oral appliance design features in the management of obstructive sleep apnea. *Am J Orthod Dentofacial Orthop*. 2010;138(5):559-76.
33. Barnes M, McEvoy RD, Banks S, et al. Efficacy of positive air pressure and oral appliance in mild and moderate obstructive sleep apnea. *Am J Respir Crit Care Med*. 2004;170(6):656-64.
34. Engleman HM, McDonald JP, Graham D, et al. Randomized cross over trail of two treatments or sleep apnea hypopnea syndrome: continuous positive pressure and Mandibular repositioning splint. *Am J Respir Crit Care Med*. 2002;166 (6):855-9.
35. Lim J, Lasserson TJ, Fleetham J, et al. Oral appliance for obstructive sleep apnoea. *Cochrane Data Base Syst Rev*. 2006;(1):CD004435.
36. Itzhaki S, Dorchin H, Clark G, et al .The effects of 1 year treatment with Herbst Mandibular advancement splint on obstructive sleep apnea, oxidative stress and endothelial function. *Chest*. 2007;131(3):740-9.
37. Sahoo NK, Jayan B, Ramakrishnan N, et al. Evaluation of upper airway dimensional changes and hyoid position following mandibular advancement in patients with skeletal class II malocclusion. *J Craniofac Surg*. 2012;23:e923-7.
38. McCarthy JG, Hopper RA, Hollier LH Jr, et al. Moulding of the regenerate in mandibular distraction: clinical experience. *Plast Reconstr Surg*. 2003;112(5):1239-46.
39. Roy Chowdhury SK, Jayan B, Menon PS, et al. Management of obstructive sleep apnea and non-apneic snoring with maxillo-mandibular distraction osteogenesis. *The Indian J Sleep Medicine*. 2007;2(3):101-8.
40. Waite PD, Shashidhar MS. Maxillo-mandibular advancement surgery: A cure for obstructive sleep apnea syndrome. *Oral and Maxillofac Surg Clin North Am*. 1995;7:327-44.
41. Prinsell JR. Maxillomandibular advancement surgery in a site-specific treatment approach for obstructive sleep apnea in 50 consecutive patients. *Chest*. 1999;116(6):1519-29.
42. Figueroa AA, Polley JW, Eilen K. Distraction osteogenesis for treatment of severe cleft maxillary deficiency with the RED technique. In: Rudolph P, Dendill J, Steln D (Eds): Craniofacial Distraction Osteogenesis, 1st edition. St. Louis: Mosby; 2001. pp. 485-94.
43. Li KK, Riley RW, Powel NB, et al. Maxillomandibular advancement for persistent obstructive sleep apnea after phase I surgery in patients without maxillo-mandibular deficiency. *Laryngoscope*. 2000;110:1684-8.
44. Cistulli PA, Palmisano RG, Poole MD. Treatment of obstructive sleep apnea syndrome by rapid maxillary expansion. *Sleep*. 1998;21(8):831-5.
45. Shepard JW Jr, Gefter WB, Guilleminault C, et al. Evaluation of upper airway in patients with obstructive sleep apnea. *Sleep*. 1991;14(4):361-71.
46. Jayan B, Vats RS, Sahu D, et al. Cranio-facial morphology, upper airway and orthodontics – the crucial connection. *India Journal of sleep medicine*. 2009;4:119-24.
47. Palmer B. The influences of breast feeding on the development of the oral cavity: a commentary. *J Hum Lact*. 1998;14(2):93-8.
48. Harvold EP, Tomer BS, Vargervik K, et al. Primate experiments on oral respiration. *Am J Orthod*. 1981;79(4):359-72.
49. Harvold EP, Chierci G, Vargervik K. Experiments on the development of dental malocclusions. *Am J Orthod*. 1972;61(1):38-44.
50. Ozbek MM, Miyamoto K, Lowe AA, et al. Natural head posture, upper air way morphology and obstructive sleep apnea severity in adults. *Eur J Orthod*. 1998;20(2): 133-43.
51. Peltomaki T. The effect of mode of breathing on craniofacial growth—revisited. *Eur J Orthod*. 2007;29(5):426-9.
52. Guilleminault C, Quo S, Haynh NT, et al. Orthodontic expansion treatment and Adenotonsillectomy in the treatment of Obstructive sleep apnea in pre-pubertal children. *Sleep*. 2008;31(7):953-7.
53. Pirelli P, Saponara M, De Rosa C, et al. Orthodontics and obstructive sleep apnea in children. *Med Clin North Am*. 2010;94(3):517-29.

54. Ozbek MM, Memikoglu TU, Gogen H, et al. Oropharyngeal airway dimensions and functional orthopedic treatment in skeletal Class II cases. *Angle Orthod.* 1998;68(4): 327-36.
55. Villa MP, Bernkopf E, Pagani J. Randomised controlled study of an oral jaw positioning appliance for the treatment of obstructive sleep apnea in children with malocclusion. *Am J Respir Crit Care Med.* 2002;165(1):123-7.
56. Schutz TC, Dominguez GC, Hallinan MP, et al. Class II correction improves nocturnal breathing in adolescents. *Angle Orthod.* 2011;81(2):222-8.
57. Cobo PJ, de Carlos UF, Maci as EE. Orthodontics and upper air way. *Orthod Fr.* 2004;75 (1):31-7.
58. Hang WA. Obstructive sleep apnea: dentistry's unique role in longetivity enhancement. *J Am Orthodontic Society.* 2007;7(3):28-32.
59. Kato T, Thie NM, Montplaisir JY, et al. Bruxism and orofacial movements during sleep. *Dental Clin North Am.* 2001;45(4):657-84.
60. Carra CM, Huynh N, Lavigne G. Sleep Bruxism: A comprehensive overview for the Dental clinician interested in sleep medicine. *Dent Clin N Am.* 2012;56(2):387-413.
61. Enlow DH, Hans MG. Essentials of Facial growth. WB Saunders Company; 1996.

CHAPTER 15

Obstructive Sleep Apnea in Children

Praveen Khilnani, Neha Sood

INTRODUCTION

Obstructive sleep apnea (OSA) is defined as a breathing disorder characterized by prolonged upper airway obstruction, partial, and/or intermittent complete. The obstruction disrupts normal ventilation during sleep and normal sleep patterns accompanied by associated signs and symptoms characteristic of the disorder[1,2] (according to American Academy of Pediatrics Clinical Practice guidelines).

Obstructive sleep apnea syndrome (OSAS) was first reported in children by Guilleminault et al. (1976) following which recognition of abnormal breathing during sleep has progressed.[3] The prevalence of OSA in childhood is around 2–3% affecting all ages with peak incidence between 2 years and 8 years.[4] Frequent snoring is reported by parents in 3–15% of children while prevalence of reported apneic events is 0.2–4%.[4]

Obstructive sleep apnea is a part of a complex of sleep disordered breathing (SDB) with a spectrum of clinical manifestations ranging from primary snoring to OSAS with upper-airway resistance syndrome (UARS) falling in between the two extremes.[5]

PRIMARY SNORING

Snoring during sleep without associated apneas, gas exchange abnormalities, or excessive arousals is defined as primary snoring. This does not progress to OSAS in young children and is known to resolve over time.[6]

Upper Airway Resistance Syndrome

Upper airway resistance syndrome is characterized by snoring, partial airway obstruction leading to increasingly negative intrathoracic pressures during inspiration. This causes arousals, sleep fragmentation but there is preservation of airflow and oxygenation. Thus, there is no evidence of apnea, hypopnea, or gas exchange abnormalities on polysomnography (PSG). Polysomnography shows snoring with marked paradoxical breathing movements or repetitive arousals. Increased respiratory effort with arousals clinches the diagnosis of UARS on esophageal pressure monitoring.[7,2]

Obstructive Sleep Apnea Syndrome

Around 1–3% children have OSAS and 40% of children referred to sleep medicine or an otolaryngologist may have OSAS. OSA is characterized by prolonged upper airway obstruction during sleep resulting in partial or complete cessation of breathing associated with reduction of oxyhemoglobin saturation or hypercarbia, or both. This may lead to obstructive apnea or obstructive hypoventilation. Obstructive hypoventilation is not seen in adults usually. It leads to paradoxical respiratory efforts, hypercarbia, and occasionally hypoxemia.[7,8]

The obstructive events resulting in hypoxia and multiple arousals contribute to metabolic, cardiovascular and neurocognitive changes.

PATHOPHYSIOLOGY

Upper airway is a collapsible tube, the patency of which is determined by the tone of the pharyngeal muscles causing dilatation as well as phasic contractions of these muscles during inspiration.[7] Pathophysiology can be arbitrarily divided into anatomical factors, control of airway patency, and obesity.

Anatomical Factors

Changes in the anatomical framework of the head and neck, affects the caliber of pharyngeal airway, which in turn contributes to increased risk of airway obstruction. The most common cause for childhood OSA is adenotonsillar hypertrophy.[8]

When MRI was used to study the airway of children with OSAS, it was found that these children had significantly enlarged tonsils and adenoids leading to smaller upper airway volumes as compared with controls. In addition, positive correlation was seen when percent difference of combined tonsil and adenoid volume between each subject and matched controls was plotted against apnea-hypopnea index.[9] Soft palate volume was also found to be more in subjects with OSA. Children with OSA have hyperplasia of lymphoid tissue in regions other than Waldeyer's ring also.

In a review of 495 children with OSA and the contribution of adenoid and tonsil size in childhood OSA and interactions between adenotonsillar hypertrophy, age and obesity was studied. They found that the effect of adenoid size on OSA decreased in adolescence. Moreover, both adenotonsillar hypertrophies together increased OSA risk more than tonsil or adenoid hypertrophy alone.[10]

Adenoidal-nasopharyngeal space is narrowest at 4.5 years of age and adenoidal mass reaches greatest size at 7–10 years of age when facial framework rapidly develops. This space gradually decreases until 12 years of age. Thus the influence of adenoid size decreases as the child reaches adolescence. However, there is no such correlation between age, tonsil size, and OSA in children.[10]

Craniofacial factors include hypoplasia or retropositioning of maxilla or mandible, large or retropositioned tongue (Box 1). Evaluation of children with craniofacial anomalies is directed toward assessing skull base shape, maxillary size and shape, tongue size and support and mandibular size and shape. OSAS in such children persists even after adenotonsillectomy (AT) and additional surgical as well as nonsurgical therapies are generally required. Infants usually

> **Box 1: Conditions associated with obstructive sleep apnea in children[8]**
>
> **Conditions with reduced upper airway patency**
> - Adenotonsillar hypertrophy
> - Obesity
> - Allergic rhinitis
> - Mucopolysaccharidoses/metabolic storage diseases
> - Macroglossia
> - Laryngomalacia
>
> **Conditions with abnormal muscle tone**
> - Down syndrome
> - Hypothyroidism
> - Prader-Willi syndrome
>
> **Craniofacial syndromes**
> - Crouzon syndrome
> - Pierre Robin syndrome
> - Apert syndrome
> - Goldenhar syndrome
> - Treacher-Collins syndrome
>
> **Neurologic disorders**
> - Cerebral palsy
> - Duchenne muscular dystrophy
> - Arnold-Chiari syndrome
> - Meningomyeloc

require tracheostomy.[9] Skeletal dysplasias such as achondroplasia may lead to "mixed apnea syndrome". Brainstem or cervicomedullary compression results in abnormal ventilatory drive and central apnea. Adenotonsillar enlargement and craniofacial factors cause obstructive sleep apnea.[7]

Control of Airway Patency

Anatomical factors are not the only determining factor leading to OSA in pediatric age group. Children with large tonsils may not have OSA. Since upper airway is a collapsible tube, the "Starling Resistor Model" has been proposed for its dynamics. According to this model, maximum inspiratory flow through a collapsible upper airway is determined by upstream (nasal) pressure changes and pressure changes surrounding the collapsible segment. This airflow is not dependent on the tracheal pressure generated by the diaphragm. The pressure outside the airway is determined by the activity of the airway dilator muscles.[7,9] The pressure at which airway collapses is termed as critical closing pressure (Pcrit) and this is a measure of airway collapsibility. Children with OSA have more airway collapsibility (Pcrit was higher or less negative) than children with primary snoring.[5]

Obesity

With increasing epidemic of obesity in children especially in developed countries and now in the developing countries too, more and more children presenting with OSA are observed to be obese. Classical presentation of a child with adenotonsillar hypertrophy and failure to thrive is now being replaced with an obese child presenting with OSA. These children may or may not have adenotonsillar hypertrophy. They usually present at a later age and the clinical profile resembles adult OSA phenotype.[9] A percentage of this group of children undergoing AT still have residual OSA following surgery.

Possible mechanisms causing OSA in childhood obesity are as follows:[7,9]

- There are alterations in mechanisms regulating upper airway patency and increased airway collapsibility in obese children
- Central obesity reduces functional residual capacity by limiting diaphragmatic descent, more during supine position. Moreover, these children have decreased lung compliance leading to hypoventilation, atelectasis, and ventilation-perfusion mismatch
- Obstructive sleep apnea can induce leptin resistance and increases ghrelin levels both of which can increase obesogenic behavior.

Three subtypes of childhood OSA have been identified:[4,11]

- Type I marked increased lymphoid tissue in upper airways in absence of obesity
- Type II milder lymphoid hypertrophy associated with obesity
- Type III Children with syndromic OSAS.

Obstructive Sleep Apnea and Inflammation

Obstructive sleep apnea leads to elevation of C-reactive protein (CRP). An animal model of intermittent hypoxia and hypercapnia leads to elevation of interleukin-6 (IL-6) level, which is a precursor of CRP.[12] Some studies demonstrated increased levels of proinflammatory cytokines tumor necrosis factor-α, IL-6, and IL-1α from OSA-derived tonsils. They postulated that recurrent vibrations of the upper airway during snoring promotes localized inflammation.[8] Goldbart et al. showed higher levels of leukotriene B4 and cysteinyl leukotriene in children with OSA. Even sputum from children with OSA exhibits neutrophilia as compared with controls.

Sequelae of Obstructive Sleep Apnea

Obstructive sleep apnea causes intermittent hypoxemia and subsequent sleep fragmentation which induces local and systemic inflammation. The combination of these inflammatory cascades and oxidative stress mechanisms lead to cell injury, dysfunction, and cell death affecting various targeted organs.

Cardiovascular System

Obstructive sleep apnea can promote cardiovascular disturbances in blood pressure regulation, ventricular remodeling, and endothelial dysfunction. Children can have a vast variety of cardiovascular symptoms including systemic and pulmonary hypertension, and cor pulmonale with heart failure.[2] Majority of children shows significant improvement in endothelial function after treatment of OSA with AT.[9,11,13]

Children with OSA have a higher diastolic BP during sleep as compared with primary snorers though elevations in systemic BP were noted even in children with primary snoring.

Overnight greater changes in brain natriuretic peptide in children with moderate to severe OSA as a result of frequent negative intrathoracic pressure swings have been demonstrated. This accounts for the ventricular dysfunction in these children.[9]

Endothelial dysfunction is known to be a precursor to atherosclerosis. Children with concomitant obesity and OSA have a greater degree of endothelial dysfunction as compared to children with only OSA. OSA severity is associated with a decrease in T regulatory lymphocytes (Tregs) in peripheral blood of children with OSA. Tregs have shown to inhibit development and progression of atherosclerosis. Gozal et al. stated that OSA in children is strongly related to changes in Tregs and their function. This in turn contributes to cardiovascular morbidity in children.[13]

C-reactive protein, an acute phase reaction protein has recently emerged as one of the powerful independent predictors of risk for future cardiovascular morbidity and is now widely used to stratify risk for ischemic heart disease. Increased CRP levels have been demonstrated in children with OSA and the level of rise in CRP levels is proportionate to the severity of OSA. However, there is significant reduction in these levels following effective treatment.[6,9]

Polverino and associates studied 101 children and found that apnea-hypopnea index (AHI) was significantly associated with Hs-CRP (high sensitivity CRP). Hs-CRP was significantly higher in children with OSA. Children with OSA and raised CRP levels are found to be at a greater risk for the development of long-term cardiovascular complications.[14]

Behavioral and Neurocognitive Impairment

Sleep disordered breathing is associated with poor learning, poor school performance, attention deficits, concentration difficulties, hyperactivity, and impulsivity. This is secondary to fragmented, nonrestorative sleep with intermittent hypoxia and its effect on the development of prefrontal cortex. Prefrontal cortex is responsible for behavioral control, working memory, organization, analysis, and self-regulation of motivation.[2,15] "Memory consolidation" occurs during REM sleep whilst growth hormone (GH) is produced in slow wave sleep. Thus sleep fragmentation occurring in OSA affects both cognition and interferes with growth. Even children with "primary snoring" (without gas exchange abnormalities) or mild OSA can present with neurobehavioral changes.[12] It has been concluded that executive dysfunction is related to nocturnal hypoxemia rather than daytime sleepiness.[15]

Gozal in 1998 performed a study in children whose school performance was in the lowest tenth percentile of their class. There was a marked prevalence of OSA in these children. Moreover, children who were treated AT showed significant improvement in school grades.[2,9,12] It has been hypothesized that neurocognitive impairment occurs as a result of changes in cerebral blood flow during sleep.[9]

It is further emphasized that not all children with OSA exhibit behavioral and cognitive deficits. Both genetic and environmental factors play a major role in phenotypic expression of these deficits. Following treatment of OSA, improvement occurs in behavior and cognition. However, early diagnosis and prompt treatment is advised as some neurocognitive changes are only partially reversed if left too long.

Metabolic Sequelae

Obstructive sleep apnea has been associated with failure to thrive. Children with OSA and primary snorers have disruption of slow wave sleep, during which GH and insulin-like growth factor (IGF-1) are secreted. Failure to thrive results from reduction of IGF-1 or insulin-like growth factor binding proteins (IGFBPs) which significantly reverses following AT.[5] Furthermore, there may be dysphagia and increased energy expenditure leading to lesser intake.[4]

In contrast to the earlier presentation of failure to thrive, more and more children presenting with OSA are now obese. Sleep fragmentation and intermittent hypoxia is associated with reduced insulin sensitivity and dyslipidemia in obese children. Fatty liver disease has been demonstrated in children with OSA and obesity. Treatment with AT followed by continuous positive airway pressure (CPAP) led to improvement in liver serum aminotransferases.[9]

Rise in low-density lipoprotein cholesterol along with lowering of high-density lipoprotein cholesterol is seen in OSA children irrespective of the presence or absence of obesity.[9]

DIAGNOSIS

Clinical Manifestations

Early diagnosis and prompt management of OSAS result in decreased morbidity and reversal of most of the sequelae of OSA. Primary snoring and OSA cannot be differentiated by history and examination alone.

Symptoms in pediatric age group are dependent on the age of the child. Nocturnal symptoms noticed by parents are seen in all age groups. They include loud, frequent snoring, choking, breathing pauses, restless sleep, arousals, and nocturnal enuresis. These children usually have unusual sleeping postures. They keep their necks hyperextended to maintain patency of upper airway. They are also known to present with paradoxical breathing, mouth breathing, nocturnal sialorrhea, nocturnal sweating, parasomnia, and bruxism[2,6,7] (Box 2).

Most of the time, daytime symptoms are more pronounced and apparent in older children. Excessive daytime sleepiness (EDS) is seen only in 7–10% of the cases. EDS is seen in children with severe OSA and obesity and is associated with higher incidence of complications (40–50%). More commonly, pediatric OSA presents as hyperactivity and inattention during the day, moodiness, and poor learning in school as explained earlier.[2,9]

Examination

First step to examining a child suspected to have OSA is to note the height and the weight of the child, because growth can be impaired in the child. A full otorhinolaryngologic examination must be conducted to establish the site of static or dynamic airway obstruction.[4,6,7,12,16]

> **Box 2: Symptoms of pediatric obstructive sleep apnea syndrome[2,8]**
>
> **Daytime symptoms**
> - Mouth breathing
> - Poor appetite/difficulty in swallowing
> - Morning headache
> - Nasal speech
> - Attention deficit/aggression/moodiness
> - Hyperactivity
> - Chronic nasal congestion/rhinorrhea
>
> **Nocturnal symptoms**
> - Snoring
> - Choking/gasping
> - Paradoxic breathing
> - Retractions (cervical or costal)
> - Abnormal sleep positions
> - Frequent awakenings
> - Enuresis
> - Sweating
> - Dry mouth
> - Bruxism
> - Parasomnia

> **Box 3: Physical examination in pediatric obstructive sleep apnea syndrome[2]**
>
> **General**
> - Obesity
> - Failure to thrive
> - Sleepiness
> - Increased neck circumference
>
> **Head and neck**
> - Tonsillar hypertrophy
> - High arched palate
> - High/large tongue position
> - Overbite
> - Posterior buccal cross bite
> - Elongated soft palate
> - Long face syndrome
> - Midfacial hypoplasia
> - Micrognathia/retrognathia
> - Deviated septum
> - Swollen nasal mucosa
>
> **Cardiovascular**
> - Systemic/pulmonary hypertension

Child suspected to be suffering from OSA will have a typical "long face syndrome". These mouth breathers have altered dentoalveolar morphology. The characteristic features include high arched palate, increased lower facial height, narrow maxilla and retrognathia[5] (Box 3).

Polysomnography

Overnight PSG in a sleep laboratory is the gold standard for diagnosis of pediatric OSAS and is the best technique to differentiate between primary snoring and OSA.[7] Accurate diagnosis of the severity of OSA will ensure the proper treatment in children and will defer unnecessary surgeries wherever not required.

American Academy of Thoracic Society, Standards and Indications of Cardiopulmonary Studies in children recommends measurement of the following parameters:[7]

- *Sleep state*: electroencephalogram, electromyogram, electrooculogram
- *Respiratory parameters*: abdominal and chest wall movements, oronasal airflow, end tidal CO_2, oxygen saturation with pulse oximetry
- *Nonrespiratory parameters*: electrocardiogram, electromyogram
- Audio video recording.

Sleep related upper airway obstruction is diagnosed in children who have evidence of significant obstructive hypoventilation or more than one obstructive apneic episode per hour. Obstructive apneic episodes in children often are shorter than 10 seconds as compared with adults where they last for more than 10 seconds. Two or more consecutive breaths with obstructive apneas or hypopneas are considered abnormal in children.[7]

The definitions of obstructive apnea and hypopnea are the same as those for adults. However, there is no international consensus for AHI cut off values to initiate treatment in children. The current accepted arbitrary cut off for AHI is more than 3 standard deviations beyond mean of normative AHI in healthy children. Children with an AHI less than 1 per hour total sleep time (TST) do not have significant OSA. On the other hand, a child with AHI more than 5 per hour TST requires treatment.[9] However, as there is no evidence-based cut-off, some children with AHI less than 5 may be symptomatic and require intervention.[2] The American Society of Anesthesiologists guidelines defines severe OSA as AHI of 10 or more.[2]

It is seen that only 10% of children with habitual snoring referred for AT actually undergo overnight sleep study. American Academy of Otolaryngology—Head and Neck Surgery (AAOHNS) published clinical practice guidelines for use of PSG before tonsillectomy in children (Box 4).[17] Many factors like the cost, inconvenience to the child and parents, expertise in pediatric sleep study, and interpretation make most of the physicians consider PSG not necessary for diagnosis.[8] Conventional numerical measures (e.g., obstructive AHI, arousal index, oxyhemoglobin desaturation index, etc.) are poor indicators of morbidity in children.[17] Additionally, many morbidities in children present after a long period of time. Children who are symptomatic, may show "normal PSG" in the presence of habitual snoring and conversely, relatively asymptomatic snoring children, may have severe respiratory disturbances in their nocturnal polysomnography (NPSG).

Box 4: AAOHNS guidelines for use of polysomnography before tonsillectomy (sleep disordered breathing)[2]

- Obesity
- Downs syndrome
- Craniofacial abnormalities
- Neuromuscular disorders
- Sickle cell disease
- Mucopolysaccharidoses

AAOHNS, American Academy of Otolaryngology—Head and Neck Surgery.

To overcome the drawbacks of using only NPSG as a diagnosing tool for the severity of OSA, several alternative methods[4,7,11] are under evaluation. These include:
- Nap PSG can be helpful if positive but it has a high false-negative rate attributed to shorter TST and lesser proportion of REM sleep in daytime nap
- Unsupervised overnight pulse oximetry gives information about desaturation but cannot rule out OSA if negative. Associated recording of end-tidal CO_2 provides additional information of cessation of airflow
- Video and audio recordings
- Multichannel devices for home recordings offer cost-effective details on sleep information in an unsupervised setting
- Flexible nasendoscopy can be used to evaluate the level of airway obstruction, lymphoid tissues, and post nasal space. Sleep endoscopy-fiber optic endoscopy is performed under artificially-induced sleep to determine the site of obstruction and plan the treatment subsequently.

TREATMENT

Surgical

Adenotonsillectomy is the first line of treatment in children with OSA and adenotonsillar hypertrophy. Combination of adenoid and tonsil surgery is considered superior and more effective in treating OSA than both alone.[8,12]

Childhood adenotonsillectomy trial has shown that as compared to watchful waiting, surgical treatment of OSA improved symptoms, behavioral changes, and quality of life.[9] AT reduces AHI to less than 1 event per hour in 25–71% children with OSA. Significant improvements are seen in quality of life, attention span, growth, behavior, school performance, and cognition.[16]

Surgery is associated with complications which are more common in high risk group.[5,9,16] The risk factors include children younger than 3 years, severe OSAS (AHI more than or equal to 10 and/or oxygen saturation nadir less than or equal to 80%), failure to thrive, obesity, cardiac complications of OSAS, craniofacial and neuromuscular disorders, and current respiratory infections.[1,2] Careful pediatric intensive care monitoring is recommended for all high risk children in the postoperative period.

According to a retrospective study, although majority of the children showed marked improvements following AT, residual OSA was prevalent in a large subset of cases. Residual OSA was seen in severe OSA cases (AHI >20/hour TST), children older than 7 years, asthmatics, positive family history of OSA, African American race, high Mallampati score, craniofacial abnormalities, chromosomal defects and neuromuscular disorders, and other obstructive causes like enlarged turbinates, deviated septum.[5] Residual OSA is seen in more than 40% of children. A repeat sleep study is recommended 6–8 weeks postsurgery in these high risk children for recurrence or persistence of OSA.

Coblation-assisted tonsillectomy is a new technique used at present, demonstrating decreased intraoperative blood loss and markedly reduced postoperative edema and pain. Conventional adenoid curettage is now being replaced increasingly with endoscopic microdebrider-assisted adenoidectomy.

Since the adenoid removal is done under direct vision, it allows complete removal of both choanal and tubal lymphoid tissue causing obstruction.

Other Surgical Options

Palatal surgery (uvulopalatopharyngoplasty, UPPP) is indicated in complicated OSAS in obese children, cerebral palsy, Down syndrome, and children with craniofacial anomalies and neurologic impairments. Kershner and colleagues demonstrated a modest improvement in oxygen saturation nadir on PSG following UPPP.[2]

Tongue-base procedures: Genioglossal advancement, radiofrequency ablation or coblation-assisted tongue base reduction, partial midline glossectomy, and lingual tonsillectomy are a list of a few procedures recommended in children with tongue base obstruction. Tongue base obstruction leading to OSA is typically seen in children with Down syndrome and Beckwith-Wiedemann syndrome.[2,12]

Other craniofacial procedures include distraction osteogenesis and mandibular distraction in children with mandibular hypoplasia and retrognathia.[2,18]

Tracheostomy is reserved for severe OSAS in children who have failed other medical and surgical therapy, children with anatomic and neuromotor issues.

Nasal surgeries like septum correction and turbinectomy are very rarely conducted in children.

Positive Airway Pressure

This is often considered as second line therapy in children with OSAS in the following clinical situations: [2]
- Persistence of symptoms (in children with other risk factors like obesity)
- Recurrence of symptoms after AT
- Adenotonsillectomy not performed or contraindicated
- Before surgery in severe OSAS.

Home nasal CPAP has been used in infants, prepubertal, and pubertal children.[2] Even though this therapy is highly efficacious adherence is particularly challenging in children. Complications of positive airway pressure devices used in children are global nasal flattening, midfacial hypoplasia, local discomfort like eye irritation, skin ulceration, and rhinorrhea.[2,5,8]

Pharmacologic therapies: Medical therapy is considered as the first line option for children with mild OSA or as an adjunct to treatment of severe OSA.

Nasal steroids: Intranasal steroids have been known to be effective in residual lymphoid tissue or adenoidal regrowth after adenotonsillar hypertrophy or in situations where surgery is not performed. Nasal corticosteroids exert lympholytic action; reduce inflammation and upper airway edema.[8] A small study with children younger than 10 years found that use of nasal fluticasone propionate decreased AHI from 10.7 ± 2.6 to 6.8 ± 2.2.[16]

Leukotriene receptor antagonists: Leukotrienes regulate inflammation in respiratory system. Both leukotrienes and their receptors are increased in adenotonsillar tissue and exhaled condensate of children with OSAS.[5] Leukotriene receptor antagonists like montelukast treat OSA through anti-inflammatory action on this pathway. Concomitant use of both montelukast and nasal budesonide for 12 weeks in children who had residual mild OSA after AT lead to significant improvement in AHI, respiratory arousal index, and nadir oxygen saturation.[9]

Other Nonsurgical Therapies

Rapid maxillary expansion devices are used to widen hard palate by opening midpalatal suture and enlarging nasal cavities in prepubertal children. After 4 months of therapy, nasal resistance decreases and there is significant improvement in OSA symptoms in children with maxillary constriction.[2,5] Oral appliances are also used which can be worn during sleep. They advance the mandible or the tongue increasing the size of the upper airway. Mandibular advancement and nasopharyngeal airways are other options in children with dysgnathia and hypotonia, respectively.

FUTURE DEVELOPMENTS

Even though sleep studies provide an objective measure of sleep disturbances, the parameters used are not predictive of OSA-associated morbidities. Home-based studies and limited multichannel studies may provide a more economical option. Moreover, identification and use of biomarker approaches requires further exploration. Some data has shown a strong association between pediatric OSA and nocturnal rise in urinary neurotransmitters. Episodic hypoxemia and arousals result in increase in sympathetic activity causing rise in urinary epinephrine and norepinephrine. Overnight changes in three neurotransmitters: gamma-aminobutyric acid, decrease in taurine, and decrease in beta-phenyl ethylamine are postulated to differentiate children with OSA with neurocognitive defects from those without.[9]

CONCLUSION

Obstructive sleep apnea is common in children and early recognition and referral is helpful in preventing long-term morbidity related to neurodevelopment and pulmonary hypertension. Risk factors such as craniofacial abnormalities, Downs Syndrome, and neuromuscular abnormalities should be identified early and addressed appropriately. A thorough evaluation of growth and development and otolaryngologic evaluation, investigations such as sleep study (PSG), and nasendoscopy are required before considering surgical options. Night continuous positive airway pressure or bilevel positive airway pressure therapy is also becoming more available in Indian setups for resistant cases of OSA not amenable to surgical correction. A clinical approach to any child with persistent snoring or episodes of apnea or hypopnea is shown in the flow diagram (Flowchart 1).

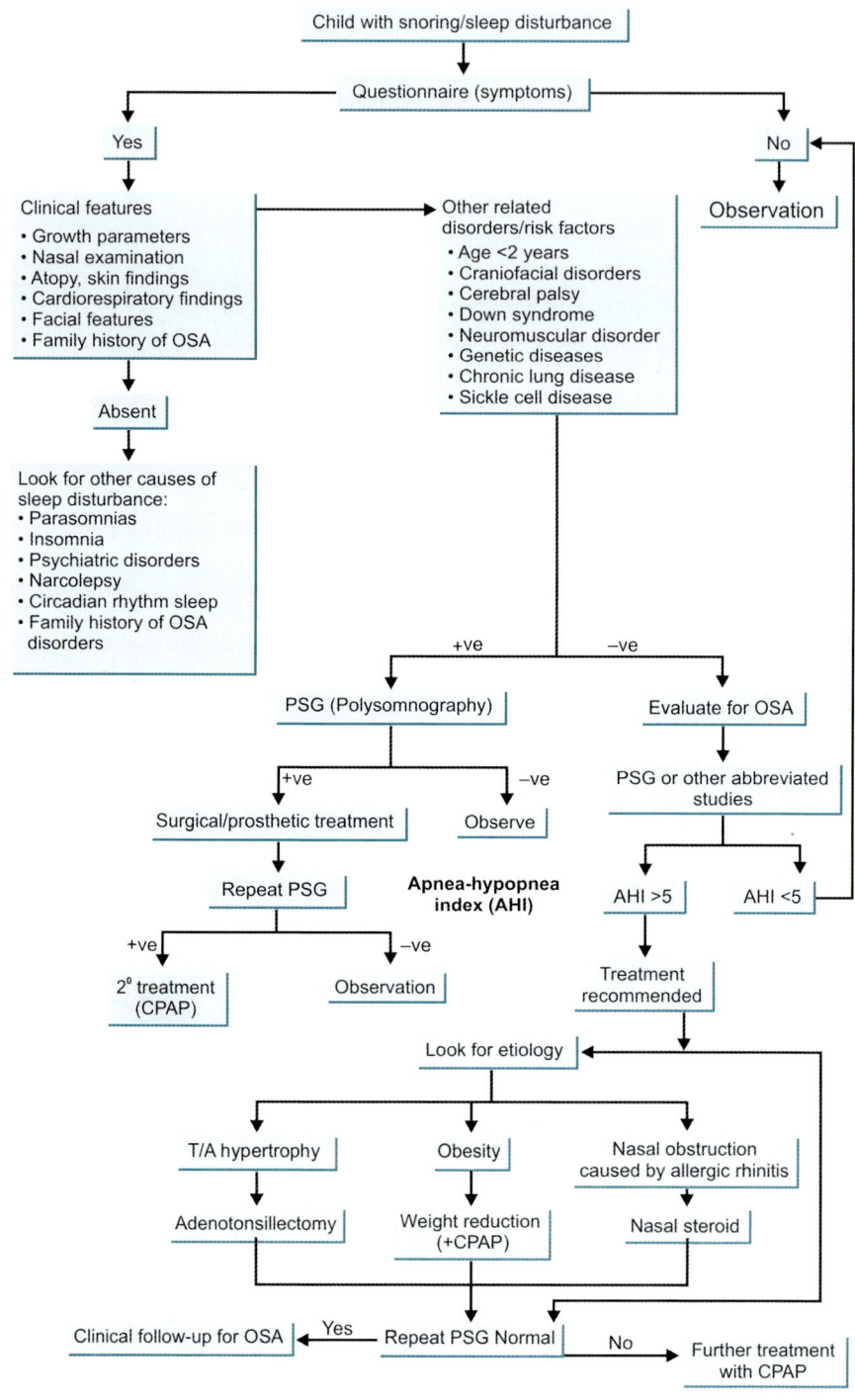

Flowchart 1: Child with snoring and sleep disturbance.

OSA, obstructive sleep apnea; CPAP, continuous positive airway pressure.

REFERENCES

1. Marcus CL, Brooks LJ, Draper KA, et al. Diagnosis and management of childhood obstructive sleep apnea syndrome. *Pediatrics.* 2012;130(3):576-84.
2. Alexander NS, Schroeder JW Jr. Pediatric obstructive sleep apnea syndrome. *Pediatr Clin N Am.* 2013;60(4):827-40.
3. Huang YS, Guillenminault C. Pediatric obstructive sleep apnea and the critical role of oral-facial growth: evidences. *Front Neurol.* 2013;3:184:
4. Facaro S, Hillard T, Henderson J. Obstructive sleep apnea in children. *Pediatrics and Child Health.* 2009;19(6):271-5.
5. Katz ES, D' Ambrosio CM. Pediatric obstructive sleep apnea. *Clin Chest Med.* 2010;31(2):221-34.
6. Kleigman RM, Staton BF, Geme JW, Schor NF, Behrman R. Sleep Medicine. Nelson Textbook of Pediatrics, 19th edition; 2011. pp. 46-55.
7. Sterni LM, Tunkel DE. Obstructive sleep apnea syndrome. Cummings Otolaryngology Head & Neck Surgery, 5th edition; 2010. pp. 2602-12.
8. Au CT, Li AM. Obstructive sleep breathing disorders. *Pediatr Clin N Am.* 2009;56(1):243-59.
9. Tan H-L, Gozal D, Gozal LK. Obstructive sleep apnea in children: a critical update. Nature and Science of Sleep. 2013;5:109-23.
10. Kang KT, Chou CH, Weng WC, et al. Associations between adenotonsillar hypertrophy, age and obesity in children with obstructive sleep apnea. 2013;8(10): e78666.
11. Nespoli L, Caprioglio A, Brunetti L, et al. Obstructive sleep apnea syndrome in childhood. *Early Hum Dev.* 2013;89 Suppl 3:S33-7
12. Urquhart DS, Starritt N. Sleep apnea in children. *Pediatrics and child health.* 2012;23(7):307-14.
13. Tan HL, Gozal D, Samiei A, et al. T regulatory lymphocytes and endothelial function in pediatric obstructive sleep apnea. 2013;8(7): e69710.
14. Lannuzzi A, Licenziati MR, Michele FD, et al. C-reactive protein and carotid intima-media thickness in children with sleep disordered breathing. *J Clin Sleep Med.* 2013;9(5):493-8.
15. Esposito M, Antinolfi L, Gallai B, et al. Neuropsychiatric Disease and Treatment. 2013;9:1087-94.
16. Cielo C, Brooks LJ. Therapies for children with obstructive sleep apnea. *Sleep Med Clin.* 2013;8:483-93.
17. Gozal D, Kheirandish-Gozal L. New approaches to the diagnosis of sleep-disordered breathing in children. *Sleep Med.* 2010;11(7):708-13.
18. Ameli F, Brocchetti F, Semino L, et al. Adenotonsillectomy in obstructive sleep apnea syndrome. Proposal of a surgical decision-taking algorithm. *Int J of Pediatric Otorhinolaryngol.* 2007;71(5):729-34.

CHAPTER 16

Perioperative Management of Sleep Related Breathing Disorders

Roop Kaw, Vivek Nangia

INTRODUCTION

The prevalence of obstructive sleep apnea (OSA) among patients undergoing elective surgery varies according to the screening or diagnostic method of the study reporting it. It has been reported to range from 0.4% (1998) and 2.7% (2007) for general surgical procedures and 0.4% (1998) and 5.5% (2007) for orthopedic procedures (from reported administrative data)[1] to 7% from a large academic registry of surgical patients undergoing anesthesia.[2] These studies have also identified some of the specific risks among patients with OSA in the surgical setting. Since patients with OSA are prone to hypoxia, especially during night, any added insults during anesthesia induction or recovery, with sedation or analgesia required in the perioperative setting can tend to exacerbate any hypoxia-related complication in the postoperative period.

PREOPERATIVE EVALUATION OF OBSTRUCTIVE SLEEP APNEA

Obstructive sleep apnea is a highly prevalent disorder which is often undiagnosed. Hence the specific symptoms and signs of OSA should be routinely asked for in all preoperative evaluations. The American Society of Anesthesiology (ASA) assigns all the signs and symptoms into three categories (Table 1); patients with signs and symptoms in two or more categories are believed to have high probability of OSA.[3] Among the quick to use screening tools an abbreviated version of the Berlin questionnaire asks only for Snoring, Tiredness, Observed apneas, and Blood pressure with comparable sensitivity and specificity. The addition of body mass index (BMI), age, neck circumference, and gender (STOP-Bang) to this tool increases the sensitivity further with a minor compromise in the specificity (STOP). For a STOP-Bang score of 5, the odd's ratio (OR) for moderate/severe and severe OSA has been shown to be 4.8 and 10.4, respectively, while for a STOP-Bang 7 and 8, the OR for moderate/severe and severe OSA was 6.9 and 14.9, respectively.[4] A STOP-Bang score more than or equal to 3 demonstrates a very high sensitivity and negative predictive value for moderate/severe OSA, hence this cut-off may be good for a surgical population with high OSA prevalence such as bariatric surgical patients. On the other hand, the patients with a STOP-Bang score of 5–8 have a high specificity to detect moderate and severe OSA. These scores may be useful in the general patient population which has a low OSA prevalence to reduce false-positive rate.

Table 1: American Society of Anesthesiology questionnaire for preoperative evaluation of obstructive sleep apnea

Category 1: predisposing physical characteristics	Category 2: history of apparent airway obstruction during sleep	Category 3: somolence
BMI >35	Two or more of the following are present (if patient lives alone or sleep is not observed by another person, then only one of the following need be present)	One or more of the following are present
Neck circumference >43 cm/17 inches (men) or 40 cm/16 inches (women)	Snoring (loud enough to be heard through closed door)	Frequent somnolence or fatigue despite adequate 'sleep'
Craniofacial abnormalities affecting the airway	Frequent snoring	Falls asleep easily in a nonstimulating environment (e.g., watching television, reading, riding in or driving a car) despite adequate 'sleep'
Anatomical nasal obstruction	Observed pauses in breathing during sleep	[Parent or teacher comments that child appears sleepy during the day, is easily distracted, is overly aggressive, or has difficulty concentrating]*
Tonsils nearly touching or touching the midline	Awakens from sleep with choking sensation Frequent arousals from sleep	[Child often difficult to arouse at usual awakening time]*

Scoring: If two or more items in category 1 are positive, category 1 is positive. If two or more items in category 2 are positive, category 2 is positive. If one or more items in category 3 are possitive, category 3 is positive. High risk of OSA, two or more categories scored as postive. Low risk of OSA, only one or no category scored as positive scored as positive.
*Items in brackets refer to pediatric type.
BMI, body mass index; OSA, obstructive sleep apnea.

On physical examination, the upper airway characteristics that predict difficult intubation (DI) should prompt strong suspicion for OSA. The Mallampati classification and Friedman tongue position assessment techniques correlate significantly with OSA severity (Figure 1).[5] After adjustment for numerous confounders, each point increase in the Mallampati score increases the risk of having OSA (OR: 2.5, 95% CI 1.2–5.0) and the apnea-hypopnea index (AHI) (coefficient 5.2 events per hour of sleep, 95% CI 0.2–10).[6]

PERIOPERATIVE COMPLICATIONS IN PATIENTS WITH OBSTRUCTIVE SLEEP APNEA

Difficult Intubation in Patients with Obstructive Sleep Apnea

Just as sleep, anesthesia also results in reductions in pharyngeal dilator muscle tone and lung volume, thereby predisposing to upper airway obstruction.[7] In patients with OSA upper airway muscular tone can be delayed (100–200 ms) or abolished during inspiration in patients with OSA[8,9] along with impaired upper airway neuromotor responses. Thus, variability in collapsibility of the upper airway between individuals cannot be explained by structural loads alone.[10]

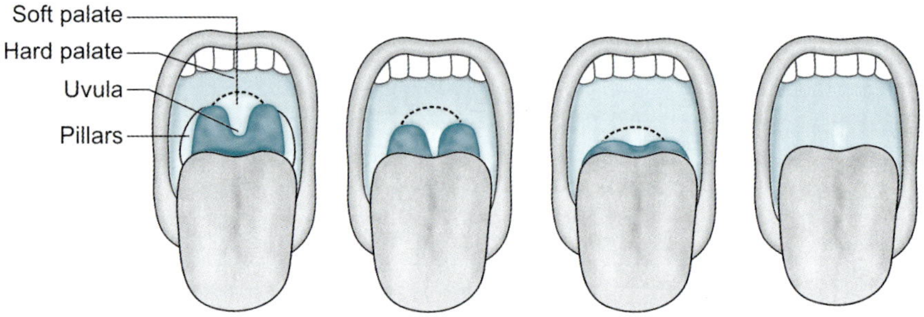

Class 1, complete visualization of the soft palate; Class 2, complete visualization of the uvula; Class 3, Visualization of only the base of the uvula; Class 4, Soft palate is not visible at all.

Figure 1: The Mallampati classifcation.

Although DI has not been specifically studied among patients with OSA, all of its major predictors such as BMI more than 30 kg/m;^{2} OSA and neck circumference more than 40 cm are the same those that predict OSA in the general population.[11] Same can be said for the clinical predictors of DI like Mallampati score and short thyromental span.[12] Indeed a close relationship has been suggested between DI and the presence of OSA.[13]

Strategies to Mitigate Difficult Intubation and/or Mask Ventilation

Passive closing pressures (PCLOSE) among anesthetized patients with OSA can be up to 9 cm H_2O higher than those among patients without OSA.[14] Proper positioning of the patient in the sitting position can decrease the PCLOSE by 6 cm of H_2O; whereas the sniffing or the ramp position will decrease the PCLOSE by 4 cm H_2O also allowing both tracheal intubation and ventilation. Awake intubation (with regional anesthesia and/or sedation) and rapid induction are preferred over slow induction when DI is suspected.[15] Pharyngeal airway closure can be prevented by application of 10 cm of positive end expiratory pressure during positive pressure ventilation in the most severe cases of OSA.

Postoperative Respiratory Failure in Obstructive Sleep Apnea

Obstructive sleep apnea can be complicated by postoperative respiratory failure. There is a fivefold increase in intubation and mechanical ventilation after orthopedic surgery (n ~ 50,000) and twofold increase after general surgery (n ~ 50,000) among patients with OSA reported.[1] A meta-analysis of nearly 4,000 patients has confirmed the high prevalence of postoperative respiratory failure (OR, 2.43; p = 0.003; Figure 2) irrespective of the kind of surgery being undertaken.[16] Higher need for emergent intubation and postoperative mechanical ventilation remains unchanged across all surgical categories.[17] The need for emergent intubation and mechanical ventilation is higher on the day of surgery or the first postoperative day compared to patients without sleep disordered breathing (SDB). Interestingly enough after adjusting for age, sex, Charleston comorbidity index, patients without SDB requiring emergent intubation had significantly worse outcomes compared to those with SDB requiring emergent intubation. This phenomenon is, perhaps,

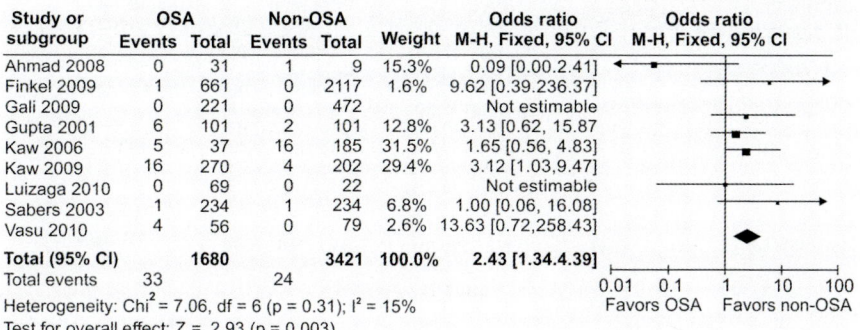

OSA, obstructive sleep apnea; CI, confidence interval.

Figure 2: Postoperative respiratory failure in patients with obstructed sleep apnea. *From:* Kaw R, Chung F, Pasupuleti V, Mehta J, Gay PC, Hernandez AV. Meta-analysis of the association between obstructive sleep apnoea and postoperative outcome. Br J Anaesth. 2012;109(6):897-906, *with permission.*

best explained by possible, rapidly reversible upper airway obstruction in the setting of opioid and sedative use in the immediate postoperative period or perhaps a lower threshold was used for intubating patients with OSA or transferring them to the intensive care unit (ICU). Early reports amongst patients with obesity hypoventilation syndrome (OHS) undergoing elective surgery shows that the incidence of postoperative respiratory failure may be even higher and that OHS is more likely to be unrecognized before elective noncardiac surgery when compared to OSA.[18] It has also been seen that OSA patients, who are on chronic opioid therapy, quite often fail continuous positive airway pressure (CPAP) therapy.[19] This has been attributed to central sleep apnea getting unmasked while using CPAP, a condition known as complex sleep apnea.

Depending upon the definition used, among the different studies reported in the literature, as well as their respective sample size, postoperative respiratory failure has not been consistently reported among patients with OSA. Moreover, some of the single center studies were originally initiated as quality improvement projects and hence by design report lesser postoperative respiratory complications than others.[20-23] Among other reasons for variations in reporting of postoperative complications between different studies are: whether OSA was diagnosed clinically, by screening or by a gold standard test; and especially among the case control studies whether the comparison was against a group of "true controls" (OSA excluded by formal polysomnography).

Unanticipated Intensive Care Unit Transfer after Surgery

Unanticipated ICU transfer after surgery has often been used as an outcome measure among patients with OSA. This measure is, however, not always easy to track as patients can often be sent to ICU for overnight observation. If the observation transfers to ICU are excluded[24] presence of OSA appears to be significantly associated with higher odds of ICU transfer (OR 2.29; 95% CI 1.62–3.24, p ≤ 0.00001), (I^2 = 57–68%, p ≤ 0.02) after surgery (Figure 3). A study using STOP-Bang score as a predictor of postoperative critical care admission

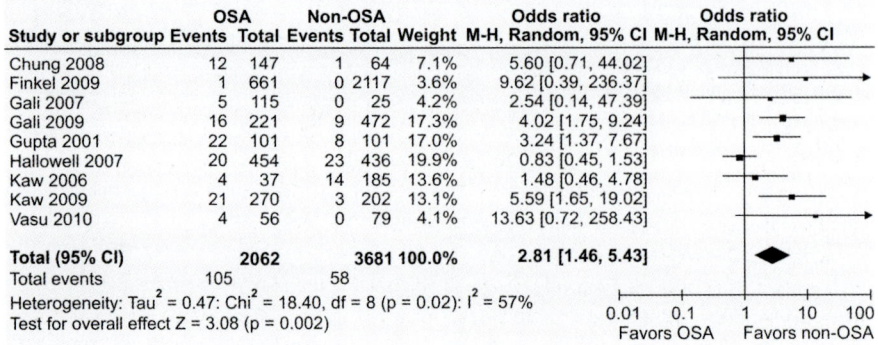

OSA, obstructive sleep apnea; CI, confidence interval.

Figure 3: Unanticipated transfer to intensive care unit after surgery among patients with obstructive sleep apnea. *From:* Kaw R, Chung F, Pasupuleti V, Mehta J, Gay PC, Hernandez AV. Meta-analysis of the association between obstructive sleep apnoea and postoperative outcome. Br J Anaesth. 2012;109(6):897-906, *with permission.*

reported OR of 2.2 (95% CI: 1.1–4.6; p = 0.037); 3.2 (95% CI: 1.2–8.1; p = 0.017) and 5.1(95% CI: 1.8–14.9; p = 0.002) for STOP-Bang scores of 4, 5, and more than or equal to 6, respectively.[25]

Postoperative Mortality

In 1997, Ostermeier et al. reported three deaths from sudden postoperative respiratory arrest associated with epidural opioids in patients with sleep apnea.[26] Sudden cardiac death (SCD) is more likely to occur during the sleep hours (12 midnight to 6.00 AM) among patients with OSA compared to those without OSA (50% compared to 21%; RR: 2.57).[27] The same group of authors has shown that among patients with OSA; the lowest nocturnal oxygen desaturation and AHI were independent predictors of SCD.[28] Few studies that have looked at postoperative mortality[17,29] did not find any association between OSA and mortality after elective surgery. This observed lack of association between postoperative mortality and OSA does not necessarily mean that death cannot be an expected sentinel event in a postoperative patient with OSA especially exposed to additional insults like failed airway; unmonitored respiratory depression opioid and or sedative administration especially with PCA infusions and others. Clearly the incidence of such events in the perioperative setting when reported from the large administrative databases is low enough to pass any statistical rigor of association.

Perioperative Risk Reduction Strategies in Obstructive Sleep Apnea

Patients with OSA present with DI and airway management issues. Practice guidelines for the perioperative management of OSA exist[3] but the recommendations are at the best cautious and mostly based on clinical consensus; although some general principles exist (Box 1). Patients with known OSA using CPAP at home should be advised to bring their machine to the hospital at the preoperative visit. Patients who are noncompliant should be encouraged to use it more consistently. In patients with previously undiagnosed OSA and

> **Box 1: General principles for perioperative management of patients with obstructed sleep apnea**
> - Symptoms and signs of OSA should be routinely asked in all preoperative evaluations
> - Refer patients for preoperative sleep evaluation if the probability of previously undiagnosed OSA is high, surgery is elective, and there is a likely need for postoperative opioids or sedation
> - Where OSA has been previously diagnosed and the patient has compliant with CPAP, ensure it is available for perioperative use
> - Where previously diagnosed but no compliant with CPAP, reinstruct in its use
> - Avoid sedative premedication
> - Use regional anesthesia and analgesia when and where possible
> - When general anesthesia is used, be prepared for difficult intubation and other difficulties in airway maintenance. Use techniques that allow early return of consciousness
> - Minimize postoperative sedation
> - Observe in a high-dependency unit with continuous monitoring of respiratory parameters (oximetry, oronasal airflow) until the patient is sentient and able to self-administer CPAP Patients requiring ongoing opioids or sedation should remain in a high-dependency area until this need abates
> - Use lateral positioning, a nasopharyngeal airway, and oxygen therapy where CPAP is refused and upper airway obstruction is problematic

CPAP, continuous positive airway pressure; OSA, obstructive sleep apnea

high clinical suspicion of OSA based on preoperative assessment, if significant use of opioids and sedation is anticipated based on the type of the surgical procedure, consideration should be given to inpatient surgery as opposed to ambulatory surgery. Wherever possible, regional anesthesia and blocks are preferred and for general anesthesia short-acting agents like desflurane, and propofol are recommended. A study on sleep apnea patients undergoing total joint arthroplasty found that patients undergoing surgery under neuraxial anesthesia had significant lower rates of major complications as compared to those receiving combined neuraxial and general or only general anesthesia.[30] When using general anesthesia, the possibility of DI should be kept in mind and preparation for induction and intubation should follow the ASA difficult airway guidelines.[31] Full reversal of neuromuscular blockade (when applicable) with use of a nerve stimulator should be verified prior to extubation.[32] These patients must be fully awake, normothermic, hemodynamically stable, spontaneously breathing with adequate respiratory rate, and tidal volume prior to breathing.

Multimodal analgesia involving the use of NSAIDS, acetaminophen, tramadol, ketamine, pregabalin, and COX-2 inhibitors should be considered to minimize the use of opioids in the postoperative setting.[33] OSA patients receiving opioids are more likely than patients receiving nonopioid analgesia to have perioperative oxygen desaturations.[34] It has been shown that in volunteers at high risk of OSA, nocturnal hypoxemia is associated with higher sensitivity to opioids, suggesting that increased potency of opioid analgesia could be a marker of its propensity to depress respiration during sleep.[35] Patients undergoing ambulatory surgeries should be observed for an extended period of time prior to their discharge home.[3] Continuous pulse oximetry monitoring is recommended in the postoperative setting in patients at risk for respiratory complications of OSA. Cautious use of supplemental oxygen is advised after extubation until the patient is able to maintain his/her baseline oxygen saturation on room air. If frequent or severe airway obstruction or hypoxemia is noted in the postoperative monitoring period, consideration should be made to initiate CPAP of noninvasive intermittent positive pressure ventilation.

Role of CPAP used perioperatively among patients with OSA has not been well-studied. Indirect evidence can be obtained from patients undergoing bariatric surgery, who happen to have higher prevalence of OSA, and have often had the chance to have a treatment plan initiated before surgery. Although some series have reported higher postoperative complication rates among bariatric surgical patients with OSA; in other studies, most patients were preoperatively diagnosed and treated with PAP therapy; the presence or severity of OSA did not lead to a higher postoperative complication rate.[36] Among patients with OSA cardioverted for atrial fibrillation, those treated with CPAP were less likely to develop recurrent atrial fibrillation within 12 months of cardioversion compared to patients without treatment with CPAP.[37] A study randomized patients with high sleep apnea clinical score (SACS) undergoing elective orthopedic surgery to standard care with auto-PAP and to standard care alone. No differences in length of stay (p = 0.65) or secondary outcomes (including unplanned ICU transfer, arrhythmia, myocardial infarction, or delirium) were observed between the two groups.[38] Some of the main limitations of this study are incomplete resolution of OSA as suggested by a median residual AHI of 13.5 events/hour, inability to distinguish central sleep apnea from OSA, and limited adherence in a hospital setting. Conclusive evidence mandating empiric use of CPAP perioperatively among patients not currently using it is still lacking. More studies are needed.

Perioperative Obstructive Sleep Apnea Protocols

At the Mayo Clinic, a clinical practice initiative has been developed, utilizing an existing tool to screen patients (the SACS), and a postanesthesia care unit (PACU) assessment looking for recurrent episodes of: (1) apnea, (2) bradypnea, (3) desaturation, and (4) pain-sedation mismatch.[23] This allows to identify patients at higher risk of postoperative respiratory complications with both tools, with highest sensitivity (OR near 20) utilizing both the preoperative and postoperative evaluations. The PACU respiratory assessment has been made a part of the electronic charting system to ensure this was done for all patients. Patients who are at high risk by preoperative screening or PACU criteria receive remote oximetry for 24–48 hours postoperatively. If positive airway pressure is necessary, patients go to a higher level of care; a step-down unit or an ICU. Patients who require PAP postoperatively are presumed to have undiagnosed OSA, seen by a sleep consult service prior to discharge allowing planning for management after discharge and follow-up recommendations. Attempts have been made to provide "just in time" hospital introduction of autopositive airway pressure used in undiagnosed patients who prove to be at high risk for OSA based on a previously verified (SACS) questionnaire.

Yet another major tertiary care institution arranges single channel home testing (oximetry) to those on CPAP to confirm the accuracy of current CPAP settings prior to surgery; whereas OSA patients with SpO_2 less than 90% for less than 10% of the time and CPAP compliance less than 4 hours/night were offered repeat testing with full polysomnography. For those with suspected OSA, full home portable testing (4 channels) is performed within 5 days of surgery.

Patients are encouraged to bring their home masks to ensure best fit although they ensure a variety of masks are available including nasal pillows, nasal masks, and full face masks. For hospital PAP devices, they chose to obtain bilevel auto devices, as these allowed them to use many modes which would be available in that device [CPAP, bilevel (S), and auto bilevel]. The group adopted their own standard for auto settings (EPAP min = 5, IPAP max = 15, PS max = 4) to allow physicians' unfamiliar with the technology have a credible starting place. IPAP max is kept low to reduce the risk of: (1) central apnea, (2) runaway pressure due to mask leak, (3) aerophagia, and (4) pressure intolerance. Hospital monitoring of PAP therapy included telemetry pulse oximetry as well as PAP downloads, is made available in real time through the computer network, facilitating sleep consultation when needed.

CONCLUSION

Clinicians taking care of patients with OSA are often intrigued and concerned about safe perioperative care. Studies till date have shown that OSA is vastly underestimated in the general population; often undiagnosed in the surgical patient and hence can lead to higher postoperative morbidity. Early clinical recognition of OSA can definitely help in designing a safer care plan for such patients.

REFERENCES

1. Memtsoudis S, Liu SS, Ma Y, et al. Perioperative pulmonary outcomes in patients with sleep apnea after noncardiac surgery. *Anesth Analg.* 2011;112(1):113-21.
2. Ramachandran SK, Kheterpal S, Consens F, et al. Derivation and validation of a simple perioperative sleep apnea prediction score. *Anesth Analg.* 2010;110(4):1007-15.
3. Gross JB, Bachenberg KL, Benumof JL, et al. American Society of Anesthesiologists Task Force on Perioperative Management. Practice guidelines for the perioperative management of patients with obstructive sleep apnea: a report by the American Society of Anesthesiologists Task Force on Perioperative Management of patients with obstructive sleep apnea. *Anesthesiology.* 2006;104:1081-93.
4. Chung F, Subramanyam R, Liao P, et al. High STOP-Bang score indicates a high probability of obstructive sleep apnoea. *Br J Anaesth.* 2012;108(5):768-75.
5. Friedman M, Hamilton C, Samuelson CG, et al. Diagnostic value of the Friedman tongue position and Mallampati classification for obstructive sleep apnea: a meta-analysis. *Otololaryngol Head Neck Surg.* 2013;148(40):540-7.
6. Nuckton TJ, Glidden DV, Browner WS, et al. Physical examination: Mallampati score as an independent predictor of obstructive sleep apnea. *Sleep.* 2006;29(7):903-8.
7. Hillman DR, Platt PR, Eastwood PR. Anesthesia, sleep, and upper airway collapsibility. *Anesthesiol Clin.* 2010;28(3):443-55.
8. Remmers JE, deGroot WJ, Sauerland EK, et al. Pathogenesis of upper airway occlusion during sleep. *J Appl Physiol Respir Environ Exerc Physiol.* 1978;44(6):931-8.
9. Strohl KP, Hensley MJ, Hallett M, et al. Activation of upper airway muscles before onset of inspiration in normal humans. *J Appl Physiol Respir Environ Exerc Physiol.* 1980;49(4):638-42.
10. McGinley BM, Schwartz AR, Schneider H, et al. Upper airway neuromuscular compensation during sleep is defective in obstructive sleep apnea. *J Appl Physiol.* 2008;105(1):197-205.
11. Kheterpal S, Martin L, Shanks AM, et al. Prediction and outcomes of impossible mask ventilation: a review of 50,000 anesthetics. *Anesthesiology.* 2009;110(4):891-7.
12. Shiga T, Wajima Z, Inoue T, et al. Predicting difficult intubation in apparently normal patients: a meta-analysis of bedside screening test performance. *Anesthesiology.* 2005;103(2):429-37.
13. Hiremath AS, Hillman DR, James AL, et al. Relationship between difficult tracheal intubation and obstructive sleep apnoea. *Br J Anaesth.* 1998;80(5):606-11.

14. Isono S. Optimal combination of head, mandible and body positions for pharyngeal airway maintenance during perioperative period: lesson from pharyngeal closing pressures. *Semin Anesth.* 2007;26:83-93.
15. Benumof JL. Management of the difficult adult airway. With special emphasis on awake tracheal intubation. *Anesthesiology.* 199;75(6):1087-110.
16. Kaw R, Chung F, Pasupuleti V, et al. Meta-analysis of the association between obstructive sleep apnoea and postoperative outcome. *Br J Anaesth.* 2012;109(6):897-906.
17. Mokhlesi B, Hovda MD, Vekhter B, et al. Sleep-disordered breathing and postoperative outcomes after elective surgery: analysis of the Nationwide Inpatient Sample. *Chest.* 2013;144(3):903-14.
18. Kaw R, Pasupuleti V, Walker E, et al. Obesity hypoventilation syndrome: An emerging and unrecognized risk factor among surgical patients. *Am J Respir Crit Care Med.* 2011;183:A3147.
19. Guillenminault C, Cao M, Yue HJ, et al. Obstructive sleep apnea and chronic opioid use. *Lung.* 2010;188(6):459-68.
20. Hwang D, Shakir N, Limann B, et al. Association of Sleep-disordered breathing with postoperative complications. *Chest.* 2008;133(5):1128-34.
21. Gali B, Whalen FX, Gay PC, et al. Management plan to reduce risks in perioperative care of patients with presumed obstructive sleep apnea syndrome. *J Clin Sleep Med.* 2007;3(6):582-8.
22. Finkel KJ, Searleman AC, Tymkew H, et al. Prevalence of undiagnosed obstructive sleep apnea among adult surgical patients in an academic medical center. *Sleep Med.* 2009;10(7):753-8.
23. Gali B, Whalen FX, Schroeder DR, et al. Identification of patients at risk for postoperative respiratory complications using a preoperative obstructive sleep apnea screening tool and post-obstructive anesthesia care assessment. *Anesthesiology.* 2009;110:869-77.
24. Liao P, Yegneswaran B, Vairavanathan S, et al. Postoperative complications in patients with obstructive Sleep apnea: a retrospective cohort matched study. *Can J Anaesth.* 2009;56(11):819-28.
25. Chia P, Seet E, Macachor JD, et al. The association of preoperative STOP-BANG scores with postoperative critical care admission. *Anesthesia.* 2013;68(9):950-2.
26. Ostermeier AM, Roizen MF, Hautkappe M, et al. Three sudden postoperative respiratory arrests associated with epidural opioids in patients with sleep apnea. *Anesth Analg.* 1997;85(2):452-6.
27. Gami AS, Howard DE, Olson EJ, et al. Day night pattern of sudden death in obstructive sleep apnea. *N Engl J Med.* 2005;352(12):1206-14.
28. Gami AS, Olson EJ, Shen WK, et al. Obstructive sleep apnea and the risk of sudden cardiac death: A longitudinal study of 10,701 adults. *J Am Coll Cardiol.* 2013;62(7):610-8.
29. Lockhart EM, Willingham MD, Abdallah AB, et al. Obstructive sleep apnea screening and postoperative mortality in a large surgical cohort. *Sleep Med.* 2013;14(5):407-15.
30. Memtsoudis SG, Stundner O, Rasul R, et al. Sleep apnea and total joint arthroplasty under various types of anesthesia: a population-based study of perioperative outcomes. *Reg Anesth Pain Med.* 2013;38(4):274-81.
31. Rosenblatt WH, Whipple J. The difficult airway algorithm of the American Society of Anesthesiologists. *Anesth Analg.* 2003;96(4):1233.
32. Murphy GS, Szokol JW, Marymont JH, et al. Residual neuromuscular blockade and critical respiratory events in the postanesthesia care unit. *Anesth Analg.* 2008;107(1):130-7.
33. Chung SA, Yuan H, Chung F. A Systematic review of obstructive sleep apnea and it's implications for anesthesiologists. *Anesth Analg.* 2008;107(5):1543-63.
34. Bolden N, Smith CE, Auckley D, et al. Perioperative complications during use of an obstructive sleep apnea protocol following surgery and anesthesia. *Anesth Analg.* 2007;105(6):1869-70.
35. Doufas AG, Tian L, Padrez KA, et al. Experimental pain and opioid analgesia in volunteers at high risk for obstructive sleep apnea. *PLoS One.* 2013;8(1):e54807.
36. Weingarten TN, Flores AS, McKenzie JA, et al. Obstructive sleep apnea and perioperative complications in bariatric patients. *Br J Anaesth.* 2011;106(1):131-9.
37. Kanagala R, Murali NS, Friedman PA, et al. Obstructive sleep apnea and the recurrence of atrial fibrillation. *Circulation.* 2003;107(20):2589-94.
38. O'gorman SM, Gay PC, Morgenthaler TI. Does auto-titrating positive airway pressure therapy improve postoperative outcome in patients at risk for obstructive sleep apnea syndrome?: a randomized controlled clinical trial. *Chest.* 2013;144:72-8.

Index

Page numbers followed by *f* refer to figure and *t* refer to table

A

Adenotonsillar hypertrophy 171
Adenotonsillectomy 178
Adenotonsillitis 155
Age related sleep alteration 1
Airflow 34
Airway grading of mallampati 155
Airway patency, control of 171
Allergic fungal rhinosinusitis 144
Allergic rhinitis 171
Allergic shiners 155
Alzheimer's disease 103
American Academy of Otolaryngology 176
American Academy of Sleep Medicine 57, 121
American Association of Dental Sleep Medicine 154
Anatomical nasal obstruction 183
Apert syndrome 171
Apnea 41
 hypopnea index 33, 56, 67, 71f, 83, 105, 117, 145
 scores 156
Arnold-Chiari syndrome 171
Arrhythmias 82
Arsenicum album 136
Arterial blood gases 70
Arterial carbon dioxide tension 67
Arterial stiffness assessment 85
Asthma severity 52f
Atrial fibrillation 31, 50, 84
Autotitrating positive airway pressure 119
Average sleep requirement 2t

B

Bariatric surgery 24, 31
Berlin questionnaire 25, 26, 31
Bilateral corpus distraction osteogenesis 161f
Bilateral sagittal split ramus osteotomy 161
Bilevel positive airway pressure 118
Blood pressure 41, 42, 88

Blood urea 85
Body habitus 41
Body mass index 24, 27, 31, 40, 67, 71, 82, 182
Brain stem pathology 61
Breathing
 cessation of 24
 disorders 182
 work of 68
Buspirone 131

C

Cardiac stress test 85
Cardiovascular disease
 burden of 81
 management of 85
Cardiovascular system 172
Carotid intima-media thickness 83, 85
Central apnea syndromes 23
Central nervous system 57
 traumatic disorders of 23
Central sleep apnea 56, 56f, 57, 57f, 59, 59t, 61, 87, 88, 88f, 117
 diagnosis of 62, 89
 epidemiology of 58
 management of 89
 treatment of 62
Cerebral palsy 171
Cerebrovascular accident 60
Chest wall disease 57
Cheyne-Stokes breathing pattern 12, 57, 58
Cheyne-Stokes respiration 23, 58, 117
Choking 48
Claustrophobia 125
Coblation tonsillectomy 145
Cold steel tonsillectomy 145
Complex sleep apnea 62, 67, 74, 90
Computed tomography 142
Congenital central hypoventilation 23, 61
Congestive heart failure 31
 atrial fibrillation 24
Continuous positive airway pressure 16, 36, 40, 46, 58, 62, 72, 98, 135, 140, 180, 187

Conventional positive airway pressure 116
Coronary angiography 85
Coronary artery disease 79, 83, 103
Corrective nasal surgical procedures 144
Craniofacial syndromes 171
C-reactive protein 172
Crouzon syndrome 171
CSA syndrome 56

D

Daytime dysfunction 48
Daytime somnolence 42
Dental sleep
   appliances 153
   medicine 151, 154
Deviated nasal septum 144
Deviated septum 175
Diabetes mellitus 79, 99
Diaphoresis 48
Diaphragmatic paralysis 72
Diathermy tonsillectomy 145
Digit span 102
Distraction osteogenesis 147
Donepezil 134
Down syndrome 103, 171, 176
Doxapram 134
Duchenne muscular dystrophy 171
Dyspnea spells 48

E

Electrocardiogram 6, 85
Electroencephalogram 3, 34, 35
Electromyogram 34, 35
Electro-oculogram 3, 34
Elongated soft palate 175
Emergent central sleep apnea, treatment of 57
Emergent sleep apnea, treatment of 62
End stage renal disease 62, 107
Endocrine disorders 59, 61
Endothelial dysfunction 81
Enlarged uvula 155
Epiglottic prolapse 14f
Epworth sleepiness scale 25, 32, 32t, 118
   scores 25, 40
Erectile dysfunction 50, 107
Estimated glomerular filtration rate 50
Excessive daytime sleepiness 22, 30, 48, 103, 174
Excessive daytime somnolence 24, 40
Excessive nocturnal sweating 24

F

Fasting blood glucose 85
Fasting lipid profile 85
Fatigue severity scale 32
Fluoxetine 131
Forgetfulness 24
Full face mask 122, 122f

G

Gasping 48
Gastroesophageal reflux 24, 48
   disease 106
Genioglossus advancement 146
Glycosylated hemoglobin 85
Goldenhar syndrome 171
Growth hormone 5

H

Heart failure 79f, 83, 84, 88f
Heart rate 88
Helicobacter pylori infection 106
High arched palate 175
Hypercapnic central sleep apnea 60
Hypertension 82, 103
Hypopharynx 14
Hypopnea syndrome 116
Hypothyroidism 72, 103, 171
Hypoventilation 23
Hypoxemia 23
   severity of 48
   syndromes 23

I

Idiopathic alveolar hypoventilation syndrome 61
Idiopathic pulmonary arterial hypertension 60
Increased upper airway resistance 40
Insomnia 24
Inspiratory positive airway pressure 118

K

Karolinska sleepiness scale 32
Kyphoscoliosis 57

L

Large tongue position 175
Laryngeal surgery 147
Laryngomalacia 171
Laser tonsillectomy 145

Lateral cephalometry 143
Leukotriene receptor antagonists 179
Long face syndrome 175
Loud snoring 24
Low forced vital capacity 71

M

Macroglossia 171
Magnetic resonance imaging 143, 158f
Mallampati classification 184f
Mandible, severe clockwise rotation
 of 155
Mandibular hypoplasia, severe 158f
Mask interfaces 121
Maxillomandibular surgical
 advancement 147, 160
Metabolic storage diseases 171
Micrognathia 175
Midfacial hypoplasia 175
Morning headache 24
Motor vehicle accidents 48
Mucopolysaccharidoses 171, 176
Muller maneuver 141, 142t
Multiple sleep latency test 6, 36

N

Nasal cavity 12f
Nasal continuous positive air pressure
 mask 122f
Nasal continuous positive airway
 pressure 43
 application of 116
Nasal inflammation systemic
 inflammation 52f
Nasal mask 121, 125
Nasal pillows 124, 124f
Nasal steroids 178
Nasopharynx 11
Neck circumference 40, 41
Neonate pharynx 153f
Neurocognitive dysfunction 103t
Neurohumoral modulator 69
Neurologic disorders 171
Neuromuscular disorders 23, 61, 176
Nicotine 135
Nocturia 24, 48
Nocturnal arrhythmias 84
Nocturnal dysrhythmias stroke 24
Nocturnal enuresis 24
Nocturnal intermittent hypoxia 103
Nocturnal polysomnography 176

Non-hypercapnic central sleep apnea 60
Noninvasive positive pressure
 ventilation 118
Non-obstructive alveolar
 hypoventilation, idiopathic 23
Non-rapid eye movement 3
Nonrefreshed and excessive daytime
 sleep 48
Nonrespiratory parameters 176
Nonrestorative sleep 48
Nonsustained ventricular tachycardia 82
Normal human sleep 1

O

Obesity 24, 31, 67, 84, 103, 171, 175, 176
 hypoventilation syndrome 67, 68f,
  71, 71f, 119, 185
 definition of 67t
Obstructed sleep apnea 185f, 187
Obstruction, levels of 140
Obstructive sleep apnea 17, 22, 24, 30,
 33, 37, 39, 46, 52f, 53, 57f, 59, 67,
 71, 79-81, 84-87, 98, 99f, 100, 101,
 103, 103t, 105-107, 116, 117, 130,
 140, 141t, 144t, 151, 169, 172, 180,
 182-184, 186, 186f, 187
 airways 10
 cerebrovascular consequences of 105
 potential consequences of 107
 prevalence of 53t
 sequelae of 172
 severe 158f
 severity of 37 71
 surgical management of 140
 syndrome 24, 40, 41, 148, 169, 170, 175
Opium 136
Oral appliance therapy 43, 156
Oral mask 123, 123f, 125
Orofacial mask 122, 122f, 125
Oropharynx 12, 13f
Orthodontic procedures 43
Oxygen desaturation index 33

P

Periodic limb movements 34
Pharyngeal manometry 144
Physiologic central sleep apnea 60
Physostigmine 134
Pierre Robin syndrome 171
Polysomnography 33, 34, 37, 71, 169,
 175

Portable sleep monitoring 36
Positive airway pressure 53, 116, 178
   devices 130
   therapy 72, 117
Posterior buccal cross bite 175
Prader-Willi syndrome 171
Primary central sleep apnea 57
Primary sleep apnea of
   infancy 57
   newborn 23
Primary snoring 169
Protryptyline 130
Psychiatric disorders 105
Psychomotor vigilance task 102
Pulmonary function tests 71
Pulmonary hypertension 23, 24, 31, 175

R

Radiofrequency assisted tonsillotomy 145
Rapid eye movement 23, 35, 60, 70, 130
Refractory hypertension 31
   treatment of 24
Renal disease 50
Respiratory disturbance index 117
Respiratory muscle function 69
Respiratory parameters 176
Respiratory system 10
Restlessness 48
Retrognathia 175
Retrograde amnesia 24
Retro-trapezoid nucleus 58
Reversed Robin Hood syndrome 105

S

Serum creatinine 85
Serum electrolytes 85
Severity of obstructive sleep apnea,
   classification of 33t
Sickle cell disease 176
Sinus surgery 144
Sleep apnea hypopnea syndrome 31
Sleep bruxism 165
Sleep disordered breathing 30, 67, 70, 119, 151
   prevalence of 163
Sleep disorders, international
   classification of 22, 39
Sleep disruption, severe 24
Sleep fragmentation 103
Sleep Health Foundation 1
Sleep Heart Health Study 82

Sleep hygiene 6
Sleep influence on endocrine system 5
Sleep magnetic resonance imaging 143
Sleep myths 7
Sleep nasoendoscopy 142
Sleep related breathing disorders 22, 79, 85t, 87, 101
   classification of 23
Sleep spindle 4
Sleep stage 3, 3f, 35t
   scoring 35
Sleep state 176
Sleep study, levels of 33t
Sleepiness 175
Slow wave sleep 3
Small nares and high and narrow nose 155
Snoring 41
Snoring and upper airways resistance syndrome 39
Snort arousals 48
Somatic functional complaints 41
Somnofluoroscopy 143
Specific tests 72
Split night polysomnography 36
Spongia 136
Stanford sleepiness scale 32
Starling resistor model 171
Steer clear performance test 102
Stroke 31, 103
Sudden cardiac death 186
Supplemental oxygen 62, 73
Swollen nasal mucosa 175
Systemic hypertension 175
Systolic heart failure 60

T

Temporomandibular joint
   ankylosis 158f
   disorders 155
Thrombosis 81
Thyroid function test 85
Tongue base procedures 178
Tongue retaining device 158f
Tonsillar hypertrophy 175
Tonsillectomy 145
Tonsils 13f
Tracheostomy 73, 148
Trazodone 132
Treacher-Collins syndrome 171
Turbinate hypertrophy 144

Turbinate reduction 144
Turbinate resection 144
Turbinectomy 43

U

Ultrasonic/harmonic scalpel
    tonsillectomy 145
Uniqueness of human pharynx 151
Upper airway dilator muscle 16
Upper airway obstruction 11
    anatomy of 11
Upper airway collapsibility of 15
Upper airway resistance syndrome 169
Upper airway respiratory syndrome 39-41
    consequences of 42
Uvulopalatopharyngoglossoplasty 54
Uvulopalatopharyngoplasty 145

V

Ventricular ectopics 82
Visual analog scale 32

W

Wakefulness test, maintenance of 6, 36
Wisconsin sleep cohort study 48